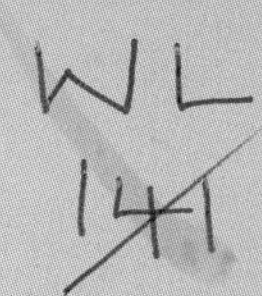

Understanding NEUROLOGY

a problem-orientated approach

John Greene

Consultant Neurologist
Institute of Neurological Sciences, Southern General Hospital, Glasgow

Ian Bone

Professor of Neurology
Institute of Neurological Sciences, Southern General Hospital, Glasgow

MANSON
PUBLISHING

Further sources of information

ASSOCIATION OF BRITISH NEUROLOGISTS
www.theabn.org
Comprehensive, good for doctors and patients, links to disease-specific websites.

PATIENT ADVICE
www.neuroguide.com
Good North American site with links to patient information sites.

THE NEUROLOGICAL ALLIANCE
www.neural.org.uk
Umbrella organization bringing together various neurological charities and interest groups.

www.theabn.org/public/patientcarer.php
Source of disease-specific information for patients and carers.

GUIDELINES
www.nice.org.uk
Applies to the NHS in England & Wales.

www.sign.ac.uk
Evidence-based guidelines, does not cover all neurological areas.

OTHER USEFUL INFORMATION
www.dvla.gov.uk/at_a_glance/content.htm
Invaluable as a source of driving regulations for all neurological conditions, not just epilepsy.

ISBN-10: 1-84076-061-3
ISBN-13: 978-1-84076-061-3

A CIP catalogue record for this book is available from the British Library.

For full details of all Manson Publishing Ltd titles please write to:
Manson Publishing Ltd, 73 Corringham Road, London NW11 7DL, UK.
Tel: +44(0)20 8905 5150
Fax: +44(0)20 8201 9233
Website: www.mansonpublishing.com

Commissioning editor: Peter Altman
Project manager: Ruth Maxwell
Copy-editor: Ruth Maxwell
Cover design: Cathy Martin, Presspack Computing Ltd
Book design and layout: Cathy Martin, Presspack Computing Ltd
Colour reproduction: Tenon & Polert Colour Scanning Ltd, Hong Kong
Printed by: New Era Printing Co Ltd, Hong Kong

Contents

Preface

While traditional neurology textbooks tend to be organized by disease process, patients, being unaware of this, arrive with a complaint, (e.g. headache, dizziness, memory problems), that requires an explanation. This multi-author book adopts a problem-oriented approach to the commonly presenting complaints seen by neurologists. We have drawn on the experience of practising clinicians in a busy department based in the Southern General Hospital, Glasgow.

The problem-based approach illustrates the manner in which clinicians, in the real world, focus on particular elements of history and examination in order to narrow down their differential diagnosis and by so doing formulate a diagnostic approach or sometimes (quite often actually) offer no more than confident professional reassurance.

This is not a comprehensive textbook of these neurological conditions in themselves, nor a manual of neuro-therapeutics. Neurology is a speciality requiring a 'good listener' and a capable examiner, no more and no less.

We hope that this book will demystify what should have never been mysterious in the first place and prove useful to medical undergraduates. It should also be of benefit to junior doctors preparing for MRCP. If trainee neurologists also derive benefit from reading it, so much the better!

John Greene and Ian Bone

Contributors

John Greene
Consultant Neurologist, Institute of Neurological Sciences, Southern General Hospital, Glasgow

Ian Bone
Consultant Neurologist and Honorary Professor of Neurology, Institute of Neurological Sciences, Southern General Hospital, Glasgow

Rod Duncan
Consultant Neurologist, Institute of Neurological Sciences, Southern General Hospital, Glasgow

Myfanwy Thomas
Consultant Neurologist, Paris, France. Formerly Consultant Neurologist, Institute of Neurological Sciences, Southern General Hospital, Glasgow

James Overell
Consultant Neurologist, Institute of Neurological Sciences, Southern General Hospital, Glasgow

Richard Metcalfe
Consultant Neurologist, Institute of Neurological Sciences, Southern General Hospital, Glasgow

Richard Petty
Consultant Neurologist, Institute of Neurological Sciences, Southern General Hospital, Glasgow

Vicky Marshall
Research Registrar in Neurology, Institute of Neurological Sciences, Southern General Hospital, Glasgow

Donald Grosset
Consultant Neurologist, Institute of Neurological Sciences, Southern General Hospital, Glasgow

Abhijit Chaudhuri
Consultant Neurologist, Essex Centre of Neurological Sciences, Oldchurch Hospital, Romford, Essex

Stewart Webb
Consultant Neurologist, Institute of Neurological Sciences, Southern General Hospital, Glasgow

John Paul Leach
Consultant Neurologist, Institute of Neurological Sciences, Southern General Hospital, Glasgow

Colin O,Leary
Consultant Neurologist, Institute of Neurological Sciences, Southern General Hospital, Glasgow

We would like to thank colleagues in Neurophysiology and Neuroradiology at the Institute for help with providing figures.

Abbreviations

ACE Addenbrooke's Cognitive Examination/angiotensin-converting enzyme
AChRAb anti-acetylcholine receptor antibody
ACTH adrenocorticotrophic hormone
AD Alzheimer's disease
AICA anterior inferior cerebellar artery
AION anterior ischaemic optic neuropathy
ALP alkaline phosphatase
ALS amyotrophic lateral sclerosis
ANA antinuclear antibody
AP antero-posterior
ARAS ascending reticular activating system
AST aspartate aminotransferase
AVM arteriovenous malformation
BIH benign intracranial hypertension
BOLD blood oxygen level dependent
BPPV benign paroxysmal positional vertigo
BSAEP brainstem auditory evoked potential
CADASIL cerebral autosomal dominant arteriopathy with subcortical infarcts and leucoencephalopathy
CAT computer assisted tomography
CBD corticobasal degeneration
CBF cerebral blood flow
CBV cerebral blood volume
Cho choline
CJD Creutzfeldt–Jakob disease
CK creatine kinase
CMAP compound muscle action potential
CNS central nervous system
COPD chronic obstructive pulmonary disease
Cr creatine
CRP C-reactive protein
CSF cerebrospinal fluid
CT computed tomography
CTA CT angiography
CTP CT perfusion
CTV CT venography
DMD Duchenne muscular dystrophy
DNA deoxyribonucleic acid
DRG dorsal root ganglion
DSA digital subtraction angiography
DWI diffusion-weighted imaging
ECG electrocardiography
EEG electroencephalogram
EMG electromyography
ENA extractable nuclear antigen
ENG electronystagmography
ERG electroretinography
ES epileptic seizure
ESR erythrocyte sedimentation rate
FBC full blood count
FLAIR (MRI) fluid-attenuated inversion recovery (MRI)
fMRI functional magnetic resonance imaging
FP-CIT fluoropropyl carboxymethoxy iodophenyl nortropane spectroscopy
GH growth hormone
GnRH gonadotrophin releasing hormone
GP general practitioner
GT glutamyl transferase
HD Huntington's disease
HIV human immunodeficiency virus
HMPAO hexamethylpropyleneamine oxime
HMSN hereditary motor and sensory neuropathy
HSV herpes simplex virus
ILAE International League against Epilepsy
INR international normalized ratio
IQ intelligence quotient
JME juvenile myoclonic epilepsy
LMN lower motor neurone
LP lumbar puncture

LSD lysergic acid diethylamide
MELAS mitochondrial encephalopathy, lactic acidosis, and stroke-like episodes
MERRF myoclonic epilepsy and ragged red fibres syndrome
MI myocardial infarction
MMSE Mini-Mental State Examination
MND motor neurone disease
MRA magnetic resonance angiography
MRI magnetic resonance imaging
MRI-ADC magnetic resonance imaging apparent diffusion coefficient
MRS MR spectroscopy
MS multiple sclerosis
MSA multiple system atrophy
MTT mean transit time
NAA N-acetyl aspartate
NART National Adult Reading Test
NCS nerve conduction study
NMJ neuromuscular junction
OCB oligoclonal band
PD Parkinson's disease
PET positron emission tomography
PICA posterior inferior cerebellar artery
PNES psychogenic nonepileptic seizures
PSP progressive supranuclear palsy
PWI perfusion-weighted imaging
RAPD relative afferent pupillary defect
RF radiofrequency/ rheumatoid factor
SAH subarachnoid haemorrhage
SCA superior cerebellar artery/spinocerebellar ataxia
SEEG stereo-EEG
SNAP sensory nerve action potential
SPECT single photon emission computed tomography
SSEP somatosensory evoked potential
SSPE subacute sclerosing panencephalitis
SSRI selective serotonin reuptake inhibitor
TCD transcranial Doppler ultrasound
TFT thyroid function test
TIA transient ischaemic attack
TRH thyrotrophin releasing hormone
TTP time-to-peak
UMN upper motor neurone
VEP visual evoked potential
VER visual evoked response
WAIS-R Wechsler Adult Intelligence Scale-Revised

Chapter 1: History Taking and Physical Examination

Ian Bone, John Greene

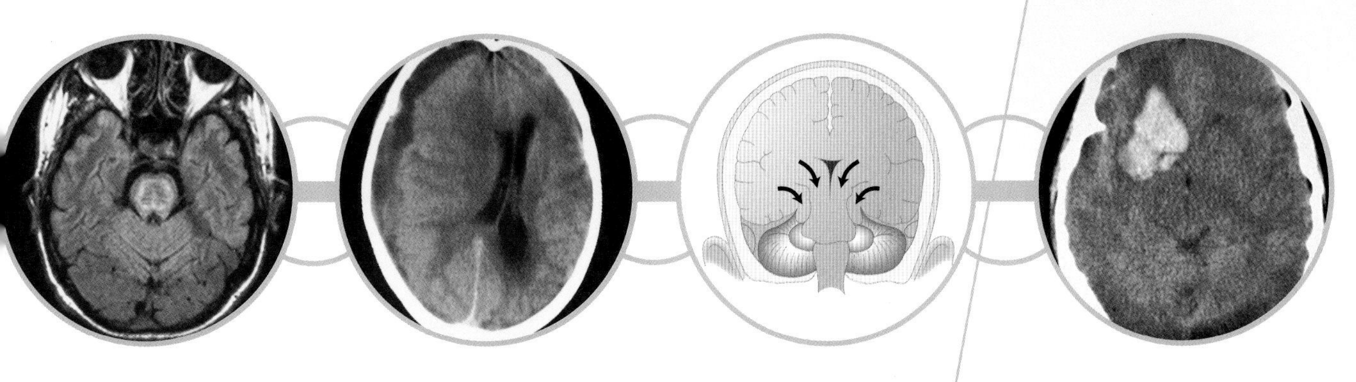

INTRODUCTION

A logical framework of history taking and examination is the basis of the discipline of clinical medicine. The increasing range, availability, and sensitivity of diagnostic tests should never replace this 'clinical acumen'. This text adopts the problem-orientated approach practised daily in clinics, surgeries, and wards worldwide. While investigative resources may vary from country to country, these diagnostic skills should not. The nature of neurological disease is such that patients are often difficult to rouse, their intellect or expression of language and memory impaired, or behaviour inappropriate. In such circumstances, history taking may be impossible and an account from a family member or friend will be essential. Specific neurological deficits, e.g. anosognosia, may result in a patient denying any symptoms (such as nondominant limb weakness). Finally, with increasing travel, a language barrier may present additional communication problems.

This initial chapter is a brief generic guide to history taking, examination, and the essentials of functional neurology (neuroanatomy). The student should use this route map not in isolation, but alongside other texts such as *Neurological Examination made easy* (1) and *Neurology and Neurosurgery Illustrated* (2).

CONCEPTS OF HISTORY TAKING

The purpose of clinical examination is to diagnose the condition responsible for the patient's symptoms, which will subsequently dictate treatment. In neurology, probably more so than in any other medical specialty, the history is vital in narrowing down the differential diagnosis.

Ideally, using a hypothetico-deductive approach, each question should be a sort of 'magic bullet' by which the differential diagnoses are eliminated, until a unique diagnosis is reached. This approach, however, takes years to develop, and a student is advised to follow a logical order of history taking, to ensure that no important parts of the history are missed. By following the same pattern of history taking time and again, it is less likely that a student will miss out an important element in a stressful situation such as an exam. The history will usually give the clinician a likely diagnosis, and physical examination may then serve merely as confirmatory.

There are two key questions to be asked: firstly, where in the neuraxis is a lesion likely to be, given the findings on history taking and examination? Secondly, what is the nature of the causal lesion inferred by the tempo of illness presentation? Insidious and progressive symptoms may be compatible with tumour or degenerative illness. A sudden onset and improving symptoms could be due to vascular disease. A subacute onset of symptoms lasting a few weeks before resolving may be due to demyelinating disease such as multiple sclerosis.

In order to answer these questions, it is important to have a good understanding of the anatomy and physiology of the nervous system. Once understood, neurology loses its mystery and is arguably the most logical of all the medical subspecialties in terms of utilizing information available from clinical examination to localize the site and nature of pathology.

TAKING THE HISTORY

THE PRESENTING COMPLAINT

Enquiry must be focused; a complaint of headache should not be met with an endless list of apparently unconnected questions about all other possible symptoms. This will tire both the patient and doctor. However, anticipating and enquiring into all potentially relevant symptoms form a vital part of history taking. For instance, memory loss, personality change, hearing loss, and double vision may accompany headache (to name but a few possibilities). Each of these additional complaints contributes importantly to defining a pathological process, anatomical localization, and targeted examination.

The pathological processes that affect the central and peripheral nervous systems are relatively few.

Pathological processes
Conditions can be *inherited*, *developmental*, or *acquired:*
Infection (e.g. meningitis)
Inflammation (e.g. multiple sclerosis)
Ischaemic (trauma and stroke)
Neoplastic (primary and secondary tumours)
Degenerative (e.g. Parkinson's disease)
Toxic/metabolic

Knowledge of these pathological possibilities leads to the first set of key questions.

Onset

Did the symptom (e.g. headache) come on suddenly (acutely), gradually (subacutely), or has it been present for weeks (chronically)? The definitions of acute, subacute, and chronic are arbitrary and reflect our understanding of the supposed disease process in hand. Several weeks of headache imply that the complaint is chronic while several weeks of memory loss or dementia indicate that this is acute. Establishing the mode of onset is not always easy. A patient complaining of weakness of the arm may recollect the day, on carrying out a specific task, that they first became aware of the problem. The manner in which weakness behaves thereafter (e.g. progressively worsening over the next year) indicates that, despite an apparently acute onset, it is actually chronic and progressive. The opinion of a family member or friend will often help clarify when a problem was first objectively noticed and the rate at which it seems to be worsening.

Age of onset should be established next. This will help separate developmental from acquired problems, e.g. weakness of the right arm and leg due to cerebral palsy from that due to stroke. Also certain disorders are more likely in specific age groups, e.g. migraine or epilepsy in childhood or adolescence, multiple sclerosis in early adult life, and stroke and dementia in later life. Age of onset is particularly important in inherited disorders, which tend to occur at the same age in families or earlier in subsequent generations (anticipation).

Duration

The length of time for which a symptom has been present helps to establish its chronicity, possible underlying pathology, and the urgency with which investigations should be sought. Duration is also of help in establishing prognosis once diagnosis is known. For example, worsening headache of short duration is more likely to be due to serious intracranial disease than headache of stable severity established over many years. Loss of consciousness due to epilepsy will normally be more prolonged than that from uncomplicated syncope. Referrals of patients to neurology clinics are commonly designated urgent, semi-urgent, or routine on the duration of history alone.

Frequency

Disorders can be divided into those in which the symptom is unremitting, those that come and go in the context of underlying progression or, finally, those which are truly intermittent with well-being in between. This latter group of paroxysmal disorders comprise a significant component of neurological outpatient practice: migraine, epilepsy/'funny turns', transient ischaemic attacks, and dizziness/vertigo. With all these paroxysmal disorders great care must be taken to consider non-neurological disorders (e.g. cardiac arrhythmias, metabolic disease, and syncope).

Associated symptoms

What else may be complained of over and above the cardinal symptom? Here 'wheat has to be separated from chaff' and the real skill of asking the correct questions and eliciting the appropriate reply comes into play. Knowledge of a list of diagnostic possibilities, even at this early stage, is needed to target the appropriate questions. With intermittent headache (migraine?) is sickness present? Does tingling occur in one arm? With weakness in the legs is bladder or erectile function disturbed? With loss of consciousness does tongue biting occur? Are involuntary movements present? The list of what could be asked is endless and narrowing these down forms the basis of the problem-orientated approach.

Aggravating or relieving factors

What makes a symptom worse and what makes it better? This applies to a host of conditions. Mechanical disorders (spinal degenerative disease, disc prolapse) produce pains that are aggravated by certain postures and improved by others. Multiple sclerosis symptoms can be exaggerated or diminished by changes in environmental and body temperature. Migraine may be worsened by certain foods, stress, or lack of sleep and improved by lying in a darkened room or catnapping. The clinician should always listen to the patient and respect that they have the complaint and are best able to judge what affects it. For instance, patients' and parents' observations on diet and its effect on behaviour or seizure frequency are so often dismissed out of hand as irrelevant when in fact they may be indicating something of fundamental importance to pathogenesis.

These five questions (onset, duration, frequency, associated symptoms, and aggravating or relieving factors) should be applied to all the possible neurological scenarios that commonly arise in practice. The common scenarios are:

- ❑ Headache.
- ❑ Visual disturbance.
- ❑ Loss of consciousness.
- ❑ Dizziness.
- ❑ Hearing loss.
- ❑ Unsteadiness.
- ❑ Memory loss.
- ❑ Speech disturbance.
- ❑ Numbness.
- ❑ Weakness.
- ❑ Bladder/bowel disturbance.

Prior medical history

This should be a standard component of all clinical history taking. However, there are certain areas where information is essential to the process of deriving the neurological differential diagnosis:

- ❑ Prior neurological symptoms or diagnosis.
- ❑ Exposure to, or possession of risk factors for neurological disease and occupational history.
- ❑ History of head injury.
- ❑ Alcohol or drug misuse.
- ❑ Psychiatric history.
- ❑ Other (e.g. clotting disorder, immunodeficiency or at risk, thyroid disease).

Family history

Many neurological illnesses have a hereditary basis. To explore this, a detailed family history is essential. Death of a parent or sibling at an early age from an unrelated cause may obscure this possibility. The genotype represents the actual genetic basis for an individual; the term phenotype refers to the outward expression of the genotype. In some disorders, the variability of the phenotype within a family may result in a significant family history being discounted. Also, with complex patterns of inheritance, tendencies and traits within a pedigree are at risk of being overlooked.

> The student should have a working knowledge of patterns of *simple inheritance* (dominant, recessive, and sex-linked) and *complex inheritance* (polygenic, multiple allelic, incomplete dominant, and sex-influenced trait).

Social history

Awareness of social activities (smoking, drinking, recreational drug use, sporting interests) may be helpful to diagnosis. For instance, the mountain biker presenting with ulnar nerve palsy (deep branch compression in the palm of the hand), the heavy drinker with seizures, or the drug user with HIV-related infection.

Employment history informs on educational achievements, behavioural and cognitive decline, stigmatization due to illness (epilepsy), or progression of physical disability (multiple sclerosis). Finally, certain employments carry inherent risks of neurological disturbance (e.g. working with solvents/petrochemicals). In patients with disability and handicap, the questioner should establish who the main carer is, what level of care is required, how independent an individual is in aspects of daily living (cooking, feeding, dressing, and bathing/showering). The following should also be documented: living circumstances (is housing appropriate to current and anticipated degree of future handicap?), provision of state benefits, social worker, and aids (wheelchairs and the like).

Current drugs and allergies

Many common complaints such as muscle pain (myalgia), tingling (paraesthesia), headache, and dizziness are recognized side-effects of commonly prescribed drugs. This is becoming increasingly recognized in the elderly who receive polypharmacy. The drug history should be ascertained in detail. Are all drugs required? Are there drug interactions that could be harmful? Does the current complaint relate in time to the commencement of a particular drug? These questions can result in the recognition of cause and halting a troublesome symptom without recourse to unnecessary investigations.

The identification of allergies is vital to avoid rechallenging the patient with a potentially harmful drug. With the widespread use of contrast dye in imaging investigations (CT and MRI), a history of prior contrast sensitivity should be sought. Finally, it is at this point that absolute or relative contraindications to investigations should be documented. Ferro-magnetic foreign bodies, pacemakers, hip replacement, breast enhancement, pregnancy, or claustrophobia must all be documented where MRI is considered necessary.

NEUROLOGICAL EXAMINATION

Anatomy of the nervous system

The nervous system is hierarchically organized. The sensory and special sensory nervous systems provide ascending input to higher centres regarding the position of the individual in the environment. This includes vision, touch, smell, joint position, pain, and hearing. Such modality-specific information is then processed and coordinated in order to provide the higher centres with a coherent model of the environment. On this basis, higher processes allow the individual to decide on and initiate a particular response to the environment. This considered response is then executed via the motor cortex, through the spinal cord and peripheral nerves to individual muscles to allow appropriate action.

Lesions to the nervous system may result in a pathological excitation, such as a focal motor seizure or, alternatively, a pathological inhibition, e.g. paralysis due to stroke. These are termed positive and negative phenomena.

Mental status

Levels of consciousness

The understanding of consciousness is made confusing by the use of terms such as stuporose or obtunded. These subjective terms are best avoided, and the following more meaningful terms should be used: *consciousness* is particularly difficult to define, but can be described as a state which allows the individual to perceive and understand the environment, and to respond to what is perceived. It requires both *arousal* and *awareness*. Arousal indicates how well a subject appears to be able to interact with the environment, e.g. whether they are awake or sleeping. Awareness, by contrast, relates to the depth and content of the aroused state. *Attention*, in turn, depends on awareness.

It is crucial for doctors to relay information regarding a patient's conscious state using reliable scales. Although the Glasgow Coma Scale was initially developed for patients with head trauma, it has proved a reliable means of assessing and reporting on patients with reduced conscious level regardless of the aetiology, and has good inter-rater reliability. It comprises three categories: eye opening, motor response, and verbal response (*Table 1*). Although the three components can be added up, e.g. GCS 9, it is best to describe the individual components, e.g. E3M4V2.

Table 1 Glasgow Coma Scale

Eye opening (E)	Spontaneous	4
	To speech	3
	To pain	2
	None	1
Motor response (M)	Obeys commands	6
	Localizes to pain	5
	Flexion withdrawal to pain	4
	Abnormal flexion of upper limbs (decorticate rigidity)	3
	Extension (decerebrate rigidity)	2
	No response	1
Best verbal response (V)	Orientated and converses	5
	Disorientated and converses	4
	Inappropriate words	3
	Incomprehensible	2
	No response	1

Anatomy of consciousness

Consciousness may be impaired by damage to the reticular formation in the midbrain and thalamus, or by bilateral damage to the cerebral hemispheres resulting in brain displacement, which thereby impairs the function of the reticular formation (**1–3**).

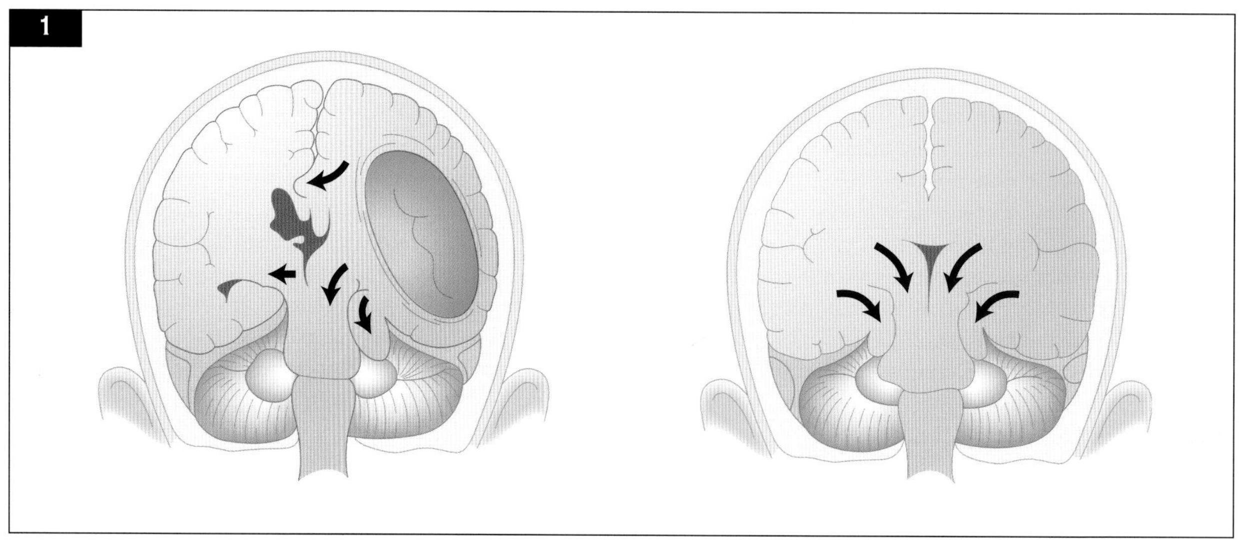

1 Diagram to show brain herniation, resulting in impaired consciousness.

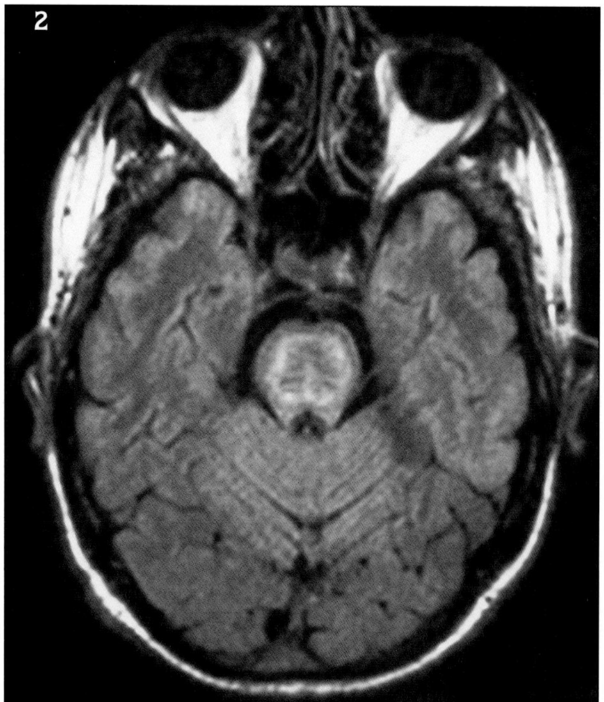

2 Magnetic resonance image illustrating central pontine myelinolysis, a brainstem cause of reduced consciousness.

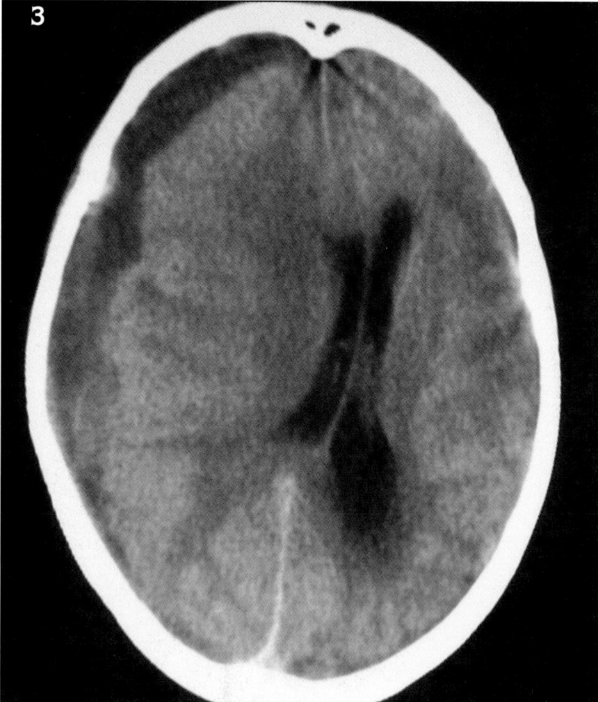

3 Computed tomography scan showing subdural collection, resulting in impaired consciousness.

Loss of awareness in the context of being awake is termed akinetic mutism, and can occur with frontal lesions (**4**).

Brainstem tests

In a patient with a reduced conscious level, it must be ascertained whether coma is due to bilateral hemispheric disease or to brainstem pathology. Utilizing brainstem reflexes can assess the integrity of the brainstem. Pupillary responses to light ascertain whether there is significant midbrain pathology. The corneal reflex tests brainstem integrity at the pontomedullary level. Gag reflex assesses the lower brainstem, while assessment of spontaneous respiratory movements indicates the integrity of the medullary respiratory centres. These four clinical assessments allow the clinician to interrogate the integrity of the brainstem (**5**). If an unconscious patient exhibits normal brainstem reflexes, then it is likely that the impaired consciousness is due to bilateral hemispheric dysfunction.

Behaviour

In the conscious patient, behaviour and cognition must be further addressed. Traditionally, behaviour is part of the psychiatric examination, and in neurology it is often neglected in favour of cognition. It is, however, worth commenting on the patient's behaviour. Mood should be noted, whether depressed, euphoric, or unduly anxious. Emotional lability may also occur, with sudden swings in mood. While taking the history, the organization and content of thought processes should also be noted. Muddled thinking may suggest a mild delirium. Thought content can highlight the presence of delusions (beliefs held which are at variance with the patient's environmental background) or illusions (misperception of stimuli, e.g. mistaking a bush in dim light for a person). These differ from hallucinations, in which the imagined object is not based on a misperceived real object (e.g. hearing voices, seeing Lilliputian figures and so on).

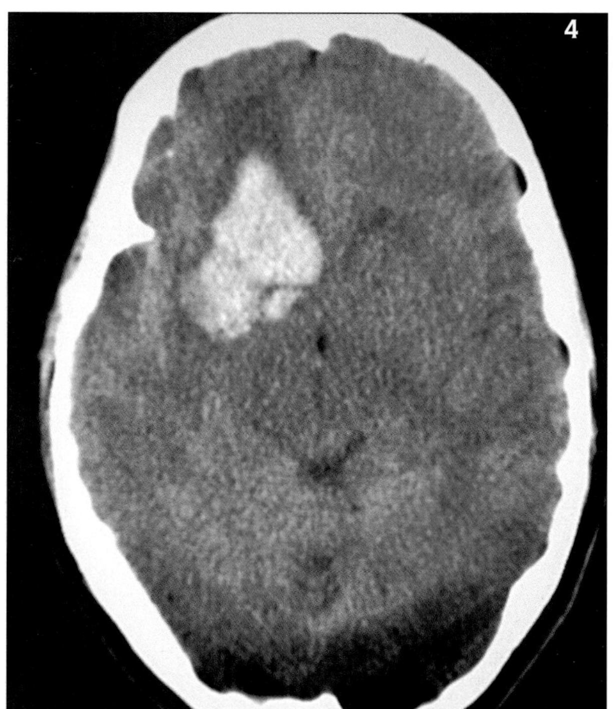

4 Computed tomography scan showing frontal haemorrhage, resulting in the patient being awake but not aware.

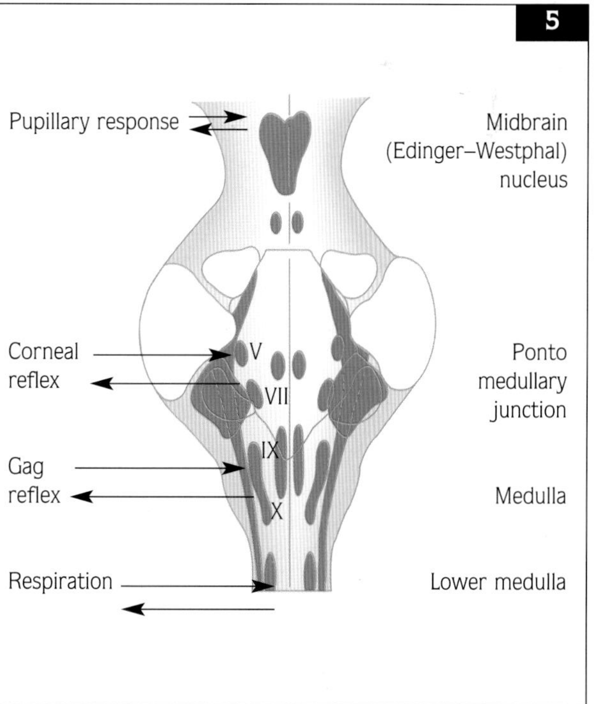

5 Diagram to illustrate the use of brainstem reflexes in assessing the integrity of the brainstem at different levels.

The degree of psychomotor activity should also be assessed. Hyperalert patients are restless and exhibit increased motor activity, including speech that may be accompanied by autonomic overactivity. By contrast, hypoalert patients may sit motionless for hours without speaking.

Cognitive function

This aspect of neurological history taking and examination was neglected for most of the twentieth century, and is still often poorly performed or even omitted. Cognition embraces many higher order activities, including attention, memory, and language. It is difficult to examine adequately these complex skills within the confines of a busy neurology clinic. However, there are brief measures for assessing cognitive function such as the Addenbrooke's Cognitive Examination (ACE). While being no match for proper neuropsychological assessment, it is a very good 'snap-shot' assessment of cognitive functions.

Cognitive functions are best divided into those that require an extensive anatomical network (distributed), and those utilizing a more localized brain area (localized) (*Table 2*). Impairment of a distributed function, such as attention, does not allow the clinician to localize the lesion, but suggests that there is a deficit somewhere in the network subserving attention, which can then be further localized with subsequent examination and investigation. By contrast, a deficit in a localized function such as language allows the lesion site to be pinpointed from history and examination alone.

Distributed cognitive functions

Attention/concentration

Attention is difficult to define, but implies concentration and persistence. Impaired attention implies inability to focus and selectively concentrate on a topic, with impersistence, distractibility, and often disorientation, e.g. as seen in the acute confusional state. Anatomically, attention requires a distributed system including neocortex (especially prefrontal), thalamus, and brainstem, linked by the reticular activating system (**6**). Attention may be disrupted by any focal lesion affecting this distributed system, or by a diffuse disturbance, such as metabolic upset or the effect of drugs.

Table 2 Cognitive functions

Distributed	Attention/concentration
	Memory
	Higher-order intellectual functions
Localized	
Dominant	Language
	Calculation
	Praxis
Nondominant	Spatially-directed attention
	Complex visuo-perceptual skills
	Constructional abilities

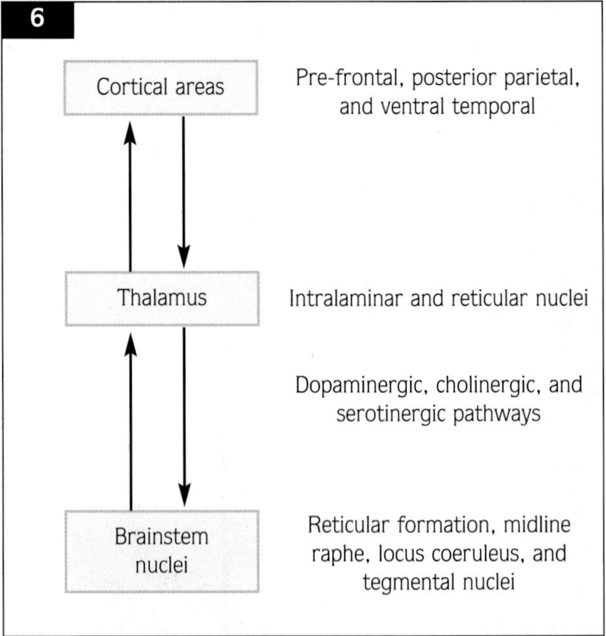

6 Schematic diagram to show the anatomy of the reticular activating system.

Bedside tests of attention/concentration include orientation, digit span (i.e. asking the patient to repeat number strings), the ability to recite months of the year backwards (not forwards as this is overlearned and not a true measure of attention), or serial sevens (i.e. asking the patient to subtract 7 from 100 and keep subtracting 7).

Higher cognitive processes

The frontal lobes are particularly involved in conceptual thinking, adaptation and set shifting (i.e. adjusting to a change in rules), planning and problem solving, and personality, motivation, and social behaviour.

Patients with frontal lobe damage show deficits in the above, in particular poor planning and goal setting, distractibility, and perseveration (i.e. being unable to discard old rules and start using new rules). Such so-called frontal behaviour can be present long before there is any supporting evidence of frontal dysfunction on neuropsychology or brain imaging (7).

In addition to the above cognitive deficits, frontal lobe damage also has behavioural consequences. Disinhibition may occur, resulting in social and sexually inappropriate behaviour. Aggression and lack of concern for others may be a feature. Loss of interest in the world also occurs, with increasing passivity.

Applied anatomy

Anatomy of the frontal lobes is described in (8). The frontal lobe syndrome may be further subdivided. Orbitomedial damage is said to result in personality and behaviour change, while dorsolateral damage tends to have more effect on executive function, such as problem solving. Such distinctions are rarely clinically apparent.

Frontal lobe function may be tested in the clinic by verbal fluency, e.g. FAS letter fluency (asking the patient to generate as many exemplars [example words] beginning with F in 1 minute, then repeating this for both A and S). Asking patients what is meant by proverbs such as ‘A rolling stone gathers no moss’ is also a measure of abstract reasoning and relies on the frontal lobes. Motor sequencing, such as the Alternating Hand Movements Test, also assesses frontal function.

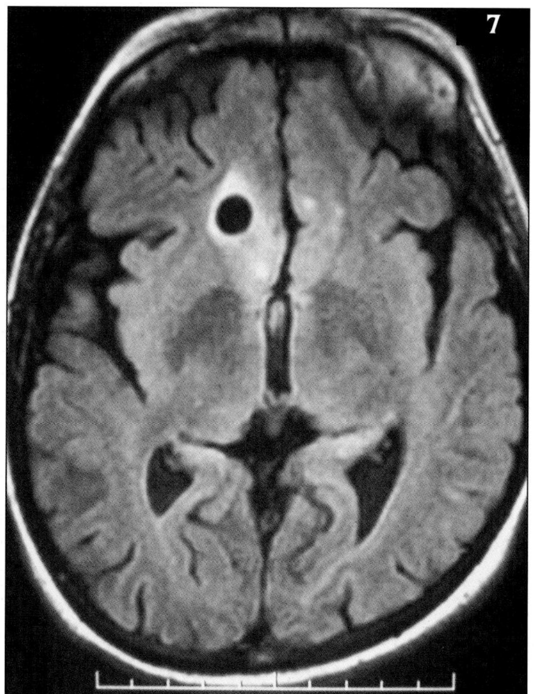

7 Magnetic resonance image of a frontal brain tumour.

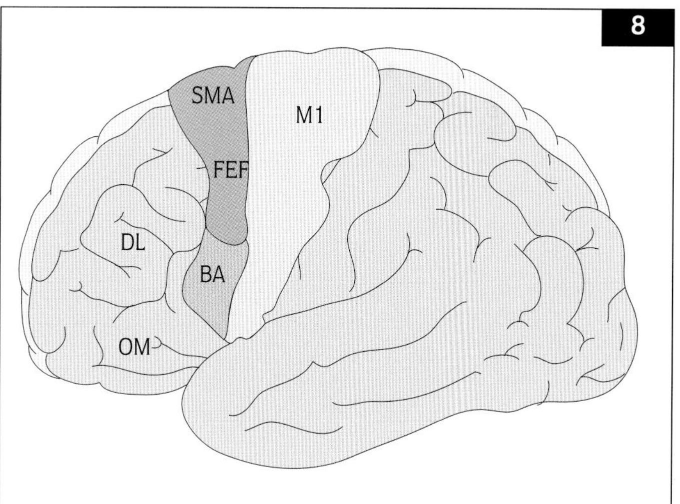

8 Diagram of the anatomy of the brain frontal lobes. BA: Broca’s area; DL: dorsolateral pre-frontal area; FEF: frontal eye fields; M1: primary motor cortex; OM: orbito-medial; SMA: supplementary motor area.

Memory

Memory is not a unitary function, but is a broad term which includes many subcomponents. For instance, episodic memory refers to the ability to learn and retain new information. Asking a patient to repeat a name and address three times, and then asking the patient to recall the name and address after at least 5 minutes can assess this. The ability to do this task is crucially dependent on the hippocampus and other limbic system structures. This is the first region of the brain to be affected in Alzheimer's disease, hence impaired delayed recall is the earliest feature found on testing patients with new-onset Alzheimer's disease.

Semantic memory, by contrast, is the database of knowledge an individual draws on to give meaning to conscious experience, e.g. knowing the capital of France or the boiling point of water. This can be tested at the bedside by category fluency (e.g. naming as many animals in the next minute, object naming [whether real objects or line drawings], and reading). Memory will be addressed more fully in the section on Memory disorders (**3.3**).

Localized cognitive functions

Dominant

Language

Language is subserved by the left hemisphere in nearly all right-handed people and in over 60% of left-handed people. Language comprehension is served mainly by the dominant temporal lobe, especially Wernicke's area (the posterior third of the superior temporal gyrus), while language expression relies on more anterior structures such as Broca's area (the posterior third of inferior frontal gyrus).

A full bedside assessment of language should include the following: spontaneous speech, naming, comprehension, repetition, reading, and writing. The nature of any language impairment (aphasia) detected by these determines the type of aphasia.

Language is more fully addressed in the section on Speech and Language Disorders (page 94).

Calculation

Pathology at the angular gyrus (the posterior Sylvian fissure straddling temporal and parietal lobes) of the dominant hemisphere can result in inability to understand or write numbers. This can be found in association with aphasia. When occurring in conjunction with the inability to write, right-left disorientation and finger agnosia (i.e. being unable to say which of the patient's or examiner's fingers is the middle one), this is termed Gerstmann's syndrome.

Praxis

Praxis refers to the ability to perform and control skilled or complex motor actions. Apraxia is the inability to execute such motor commands in the context of good comprehension and cooperation, together with functioning motor and sensory systems. Apraxia is further subdivided into ideomotor and ideational apraxia, terms that can generate confusion.

Ideomotor apraxia is the inability to carry out motor acts to command, yet with preserved ability to carry these out spontaneously, e.g. lighting a match. It is thought that ideomotor apraxia occurs due to stored programmes for specific motor acts, called engrams, being damaged or disconnected. It is usually due to dominant hemisphere, inferior parietal or prefrontal pathology.

Ideational apraxia is the inability to synthesize the individual components of a complex motor act into one unified operation, with retained ability to perform each component, e.g. able to open a matchbox to command, strike a match to command, yet be unable to effortlessly carry out the entire motor repertoire seamlessly. It can occur with extensive left hemisphere disease or lesions affecting the corpus callosum (the fibres connecting the cerebral hemispheres).

Apraxia may affect only selected movements. For example, orobuccal apraxia results in difficulty performing motor commands involving buccal areas (such as whistling, chewing) and occurs with inferior frontal or insular lesions. Asking the patient to mime certain actions, such as whistling, waving goodbye, and pouring tea may test praxis.

Right hemisphere function

Visuo-spatial and perceptual function rely heavily but not exclusively on the nondominant hemisphere. These are required for visual attention, i.e. the ability to attend to the visual environment. The ability to dress, construct objects, and ability to understand what one is seeing may be impaired with right hemisphere damage. Such patients may fail to recognize objects or people. They tend to ignore objects to their left side and may fail to identify objects or faces despite intact vision. Visuo-spatial and perceptual function may be tested at the bedside by asking the patient to draw a clock face, overlapping pentagons, or a three-dimensional cube.

Damage to the right hemisphere can impair spatially directed attention leading to the disorder of neglect, where patients attend less to left hemispace (**9**). This may amount to a complete denial of the left side (**10**), or lesser states such as sensory extinction where a visual or tactile stimulus, when administered bilaterally, fails to be perceived on the left side. Neglect usually occurs due to right inferior parietal or prefrontal pathology, but occasionally results from damage to the thalamus, basal ganglia, or cingulate gyrus.

That neglect occurs almost always to the left may be due to the left hemisphere monitoring right hemispace, while the right hemisphere monitors both hemispaces. Thus a right hemisphere lesion means that only right hemispace is monitored, while the converse does not apply with a left hemisphere lesion.

Dressing apraxia is not an apraxia as such, but a visuo-perceptual disorder in which the patient is unable to dress (becoming entangled in clothing), despite there being no motor disorder. It usually occurs due to right posterior parietal damage.

The ability to copy a shape, e.g. overlapping pentagons or a cube, requires vision, perception, and visuo-motor output. Difficulties copying usually reflect right parietal dysfunction. Patients with right-sided lesions tend to produce drawings with grossly altered spatial arrangements, while patients with left-sided lesions make over-simplified drawings.

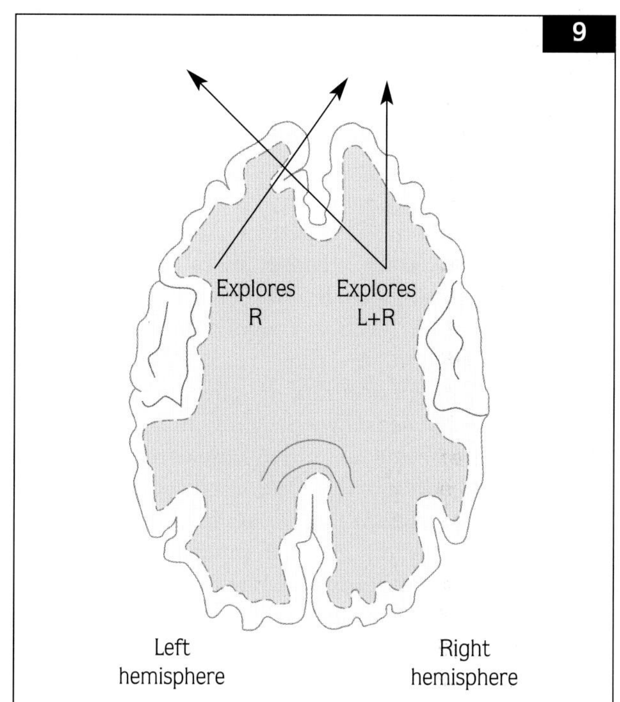

9 Diagram to show the dominance of the right hemisphere for directed attention.

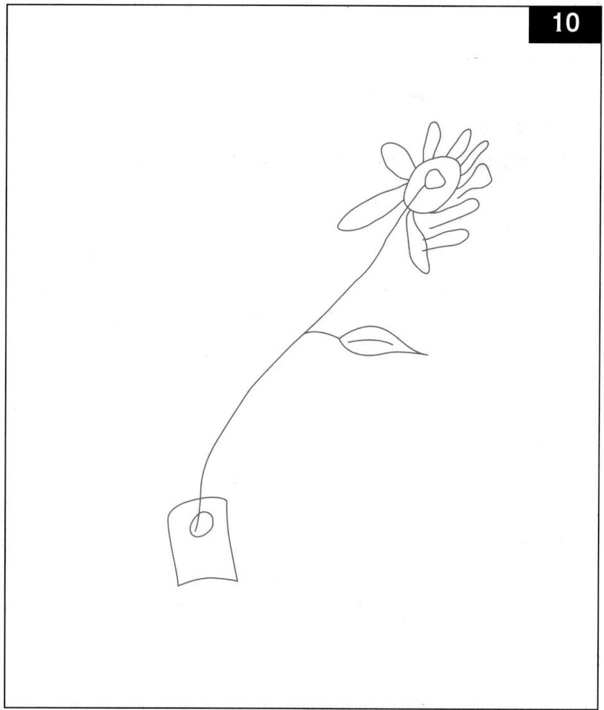

10 Unilateral visual neglect analysis. The patient neglects the left hemispace due to a right hemisphere stroke. (The original drawing was of a double-headed daisy.)

Difficulties in higher order visuo-perceptual skills may occur in right hemisphere damage. In visual object agnosia, the patient is unable to identify an object visually despite having normal basic perception. This does not represent a general semantic memory loss about the object, as identification through tactile or auditory modalities results in access to full semantic information about the object. The deficit in access is therefore modality-specific, i.e. inability to access semantic information about an object when this is presented visually.

This deficit can apply specifically to person recognition. In prosopagnosia, the patient is unable to recognize familiar faces. Knowledge about the person is not lost, however, as gait, voice, and so on cause the patient to identify the person whose face is not recognized. It is usually due to bilateral inferior occipito-temporal lesions.

Cognitive history taking

Although cognitive history taking broadly follows the general principles of history taking, the presence of cognitive deficits (not always noticed by the patient while causing them inexplicable distress) means that there are differences in the conduct of this part of the examination. It is worthwhile trying to interview both patient and informant alone at some point; this allows any sensitive issues to be mentioned by the patient, and also allows the informant to give a clear history of the nature of the presenting complaint without risk of offending the patient. In view of the possible lack of insight, it is worth asking the patient if they know why they have been referred to the clinic. In addition to the presenting complaints themselves, it is useful to ask how these difficulties are impacting on daily living activities.

A complaint such as 'poor memory' cannot be accepted simply at face value, but the nature of the complaint must be determined further. Patients may use the term 'poor memory' to represent many problems, including failing to keep appointments or retain new information (true episodic memory impairment), forgetting objects' and people's names (anomia, usually in keeping with semantic memory impairment), or forgetting where they have left their keys or why they have gone into the kitchen (often simply slips of attention or concentration). Enquiries about anterograde memory (i.e. ability to retain new information), retrograde memory (ability to retrieve knowledge about previous holidays and so on), and semantic memory (factual knowledge, knowing what objects are used for) are important.

For language, in addition to asking whether patients have difficulty expressing themselves or in understanding others, it is also worth asking whether there has been any impairment of reading or writing. Difficulties with dressing, finding one's way around the house or the town, or difficulties constructing objects suggest a visuo-spatial problem.

The informant interview

When speaking to the informant alone, information on what was the initial symptom, and how symptoms have changed with time is important. For example, initial symptoms of no longer being able to retain new information indicate an anterograde episodic memory deficit, which could be the beginnings of Alzheimer's disease. By contrast, an initial symptom of word-finding difficulty and forgetting the function of objects suggests a semantic memory deficit such as can occur in fronto-temporal dementia. The tempo of evolution of symptoms can help to determine the underlying pathology. Sudden-onset symptoms with subsequent improvement suggest a vascular cause. Insidious-onset progressive symptoms are more in keeping with neurodegenerative disease, or perhaps a slow-growing tumour.

Examples of how the cognitive deficit affects the patient in the real world should be sought, such as work, cooking and general household tasks, driving and so on. The informant may well be able to provide further history, which the patient cannot. Past history should enquire as to whether there have been any previous neurological or psychiatric illnesses, or whether there has been any significant head trauma (i.e. sufficient at the time to result in loss of consciousness). An accurate drug history is essential, particularly as sedating drugs can be an easily reversible cause of cognitive impairment. Family history must be thorough, and diagnoses should not necessarily be taken at face value; institutionalization or 'nervous breakdown' may indicate a previously undetected neurological disease, while depression may be secondary to a neurodegenerative process. Social history provides the patient's occupation, which is of use in estimating premorbid IQ. Alcohol habits are particularly relevant here.

Physical examination

In a busy clinic, the clinician may be hard pushed to obtain a history from both patient and informant, perform bedside cognitive testing, and also conduct a physical examination. A detailed neurological examination is not routinely necessary, but the following features may be of particular relevance.

Visual field deficits may not be noticed by the patient or relative, and can easily be screened for by confrontation, preferably using a redheaded pin, but if necessary using a wiggling finger. Eye movements, both saccades (voluntary rapid movements) and pursuit (tracking the examiner's finger) should be checked. For example, inability to look down to command can occur in progressive supranuclear palsy, while impaired pursuit movements can occur in basal ganglia disorders such as Huntington's disease.

Specific signs of frontal disease can include the presence of so-called primitive reflexes such as grasp reflex (grip occurring due to stroking palm), pout reflex (puckering of lips when lips lightly tapped), and palmo-mental reflex (chin quivering when palm stroked) (**11**). Involuntary movements such as fidgeting, which could indicate Huntington's disease, can be easily overlooked unless consciously looked for. Gait analysis can also be useful. The stooping festinant gait of Parkinson's disease or the 'feet glued to the floor' sign of normal pressure hydrocephalus can be diagnostic.

Bedside cognitive testing

The assessment of higher cerebral function is carried out during the neurological examination, but may also be supplemented by a more detailed assessment of cognitive function performed by a neuropsychologist (if available). The extent to which the clinician is able to assess cortical function depends on the time available in clinic, and also whether the clinician has the backup of a neuropsychologist, as these services are not universally available. The clinician should be able to sample various aspects of cognitive function, such as general functioning, frontal function, memory, language, and visuoperceptual function.

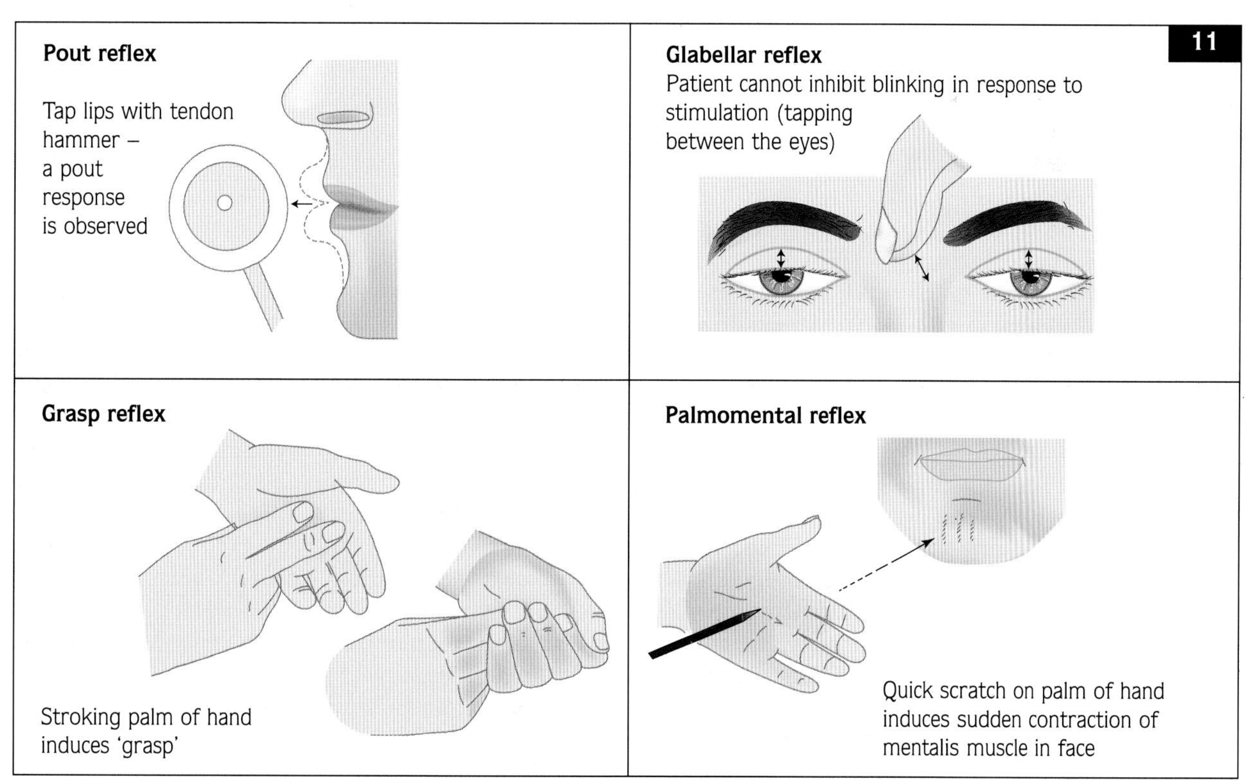

11 Diagram to illustrate primitive reflexes.

A standardized test such as the Mini-Mental State Examination (MMSE) can be used to test aspects of cognitive function. Although this was originally devised to be used as a screening tool for dementia, it is of some use for a brief cognitive overview.

Some criticisms of the MMSE are that the language and visuo-perceptual items are too easy, there is not a proper test of delayed recall, and there is no timed test to assess subcortical cognitive slowing. In an effort to address these issues, the Addenbrooke's Cognitive Examination (ACE) includes the 30 points of the MMSE, but the additional 70 points improve the assessment of memory and language and include timed fluency tasks which are sensitive to subcortical dysfunction.

CRANIAL NERVE EXAMINATION

CRANIAL NERVE I (OLFACTORY NERVE)

The patient should be asked if taste and smell are affected. Further testing is not necessary unless the patient concurs or there is a special reason to test olfaction. Before testing, the airway should be checked that it is clear. Each nostril is tested with an odour such as camphor or peppermint. Loss of smell is termed anosmia. If nasal disease is excluded, a lack of smell may be due to closed head injury or anterior cranial fossa disease but is also a feature of certain neurodegenerative disorders such as Parkinson's disease.

CRANIAL NERVE II (OPTIC NERVE)

The basic tools for assessment are a bright light, an ophthalmoscope, coloured pins, and a vision reading chart (e.g. Snellen). First assess visual acuity. The patient is asked if they are aware of reduced vision in either or both eyes. Visual acuity should be tested wearing glasses if prescribed. Each eye is covered in turn and its neighbour tested separately. When using the Snellen chart, the patient stands 3–6 m from the chart and reads from largest to smallest print, visual acuity being measured as the distance from the chart (3 or 6 m) over the distance at which the letters should normally be seen, e.g. 6/6 for normal and 6/60 for poor vision. Alternatively, a near vision chart is held 30 cm from the patient and again they are asked to read the smallest print possible with each eye in turn. Results are expressed as N6 and so on.

Visual fields testing requires a 7 mm coloured (red) pin. The patient is asked if they are aware of a gap or 'blindspot' in either eye and the clincian establishes that the red pin target is visible to each eye. The patient should then look into the examiner's eyes, standing 1 m away. The field of vision of the examiner can then be compared with that of the patient (confrontation). The extent of visual field can be ascertained by testing each eye from each quadrant, asking the patient to state as soon as they can see the pinhead at all (regardless of colour). Whether the patient can see red in central vision should also be checked.

The following findings may be demonstrated:

- ❑ Constricted fields of vision, e.g. chronic papilloedema, glaucoma, and functional illness (tunnel vision).
- ❑ Central field defect (scotoma), e.g. optic neuritis, retinal haemorrhage.
- ❑ Altitudinal (vertical) field defects in one eye, e.g. retinal infarction.
- ❑ Hemianopia.
- ❑ Bitemporal (defect in the temporal fields in both eyes), e.g. pituitary disease.
- ❑ Homonymous (defect to the same side in both eyes), e.g. parietal, temporal, or occipital lobe disease.

Quadrantanopia, congruous, and incongruous field defects further localize defects (see page 104).

Fundoscopy

The ophthalmoscope is used to examine the fundus of each eye separately, while the patient fixates, in a darkened environment, into the distance. The ophthalmoscope should be adjusted for the clinician's own vision. If myopic, the lens is turned anticlockwise (red), if long-sighted clockwise (black). The patient's eye is then approached approximately 15° from the line of fixation and the disc, blood vessels, and retina are assessed and findings documented accordingly.

> The student should be aware of the following fundoscopic findings:
> Optic disc: normal, pale, swollen.
> Blood vessels: normal, attenuated, swollen, nipped, absent, containing emboli, cholesterol.
> Retina: infarcts, haemorrhages, exudate, retinopathy.

Cranial nerves III, IV, and VI (Oculomotor, trochlear, and abducent nerves)

These nerves are responsible for all eye movements. The clinician should inspect for ptosis (drooping eyelid), pupil size, strabismus (squint), and proptosis (protuberance of the globe of the eye). If proptosis is suspected, the eye should be inspected from above, tilting the head back to contrast the prominence of each eye. The pupil light reaction should be tested in each eye separately, checking both the direct (illuminated eye) and indirect (nonilluminated eye) responses. The pupils' reaction to converging (when looking at the end of the nose the pupils constrict) should also be assessed. The patient should be asked if double vision is present; if so, confirmation that the double vision is binocular (requires both eyes to be present) can be obtained by covering one eye at a time. The patient should be asked whether the two images are separated vertically or horizontally, and in which direction the two images (true and false) maximally separate. The range of slow-pursuit horizontal and vertical eye movements is assessed by asking the patient to follow the clinician's moving finger or similar object. If double vision is present, in which direction of gaze double vision is maximal should be determined.

> The following rules help assessment:
> Double vision is worse (maximal) in the direction of the affected muscle.
> The false image is always the outermost one.
> The false image is the product of the affected eye.

When evaluating eye movements:

- ❏ The position of the head should be noted (patients with double vision will often tilt the head to minimize this).
- ❏ The eyes should be checked in the primary position (at rest) and ptosis or pupillary asymmetry noted.
- ❏ The eyes should be assessed following an object. Are abnormal movements (nystagmus) present? Is there paralysis of one or more muscles? All directions of gaze must be tested and knowledge of the specific muscle innervation is essential.
- ❏ Nystagmus is defined as a slow drift of the eyes to one side with a fast corrective movement in the opposite direction. While physiological when watching an object moving rapidly by, these movements are generally abnormal and inform on the presence of brainstem/cerebellar disease.

The patient should be asked to follow a moving finger and any jerky movements observed. Nystagmus can be:

- Vertical. Upbeat: upper brainstem, e.g. pontine infarction. Downbeat: cervico-medullary junction, e.g. Arnold–Chiari malformation.
- Horizontal. Ataxic: greater in the abducting (looking outwards) rather than adducting (looking inwards) eye, e.g. multiple sclerosis.
- Multi-directional. Present in all directions of gaze (though maximal in one), e.g. drug-induced.
- Unidirectional. Peripheral: labyrinthine disease. Central: unilateral cerebellar disease.

Cranial nerve V (Trigeminal nerve)

The patient is asked if they are aware of altered facial sensation, and sensation of light touch with cotton wool is tested in each of the three sensory divisions (ophthalmic V1, maxillary V2, and mandibular V3). The corneal reflex (V1&V2) is tested with a wisp of cotton wool, touching cornea not sclera. Next, the three divisions are tested with a pin. When defining the territories of sensory loss, the clinician should always move from the abnormal to the normal.

Evidence of wasting (temporalis muscles) should be noted and motor function assessed. The pterygoids are tested with the jaw open wide (thus avoiding any minor deviation due to temperomandibular joint asymmetry), then jaw opening resisted by pressing against the joint. In order to test the jaw jerk, the patient is asked to let the jaw hang loosely open and a tendon hammer is used to percuss on the clinician's finger placed on the patient's chin.

Cranial nerve VII (Facial nerve)

The nasolabial folds (from the corner of the mouth to the sides of the nose) should be observed and spontaneous movements such as blinking and smiling noted. The following muscles are tested using the instructions described: *frontalis*: 'wrinkle the forehead'; *orbicularis oculi*: 'screw up the eyes'; *buccinator*: 'blow out the cheeks'; and *orbicularis oris*: 'show the teeth'. Ptosis (drooping of an eyelid) is not due to weakness of facial nerve muscles, and facial asymmetries without weakness is common so the clinician should not be misled. The patient should be asked about taste (absence or distortion) and tested with a sugar or salt solution applied by a cotton bud to the anterior two-thirds of the tongue.

The facial nerve also supplies the muscle to the stapedius and the parasympathetic supply to the lachrymal gland, though neither is tested at the bedside. Four types of disturbance are found:

- Unilateral lower motor neurone, e.g. Bell's palsy.
- Bilateral lower motor neurone, e.g. myasthenia gravis.
- Unilateral upper motor neurone, e.g. hemisphere stroke.
- Bilateral upper motor neurone, e.g. brainstem stroke (pseudobulbar palsy).

Loss of emotional expression is a feature of Parkinson's disease, while excessive emotional expression (emotional incontinence) occurs in pseudobulbar palsy.

Distinction between unilateral upper and lower motor neurone facial weakness is simple. In upper motor neurone (UMN) weakness, forehead and eye closure is relatively spared (bilateral supranuclear innervation) while these are affected with lower motor neurone (LMN) lesions (the final common pathway for all that travels to the facial nucleus).

Cranial nerve VIII (Auditory and vestibular nerves)

Assessment requires a 256 or 512 Hz tuning fork and an auroscope. First, the patient is asked if they have noticed any problem with their hearing. The clinician then speaks in a whisper (counting in numbers) at arm's length from the patient, while occluding the nontested ear with the hand and notes if hearing loss is reported or demonstrated.

Weber's test involves striking a 256 or 512 Hz tuning fork on the examiner's knee and placing it on the patient's forehead. Normally this should be heard in the middle of the head and should not lateralize. When the sound does lateralize, it does so to the side of greater conductive loss or that with the intact cochlea (to the opposite side) in sensori-neural hearing loss.

The Rinne test again utilizes the vibrating tuning fork. The tuning fork is applied firmly to the mastoid process behind the ear and is then held in front of the external auditory meatus. The patient is asked which they hear loudest. Patients with normal middle ear function hear well by air rather than by bone conduction. Those with conductive deafness experience the reverse. The external auditory meatus and tympanic membrane are examined with the auroscope. Conductive deafness is common (wax, middle ear disease). Sensori-neural deafness is less common and takes three forms:

- Cochlea, e.g. noise, Ménière's disease.
- Nerve lesion, e.g. meningitis, acoustic neuroma.
- Brainstem, e.g. vascular, demyelinating disease.

Examination of the vestibular nerve includes testing gait, nystagmus, and caloric testing (see Chapter 2).

Cranial nerve IX (Glossopharyngeal nerve)

Sensation on the posterior wall of the tonsillar fossa is examined with an orange stick. The motor (stylopharyngeus) and autonomic (parotid glands) components are not tested.

Cranial nerve X (Vagus nerve)

Articulation, cough, and ability to elevate the soft palate ('saying Ah!') are tested. Touching the posterior pharyngeal wall on each side with a throat swab and comparing each response tests the gag reflex. The autonomic and sensory (external auditory meatus/external ear) are not tested at the bedside.

Cranial nerve XI (Accessory nerve)

The sternocleidomastoid muscle is tested by tilting the head to the opposite side while applying resistance against the examiner's hand, pressing on the angle of the jaw. The muscle belly can be observed to stand out. Asking the patient to shrug the shoulders against resistance also tests the trapezius muscle.

Cranial nerve XII (Hypoglossal nerve)

The tongue at rest on the floor of the mouth is examined for wasting and fibrillation. The patient is asked to protrude the tongue and any deviation noted. The tongue should also be observed for reduced movement as seen in UMN lesions.

Multiple cranial nerve palsies

Patterns of multiple cranial nerve palsies due to extra-axial lesions reflect their anatomical relationships (*Table 3*).

Table 3 Relationship between cranial nerve palsies and location of extra-axial lesions

III, IV, VI, V1	Superior orbital fissure or (anterior) cavernous sinus
III, IV, VI, V1, V2	Posterior cavernous sinus
V, VI	Apex of petrous temporal bone
VII, VIII	Internal auditory meatus or cerebello-pontine angle
IX, X, XI	Jugular foramen
IX, X, XI, XII, and sympathetic	Below the base of the skull (retropharyngeal space)

MOTOR EXAMINATION

Evaluation of patterns of limb weakness is essential for localizing disease. Weakness may affect a single limb (monoplegia), arm and leg on the same side (hemiplegia), or all limbs (tetraplegia). Weakness may be proximal (muscle disease or inflammatory neuropathy) or distal (axonal neuropathy). Observations on muscle wasting, abnormal movements, tone, and reflex state help to differentiate UMN from LMN disorders. Finally, weakness that does not follow a recognizable organic pattern may be psychologically based. The components of assessment are:

Observation

- ❑ Involuntary movements, e.g. extrapyramidal disease, fasciculation, myokymia.
- ❑ Muscle symmetry.
- ❑ Left to right (mononeuropathy, e.g. carpal tunnel).
- ❑ Proximal versus distal, e.g. myopathy or neuropathy.

Examination of muscle tone

The patient is asked to relax and the upper and lower limbs are tested. The patient's fingers, wrist, and elbow are flexed and extended. Similarly, the patient's ankle and knee are flexed and extended. Normally, a small, continuous resistance to passive movement is felt, and decreased (flaccid) or increased (rigid/spastic) tone should be noted. Failure to relax is a common problem. A flaccid (weak) limb suggests a LMN disorder, while a spastic (weak) limb suggests UMN problems. Rigidity occurs in extrapyramidal disease and fluctuating stiffness (paratonia or Gegenhalten) with diffuse frontal lobe disturbance.

Examination of muscle strength

Muscle strength is under corticospinal (UMN) and anterior horn cell/nerve root/nerve plexus/peripheral nerve/neuromuscular junction (LMN) control. The target of all pathways is the muscle itself. Muscle strength is tested by having the patient move against the examiner's resistance. One side is always compared with the other and strength is graded on a scale from 0–5/5 (*Table 4*).

When testing, the following should be considered: the overall distribution (proximal versus distal), the pattern (flexor versus extensor), and the grouping (single root versus multiple roots versus plexus versus single nerve versus multiple nerves). There is no avoiding knowing the detailed innervation of muscles. In a minimal examination the following should be tested:

Table 4 Grading of motor strength

Grade	Description
0/5	No muscle movement
1/5	Visible muscle movement but no movement at the joint
2/5	Movement at the joint, but not against gravity
3/5	Movement against gravity, but not against added resistance
4/5	Movement against resistance, but less than normal
5/5	Normal strength

Upper limbs

- ❑ Flexion at the elbow (C5, C6, biceps).
- ❑ Extension at the elbow (C6, C7, C8, triceps).
- ❑ Extension at the wrist (C6, C7, C8, radial nerve).
- ❑ Finger abduction (C8, T1, ulnar nerve).
- ❑ Opposition of the thumb (C8, T1, median nerve).

Lower limbs

- ❑ Flexion at the hip (L2, L3, L4, iliopsoas).
- ❑ Adduction at the hips (L2, L3, L4, adductors).
- ❑ Abduction at the hips (L4, L5, S1, gluteus medius and minimus).
- ❑ Extension at the hips (S1, gluteus maximus).
- ❑ Extension at the knee (L2, L3, L4, quadriceps).
- ❑ Flexion at the knee (L4, L5, S1, S2, hamstrings).
- ❑ Dorsiflexion at the ankle (L4, L5).
- ❑ Plantar flexion (S1).

Pronator drift

The patient is asked to stand for 20–30 seconds with both arms straight forward, palms up, and eyes closed, keeping the arms still while the examiner gently taps downwards. In pronator drift, the patient fails to maintain extension and supination (and the limb 'drifts' into pronation). Pronator drift is seen in UMN disease.

Reflexes

The tendon reflex comprises a stretch sensitive afferent (from muscle spindles) via a single synapse (anterior horn cell region) to the efferent (motor) nerve. These reflexes are accentuated in UMN disease and diminished or absent with LMN disorders.

Deep tendon reflex

Patients must be relaxed and positioned properly before starting the test. No more force with the tendon hammer should be used than is required to provoke a definite response. Reflexes can be 'reinforced' by asking the patient to perform isometric contraction of other muscles groups (clenched teeth, upper limbs or pull on hands, lower limbs). Reflexes should be graded on a 0 to 4 'plus' scale (*Table 5*).

The following reflexes should be tested:

- ❑ Biceps (C5, C6): examiner's thumb or finger is placed firmly on the biceps tendon and the examiner's fingers are struck with the reflex hammer.
- ❑ Triceps (C6, C7): the patient's upper arm is supported and the patient's forearm is allowed to hang free; the triceps tendon is struck above the elbow.
- ❑ Brachioradialis (C5, C6): the patient's forearm rests on their abdomen or lap and the radius is struck about 3–5 cm (1–2 inches) above the wrist.
- ❑ Abdominal (T8, T9, T10, T11, T12): a blunt object is used to stroke the patient's abdomen lightly on each side in an inward and downward direction above (T8, T9, T10) and below the umbilicus (T10, T11, T12), while noting contraction of the abdominal muscles with deviation of the umbilicus towards the stimulus.
- ❑ Knee (L2, L3, L4): the patient sits or lies down with the knee flexed and the patellar tendon is struck just below the knee.
- ❑ Ankle (L5 S1): the patient's foot is dorsiflexed at the ankle and the Achilles tendon struck.

Clonus

If the reflexes are hyperactive, clonus is tested for. This can be done at any joint but is usually performed at the ankle. The knee is supported in a partly flexed position and the foot then quickly dorsiflexed. Clonus is manifest by rhythmic sustained oscillations.

Plantar response (Babinski)

A positive Babinski sign indicates UMN disease while a negative test is normal. The lateral aspect of the sole of each foot is stroked with the end of a reflex hammer and movement of the toes noted. The normal movement is that of plantar flexion. Extension of the big toe with fanning of the other toes is abnormal, a positive Babinski.

Table 5 Tendon reflex grading scale

Grade	Description
0	Absent
1+ or 1++	Hypoactive
2+ or 2++	Normal
3+ or 3++	Hyperactive without clonus
4+ or 4++	Hyperactive with clonus

SENSORY EXAMINATION

This is the most exacting and potentially misleading part of the neurological examination. There are five categories of sensation to test: pain, temperature (small fibre/spinothalamic tract/thalamus/diffuse + frontal cortex), vibration, joint position, and light touch (large fibre/dorsal column/medial lemnisci/ parietal cortex). These anatomically separate pathways explain why sensory loss is often incomplete (dissociated).

The examination requires a cooperative patient and an alert examiner! Each test should be explained to the patient before it is performed. The patient should have their eyes closed during testing. Symmetrical areas both sides of the body are compared as well as distal and proximal areas of each limb. Where an area of sensory abnormality is found, the boundaries should be mapped out in detail, moving from the abnormal to the normal area.

- ❑ Distal and symmetrical impairment in limbs suggests sensory neuropathy.
- ❑ A level on the trunk below which sensation is lost localizes spinal cord disease.
- ❑ An area on the trunk or limbs confined to one side suggests nerve root or single peripheral nerve disturbance.

The five components of sensation are tested as follows:

VIBRATION

A low-pitched (128 Hz) tuning fork is used to test awareness at bony prominences such as wrists, elbows, medial malleoli, patellae, anterior superior iliac spines, spinous processes, and clavicles. Vibration is normally lost at the ankles in those over 60 years. The patient must understand that it is the sensation of vibration rather than the sound from the fork that is being tested.

SUBJECTIVE LIGHT TOUCH

Cotton wool is used to touch the skin lightly on both sides. Sometimes when a stimulus is presented simultaneously on both sides it is not felt on one side, yet it is felt on that side when the stimulus is presented separately (sensory inattention, suggesting parietal lobe disease). Several areas on both the upper and lower extremities are tested and the patient is asked if there is a difference from side to side.

POSITIONAL SENSATION

The patient's big toe is held away from the other toes to avoid 'cueing' and is moved to demonstrate to the patient what is meant by 'up' and 'down'. The examiner then moves the toe and asks the patient to identify the direction the toe has moved with eyes closed. If position sense is impaired the ankle joint is then tested and then the fingers in a similar fashion. The examiner should then move proximally to test the metacarpophalangeal joints, wrists, and elbows.

PAIN

A suitable sharp disposable object is used to test 'sharp' sensation. The following areas are tested:

- ❑ Shoulders (C4).
- ❑ Inner and outer aspects of the forearms (C6 and T1).
- ❑ Thumbs and fingers (C6 and C8).
- ❑ Front of both thighs (L2).
- ❑ Medial and lateral aspect of both calves (L4 and L5).
- ❑ Little toes (S1).

Remembering these particular dermatomal areas is helpful. Pinprick examination is critical to defining a 'level' when localizing spinal cord disease.

TEMPERATURE

This is omitted if pain sensation is normal, but is helpful in confirming the presence and distribution of pinprick loss. A tuning fork heated or cooled by water is used and the patient asked to identify 'hot' or 'cold'. Similar areas as above are tested. Temperature loss is much less helpful when defining a precise spinal cord level.

DISCRIMINATION

Tests of discrimination are dependent on intact touch and position sense; they cannot be performed where these are clearly abnormal. These tests assess cortical (parietal) sensation.

Graphaesthesia

With the blunt end of a pen or pencil, a large number is 'drawn' in the patient's palm and the patient asked to identify the number.

Stereognosis (an alternative to graphaesthesia)

A familiar object is placed in the patient's hand (coin, paper clip, pencil) and the patient then asked to name the object.

Two point discrimination

An opened paper clip or divider is used to touch the patient's finger pads, alternating irregularly between one point touch and touch in two places simultaneously. The patient is asked to identify if they feel 'one' or 'two' points. The minimum distance at which the patient can discriminate is identified.

COORDINATION

These tests assess cerebellar function and require relatively intact motor power. To test for lack of coordination with weakness present is unsound, as such tests cannot be performed to a level that allows accurate interpretation. Associated signs, dysarthria, and nystagmus are further pointers to cerebellar disease.

Rapid alternating movements

The patient is asked to slap rapidly the palmar and dorsal surface of the hand alternately on the thigh. In the lower limbs, the patient taps the examiner's hand with the sole of each foot.

Limb coordination

This is assessed by 'point-to-point' tests. The patient is asked to touch the tip of the examiner's finger and then their own nose. The accuracy in approaching each target and the smoothness of movement between the two targets is recorded (deficits being termed past-pointing and dysmetria, respectively). In the lower limbs, the patient is asked to touch the front of the shin with each heel, and then to run the heel up the front of the leg to the knee and similar observations are made.

STANCE AND GAIT

General

The patient is asked to stand with feet together and, once they feel comfortable, to close the eyes. If the patient cannot balance well with eyes open, they should not be asked to close the eyes. The clinician stands close to the patient and must be ready to support them should they fall to either side. Instability with eyes open suggests cerebellar disease, and with the eyes closed afferent (sensory ataxia) disturbance. Unsteadiness only on eye closure is a positive Romberg test.

Postural stability (the retropulsion or forced pull-back test)

The patient is asked to stand with eyes open and feet apart. The clinician stands behind the patient and warns that the patient will suddenly be pulled backwards. An abnormal response should be anticipated and the clinician must be prepared to catch the patient! An abnormal reaction is seen in extrapyramidal disorders (e.g. Parkinson's disease) with retropulsion (taking several steps backwards and being unable to maintain stability).

> The student should be able to recognize certain walking disorders: the hemiplegic, ataxic, extrapyramidal, and myopathic gaits; also the high 'steppage' gait of unilateral or bilateral footdrop.

REFERENCES

1 Fuller G (2004). *Neurological Examination Made Easy.* Churchill Livingstone, London.

2 Lindsay K, Bone I (2004). *Neurology and Neurosurgery* Illustrated. Churchill Livingstone, London.

CHAPTER 2: NEUROLOGICAL INVESTIGATIONS

Ian Bone, John Greene

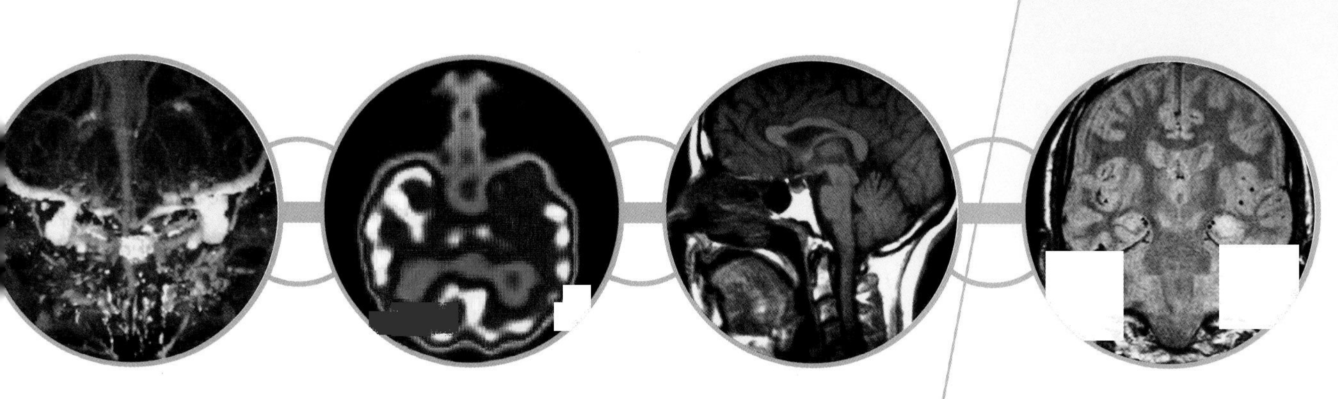

INTRODUCTION

The evaluation of a clinical presentation often, though not invariably, leads to the formulation of an 'investigative pathway'. Thoughtful and thorough history taking and examination are central to deciding not only 'whether to investigate' but also 'where to look'. Once the decision to investigate has been reached the clinician must ask 'Is it in the head, the spine, in nerve, or muscle?' The answer is crucial as each of these sites or levels has specific investigations. Getting it right is not always easy. For example, the complaint of a 'foot drop' can indicate cerebral, spinal, or peripheral nerve disease, the skill being to decide from the history and examination where the culprit lies and to investigate accordingly.

In this chapter the student will be introduced to the basics of neurological investigation as an aid to the problem-oriented text that follows. Rather than list and describe these in order of complexity, cost, or availability, each compartment (head, spine, nerve and muscle) will be addressed separately. Obviously some disease processes will be multifocal, multi-system, and straddle compartments (e.g. the craniocervical junction) or medical disciplines (e.g. the orbit and ear), and resultant investigations will be more complex and diverse. What follows is therefore a 'rough guide' to introduce the student to techniques, indications, sensitivity, specificity, and potential complications of the tools used to diagnose and help treat neurological disease.

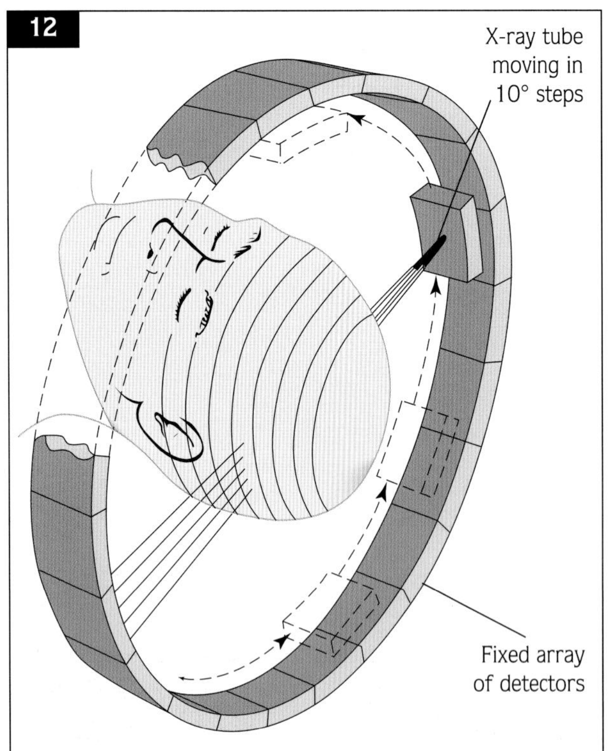

12 Diagram to illustrate a computed tomography gantry.

INVESTIGATING THE HEAD

A computed tomography (CT) or magnetic resonance imaging (MRI) scan is now indicated in most work-ups of suspected intracranial disease. Indeed, it is difficult to imagine practice without such imaging. Before the 1970s, the ability to image the brain depended on isotope studies, invasive injection of air (air encephalography), or contrast (angiography/ myodil ventriculography). These techniques showed no more than outlines and shadows and were risky. As a result the clinician was much more conservative and circumspect as to which patients were subjected to such tests. The advent, easy availability, and low risk of cross-sectional imaging have undoubtedly diluted clinical skills but the advances in diagnosis and improved patient care are well worth this price. The current danger is that of over-investigation and that clinical skills are reduced such that investigations are targeted to the wrong site or incidental imaging findings are mistaken as relevant.

COMPUTED TOMOGRAPHY

Also referred to as CAT (computer assisted tomography) scanning, this revolutionary technique was introduced into clinical practice in 1973. It is the most commonly used form of cranial imaging, being available on a 24 hour basis in almost all hospitals. The word tomography refers to imaging of slices of the brain (or indeed any other organ). The patient is placed in a gantry (**12**) and a thin beam of X-rays, created by a collimator, traverses each 'slice' to a multichannel ionization detector.

The path from collimator to detector establishes a single 'beam' passing though a patient's tissues. During the scan the computer takes brief readings from all detectors. In the earlier scanners both collimator and detector rotated around the patient whereas in modern third and fourth generation units the detectors are fixed with only the X-ray source moving. Computer processing with multiple beams and detectors completely encircling the head allows absorption values for blocks of tissue (voxels) to be established. Reconstruction of this by two-dimensional display (pixels) results in the eventual CT appearance (**13**). Slices studied can be varied in thickness (1–10 mm) and can be rendered parallel to the orbitomeatal line (a reference line drawn through the orbit and ear), to allow anatomical interpretation and reproducibility for repeated studies. 'High definition' (1–2 mm) scans give greater anatomical detail, take longer to acquire, and are reserved for examination of specific sites (orbit, Circle of Willis, pituitary). Alteration of window level will change the contrast appearance and allow more detailed assessment of bony structures or help visualize subtle differences in tissue contrast, such as with an acute cerebral infarct.

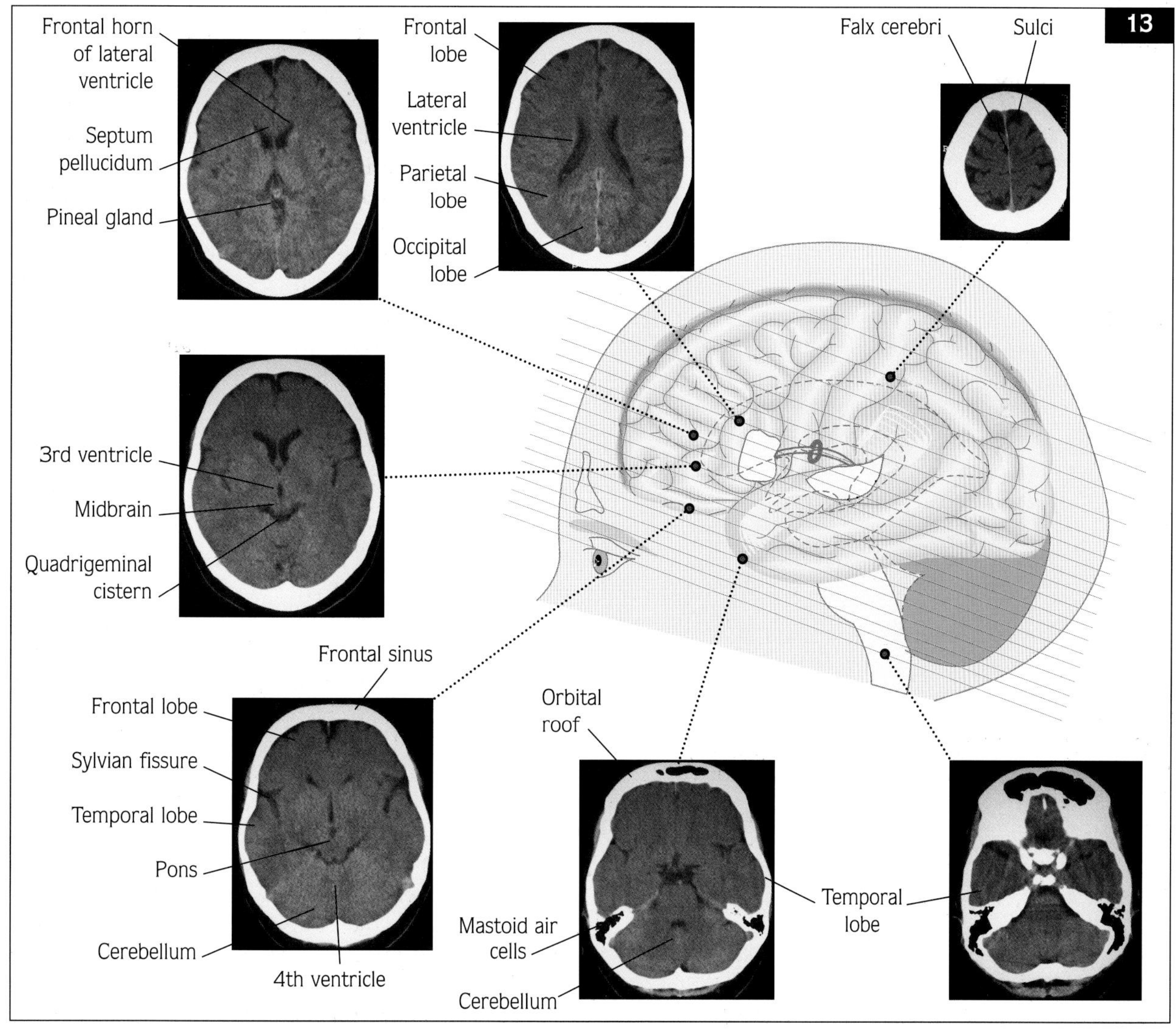

13 Computed tomography of normal brain, illustrating landmark anatomical details.

Knowledge of the display and normal appearance along with anatomical structures is essential.

Because each slice is oriented along the orbitomeatal line, with the head tilted backwards, lesions appear more posterior than is the case. Scans can be displayed in coronal (ear to ear) or sagittal (forehead to occiput) planes to look at specific regions (e.g. orbits or foramen magnum).

Intravenous contrast medium should not be given routinely but only where a noncontrast scan has shown an abnormality and clarification is required (e.g. a possible abscess, metastatic tumour, or vascular anomaly). Reactions occur in 5% of examinations, this being dose-dependent. Contrast will show up areas of high vascularity and regions of breakdown of the blood–brain barrier, and will demonstrate areas of altered blood perfusion (see later). A contrast-enhanced scan also highlights up all the major intracranial vessels (**14**).

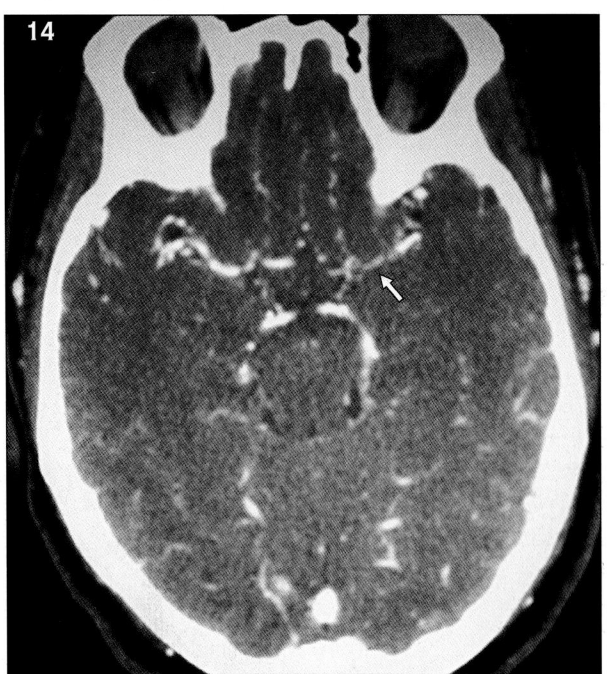

14 Contrast computed tomography scan showing left middle cerebral artery stenosis (arrow).

The patient requires no special preparation for CT other than reassurance that the procedure is safe. Metal should be removed from the head (hairpins, dental bridgework) as this will cause signal scatter and result in artefacts. If contrast is to be given, the clinician must enquire after a history of previous reaction to injected contrast. Radiation dose is comparable to a routine skull X-ray (now rarely performed). Pregnancy is not a contraindication as only a very small quantity of radiation 'scatters' in the direction of the abdomen and uterus. The limitations of CT are listed below.

Helical CT (spiral CT) is performed by 'pulling' the patient though the scan field of the rotating X-ray source. This allows faster scanning time, better image reformation, and the ability to perform newer techniques such as CT angiography (CTA).

Limitations of CT imaging

- ❏ Uses ionizing radiation.
- ❏ Visualization of posterior fossa structures (e.g. brain stem or cerebellar pontine angle) inferior to MRI.
- ❏ Less sensitive than MRI to acute changes (e.g. early infarction).

CT angiography

This examination uses X-rays to visualize blood flow in arterial vessels. CT venography (CTV) studies similar flow through veins (**15**). An automatic injector controls the timing and rate of injected contrast, continuing through the initial image recording. The rotating scanner spins in a helical manner around the patient, creating a fan-shaped beam of X-rays. As many as 1000 of these pictures may be recorded in one turn of the detector. Once acquired, processing these images requires a powerful computer programme making it possible to display cross-sectional slices or three-dimensional 'casts' of the blood vessels.

CTA is used to study blood vessel wall disease (narrowing [**16**], dissection, atheroma, inflammation, and aneurysm). Both extracranial (aortic arch and branches) and intracranial vessels (Circle of Willis and branches) can be studied. Intracranial aneurysms sized ≥3 mm can be detected.

CT perfusion

CT perfusion (CTP) has been proposed as a method of evaluating patients suspected of having an acute stroke where thrombolysis is considered. It may provide information about the presence and site of vascular occlusion, the presence and extent of ischaemia, and tissue viability. CTP provides accurate measures of local cerebral blood volume (CBV), blood flow (CBF), and mean transit time (MTT).

Magnetic resonance imaging

The millions of water molecules within the human body contain hydrogen ions which themselves have protons which act as microscopic magnets. When placed in a magnetic field, the protons within an individual will align in part to that field. If a radiofrequency (RF) pulse is then applied, these protons become excited, start spinning and 'flip' their orientation. When the RF field is turned off, the spinning protons revert to their prior state (or alignment), releasing energy. These microscopic magnets, and the vectors that they set up by realignment, form the basis for generating images. Variability of these ions from tissue to tissue as well as their response to applied electromagnetic pulses creates images of organs (brain and spine) in health and disease.

> The student should understand two simple terms. The time it takes for a proton to recover most of its longitudinal alignment (or magnetization) is referred to as T1 or spin-lattice relaxation time. The time it takes for the proton to lose most of its transverse alignment (or magnetization) is referred to as T2 or spin-spin relaxation time.

A bewildering variety of RF pulse sequences (spin echo, gradient echo, inversion recovery, and saturation recovery) can be used, often with a specific purpose (e.g. gradient echo to show previous haemorrhage). The introduction of magnets with increasing field strength (>1.5 Tesla) allows a better signal to noise ratio, and faster scanning with a reduction of imaging time. By acquiring data more rapidly, these MRI scanners can perform MR angiography and gain functional information on diffusion and perfusion, as well as images of those acutely ill patients whose physiological instability previously precluded lengthy investigations.

15 Computed tomography venogram illustrating cerebral venous drainage.

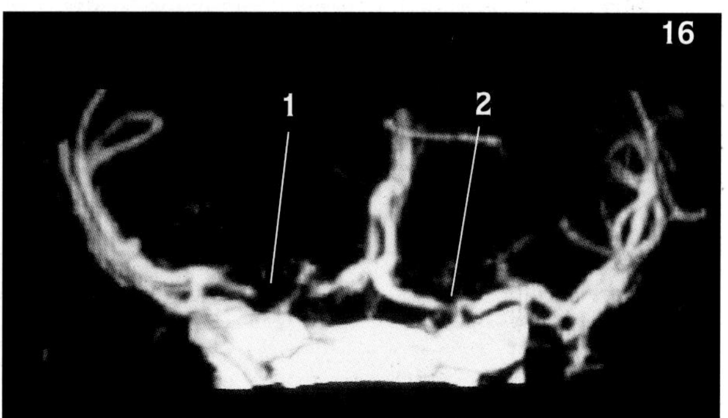

16 Computed tomography angiogram illustrating left middle cerebral artery occlusion (**1**) and right middle cerebral artery narrowing (**2**).

Advantages and disadvantages of MRI (compared to CT)

Advantages

- ❑ Select any plane, e.g. oblique.
- ❑ No ionizing radiation.
- ❑ More sensitive (early ischaemia/demyelination).
- ❑ No bony artefacts (looking at sites adjacent to bone).

Disadvantages

- ❑ Cannot use with any ferromagnetic implant, e.g. pacemaker.
- ❑ Claustrophobic.
- ❑ Does show bony artefact.
- ❑ Long-term hazards not known.

T1 and T2 images can easily be distinguished. On T1, CSF is black (hypointense) while on T2 it is white (hyperintense). *Table 6* will help interpretation of MR images (increase or decrease in signal is defined in relation to normal grey matter). Figures 17–20 present MRI images.

Paramagnetic enhancement

The intravenous agents used (e.g. gadolinium) induce a strong local magnetic field effect that will shorten T1 signals. This will result in enhancement of the image in areas of contrast leakage (across a damaged blood–brain barrier) or within the vascular compartment (arteries, microcirculation, and veins). Gadolinium and other such agents highlight ischaemia, infection, and demyelination and can help distinguish tumours from surrounding oedema.

Table 6 Guide to identifying the MRI sequence

T2-weighted image

- ❑ CSF bright.
- ❑ Grey matter brighter than white matter.

Perfusion-/diffusion-weighted image

- ❑ CSF grey.
- ❑ Grey matter brighter than white matter.

T1-weighted image

- ❑ CSF dark.
- ❑ White matter brighter than grey matter.

CSF: cerebrospinal fluid.

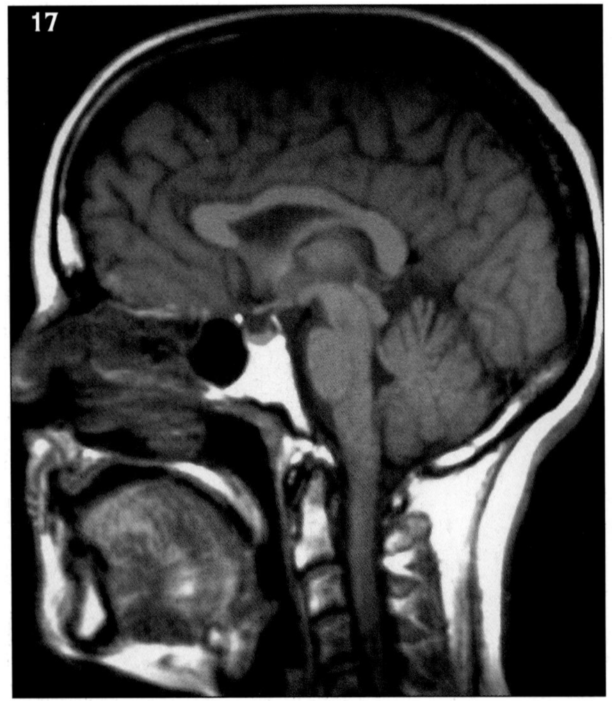

17 T1 sagittal magnetic resonance image of the brain.

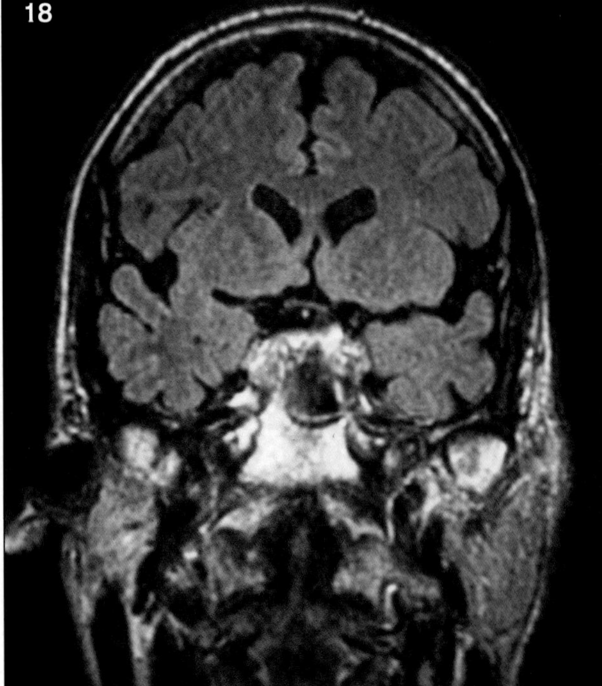

18 T1 coronal magnetic resonance image of the brain.

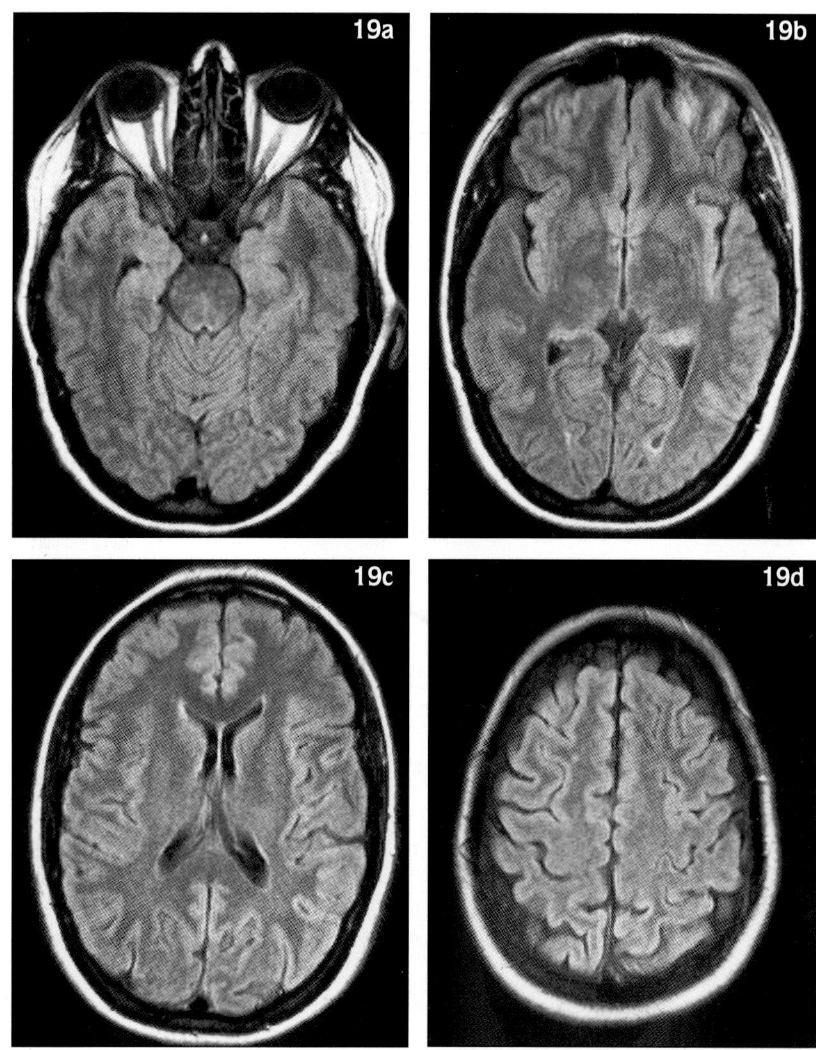

19a–d Axial magnetic resonance image (MRI) of the brain illustrating the superiority of MRI over computed tomography.

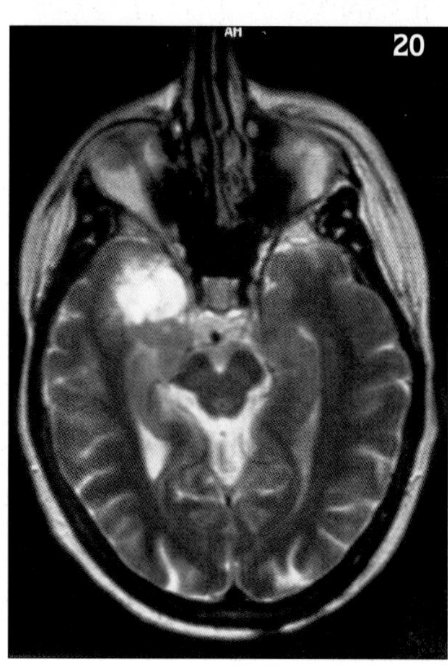

20 T2 magnetic resonance image showing a primitive neuroepithelial tumour in the right anterior temporal lobe.

Fluid-attenuated inversion recovery

Fluid-attenuated inversion recovery (FLAIR) MRI depicts areas of tissue T2 prolongation while suppressing the signal from neighbouring cerebrospinal fluid (CSF). It is helpful in assessing lesions that are adjacent to CSF, such as at periventricular and superficial cortical sites (**21, 22**).

Magnetic resonance angiography

Magnetic resonance angiography (MRA) can be based on either time-of-flight methods (measuring the contrast enhancement produced by inflowing blood), or phase contrast methods, which utilize the flow-induced variations in signal induced by the motion of blood alone. Time-of-flight measurements are better suited for imaging arterial wall morphology. MRA can demonstrate extracranial and intracranial stenosis (narrowing) noninvasively, but tends to overestimate the degree of a stenosis and consequently misinterprets low flow through a tight stenosis as an occlusion. It is usually used in conjunction with ultrasound (or CTA) for the presurgical evaluation of carotid artery stenosis (**23**). MRA is used to screen for intracranial aneurysms but will not show all of those seen on intra-arterial digital subtraction angiography (see later). By selecting a specific flow velocity, veins can also be imaged (MRV) (**24**).

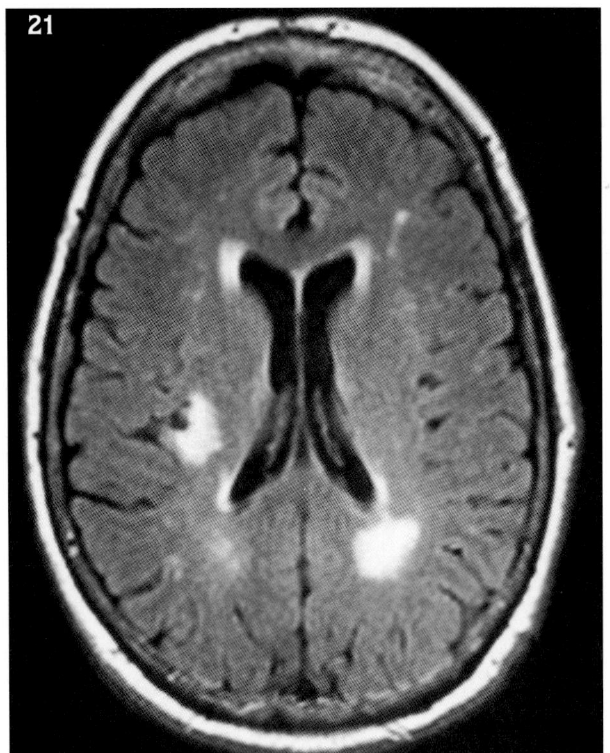

21 Fluid-attenuated inversion recovery (FLAIR) magnetic resonance image showing the white matter changes of multiple sclerosis. Note that cerebrospinal fluid (CSF) is dark on FLAIR unlike the bright CSF seen on T2.

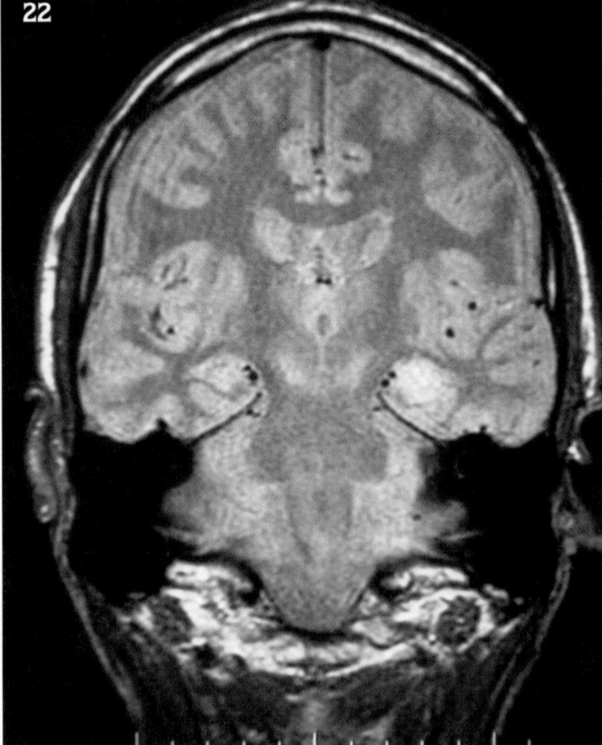

22 Fluid-attenuated inversion recovery (FLAIR) magnetic resonance image showing left mesial temporal sclerosis causing epilepsy.

Diffusion and perfusion MRI

MR scanning is superior to CT scanning in the diagnosis of acute stroke. However, conventional MRI does not demonstrate early acute cerebral ischaemia particularly in a period when therapy may reverse or limit the permanent brain injury. T2 sequences require at least several hours from the onset of the stroke before demonstrating signal change abnormalities. Water diffusion has been introduced as an additional contrast parameter in the MR imaging of acute stroke. Diffusion-weighted imaging (DWI) can demonstrate altered cellular metabolism and the reduction in the microscopic water molecule motion (Brownian motion) in acute and subacute stroke. Damaged tissue may be visualized as early as 5–15 minutes after the onset of stroke.

Perfusion-weighted imaging (PWI) allows assessment of perfusion of the brain microvasculature. PWI requires intravenous gadolinium contrast (bolus tracking) that causes a paramagnetic susceptibility effect. Thus, MRI signal declines as gadolinium travels through the microvasculature. PWI is used to complement the information obtained by DWI in acute stroke patients. PWI may show reduced perfusion in a larger area of tissue than that shown on DWI. This indicates a significant area of tissue at risk of infarction, a diffusion–perfusion mismatch. Using PWI, various perfusion properties of the contrast bolus can be calculated, such as CBV, CBF, MTT, and time-to-peak (TTP) of contrast arrival. A very low CBV implies irreversible ischaemia.

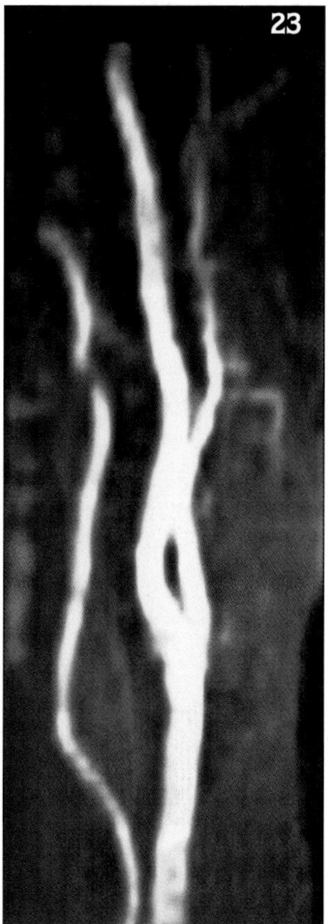

23 Magnetic resonance angiogram of the carotid arteries.

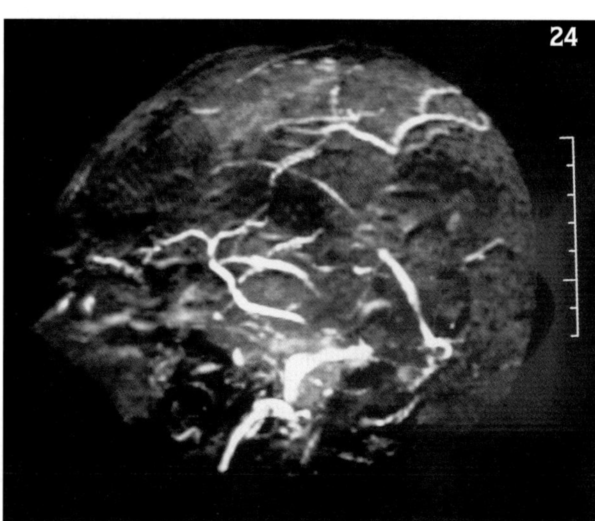

24 Magnetic resonance venogram showing superior sagittal thrombosis.

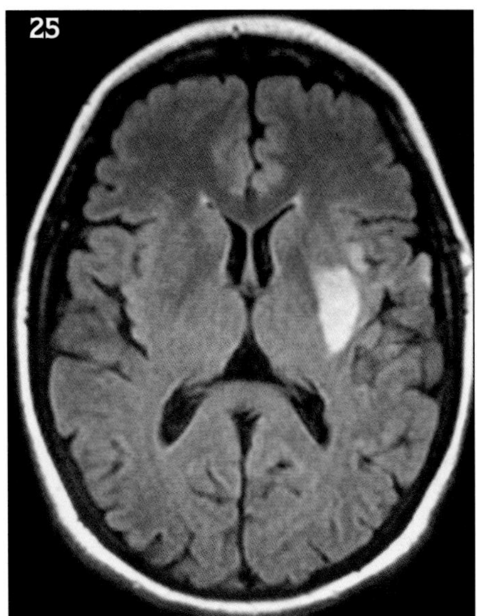

25 T1 magnetic resonance image of a subcortical infarct.

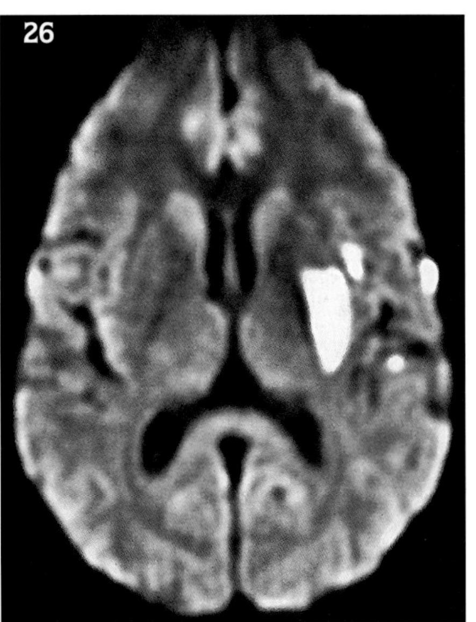

26 Diffusion-weighted imaging (DWI) magnetic resonance image of the same subcortical infarct shown in **25**.

The combination of MRA to visualize vessels, and DWI and PWI to define early infarction and 'tissue at risk' ('the ischaemic penumbra') represents an ideal 'package' to help plan acute stroke treatments (25–27).

Functional MRI

MRI is able to map functional cortical activity during the performance of tasks. This is achieved by detecting regional cortical tissue changes in venous blood oxygenation. This technique is known as blood oxygen level dependent (BOLD) imaging or simply functional MRI (fMRI) (28). The key to fMRI is that oxyhaemoglobin is diamagnetic whereas deoxyhaemoglobin is paramagnetic. The role of fMRI is mainly in research. It has, however, been used to guide surgical resection of brain in or adjacent to eloquent areas.

MR spectroscopy

Proton MR spectroscopy (MRS) is a noninvasive method used to obtain a biochemical profile of brain tissue (a biochemical biopsy). Although 31 phosphorous (^{31}P) spectra are sometimes used, MRS studies are usually obtained by proton spectroscopy with water suppression (protons are abundant in brain tissue and have high nuclear magnetic sensitivity compared with other magnetic nuclei). Single voxel spectroscopy can be performed in many clinical 1.5T MR units using commercially available software. Two types of MRS finding are encountered. Either the spectrum reveals a metabolite that is not normally present or, more commonly, an abnormal quantity of a normal metabolite is present. Metabolites studied are N-acetyl aspartate (NAA), choline (Cho), creatine (Cr), glutamate, and lactate. NAA is present exclusively in neurones and declines with neuronal and axonal damage and death. Choline is important in the myelination of nerves and is altered by demyelinating diseases. Lactate is a marker of anaerobic respiration and increases in hypoxic ischaemic states. In the future it is hoped for a diagnostic 'biochemical biopsy' for specific tumour types and other pathologies.

Single photon emission computed tomography

Single photon emission computed tomography (SPECT) utilizes a gamma camera that can rotate and computer reconstruction similar to CT, to produce a two-dimensional image. Compounds labelled with gamma-emitting tracers (ligands) have been developed to study blood flow, map receptors, and evaluate

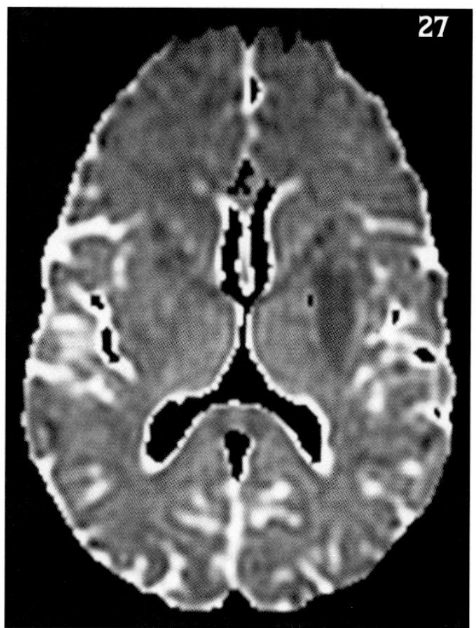

27 Apparent diffusion coefficient (ADC) magnetic resonance image of the same subcortical infarct shown in **25**.

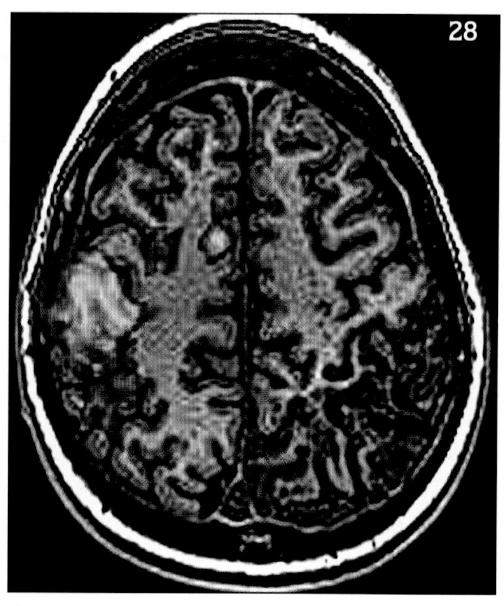

28 Functional magnetic resonance image of a patient performing left finger tapping, activating right motor cortex.

29 Ictal hexamethylpropyleneamine oxime (HMPAO) spectroscopy (axial slice in the long axis of the temporal lobe) with injection 25 seconds after the onset of a right mesial temporal lobe seizure, showing hyperfusion of the whole temporal lobe.

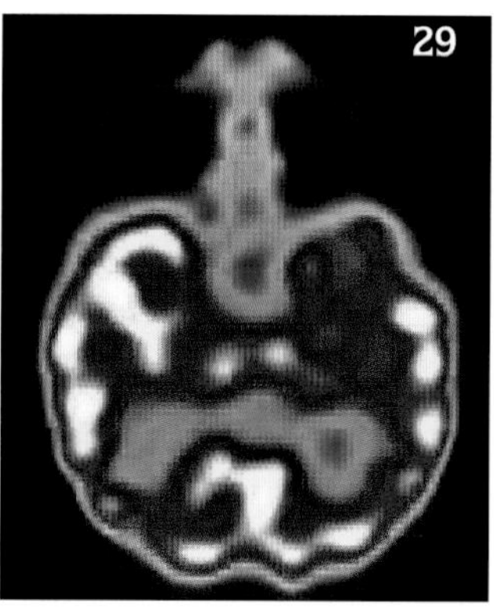

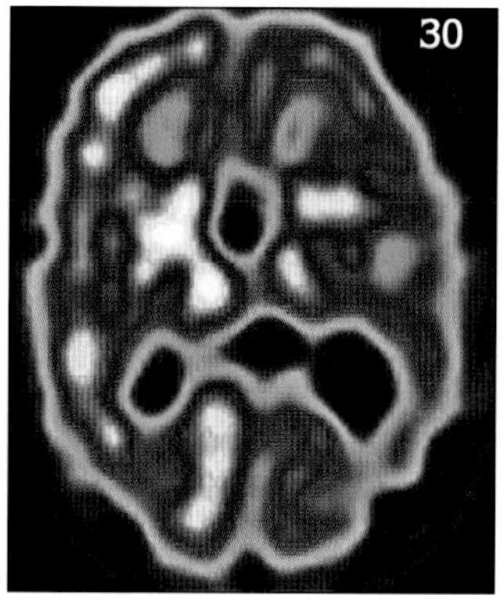

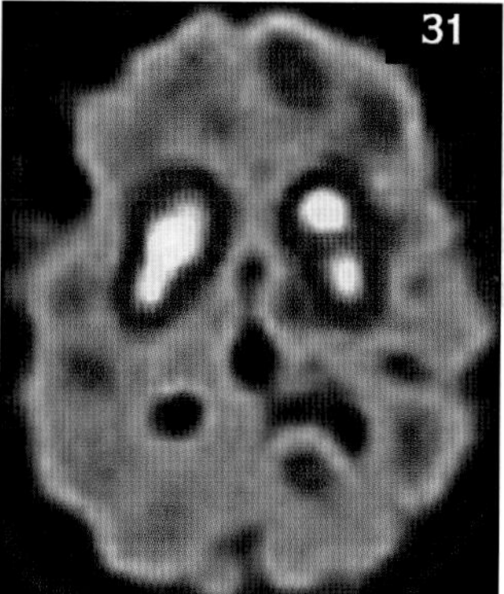

30 SPECT imaging showing reduced left hemisphere perfusion in primary progressive aphasia.

31 Fluoropropyl carboxymethoxy iodophenyl nortropane spectroscopy (FP-CIT) showing reduced dopamine transport in corticobasal degeneration.

tumour growth. While a rotating scanner is most commonly used, fixed multidetector systems produce better image definition as well as axial, coronal, and sagittal views. Ligands are labelled with radioactive iodine or thallium and are given intravenously. Radiation dose limits repeated investigations. SPECT scans are interpreted visually, usually in conjunction with structural imaging (CT or MRI), as an anatomical abnormality will influence ligand uptake.

SPECT scanning is used to study cerebral blood flow (in stroke, dementia, and seizures). CNS receptors include benzodiazepine (epilepsy), glutamate (stroke), and dopamine (Parkinson's disease and other movement disorders). Rates of tumour growth can also be studied (high-grade thallium, low-grade tyrosine). The following figures illustrate the clinical applications of SPECT imaging (**29–31**).

Positron emission tomography

The positron emission tomography (PET) technique uses positron-emitting isotopes (radionuclides). These have a short half-life and have to be generated on-site by a cyclotron. Imaging and display also involve cross-sectional data acquisition and reconstruction, much like CT scanning. When a positron encounters an electron (which will be almost immediately it is emitted from the source) mutual annihilation occurs, with the emission of photons (gamma rays). Multiple detectors enable detection and quantification of radioactivity. Labelled oxygen, fluorine, or carbon is used given by intravenous bolus or by inhalation. As well as studying receptor sites and receptor binding, this technique can quantify CBF, CBV, and glucose and oxygen metabolism. Lack of availability and complexity have limited the wider application of PET; however, it may be particularly helpful in detecting small tumours (e.g. small cell lung cancer in paraneoplastic syndromes).

Cerebral angiography

Angiography remains the 'gold standard' choice in the evaluation of arterial and venous occlusive disease, aneurysm (**32**), and arteriovenous malformation (AVM). It is also useful in defining the blood supply of some tumours (e.g. meningioma). Finally, it is necessary for interventional neuroradiologic procedures such as coiling aneurysms, stenting stenosis, and delivering intra-arterial thrombolysis. Contrast is injected via a flexible catheter introduced by the femoral artery, and rapid film changers are used to capture its flow through extra- and intracranial vessels.

Advances in the development of high-quality digital subtraction units provide instantaneous images for view on a cathode ray tube. This digital subtraction angiography (DSA) utilizes analogue to digital image conversion with digital image display. Iodine-containing, water-soluble media provide the necessary density to allow the visualization of the cerebral arterial, capillary, and venous systems. The

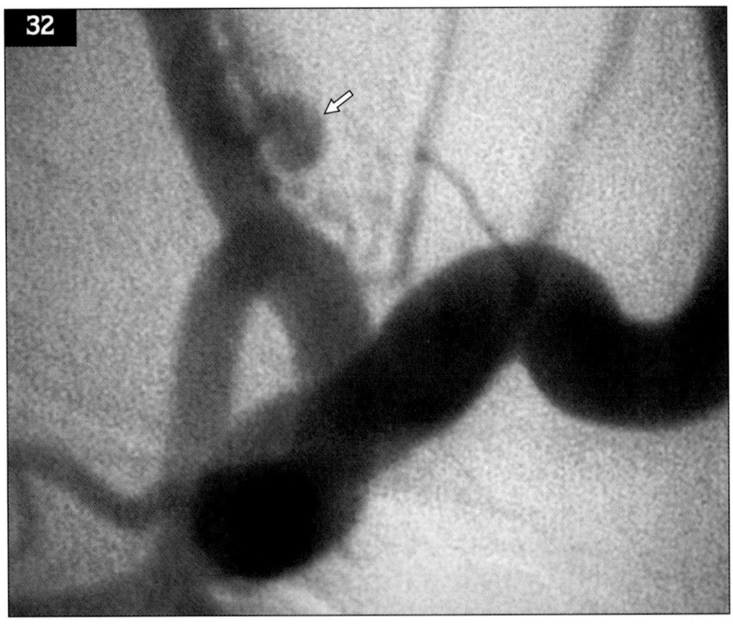

32 Angiogram showing intracerebral aneurysm (arrow).

major complication of cerebral angiography is stroke, either from damaging the vessel wall (dissection) or dislodging thrombus (embolism). Meticulous care to detail is mandatory. With ectatic and tortuous arteries it may be difficult to catheterize these selectively, and injections at the origin of such vessels may be safest.

Once the procedure is over, general care is important, particularly with regard to blood pressure. Elderly patients following a large contrast load may become hypotensive, and with haemodynamically significant carotid artery stenosis, relative hypoperfusion will cause ischaemia and 'watershed' infarction. Systemic reactions to contrast occur, ranging from urticaria to bradycardia and laryngeal spasm. Local complications include haematoma at the catheter site, femoral nerve damage, and arterial thrombosis with distal embolism.

The appearances of a normal examination should be noted with regard to major vessels and their divisions. Oblique views may be used in assessing aneurysms and cervical views for evaluation (and precise measurement) of internal carotid and vertebral artery disease.

Interventional angiography

Recent advances in endovascular procedures now play an important part in patient management. Tumours, aneurysms, fistulas (acquired openings between arteries and veins), AVMs, and narrowed intracranial arteries can be treated by an array of particles, glues, balloons, coils, and stents.

Ultrasound

This noninvasive technique utilizes a probe (transducer) that emits ultrasonic waves, usually at frequencies of 5–10 MHz. When held over a blood vessel these ultrasonic waves are reflected back to the probe, which also doubles as a detector. Reflected waves can then be displayed as a two-dimensional image (B-mode). When the probe is held over a moving column of blood, the frequency shift of reflected waves (Doppler effect) informs on the velocity of the column. There are four types of Doppler ultrasound:

- *Continuous wave Doppler* measures how continuous sound waves change in pitch as they encounter blood flow blockages or narrowed blood vessels. This is performed at the bedside and provides a quick, rough guide of damage or disease.
- *Duplex Doppler* produces a picture of a blood vessel and the organs that surround it. A computer converts the Doppler signals into a graph that provides information about the speed and direction of blood flow through the blood vessel being examined.
- *Colour Doppler* is computer assisted and converts the Doppler signals into colours that represent the speed and direction of flow through the vessel.
- *Power Doppler* is a new technique being developed that is up to five times more sensitive than colour Doppler and is used to study blood flow in vessels within solid organs.

Ultrasound is used to assess extracranial (carotid) arterial disease (33).

Transcranial Doppler ultrasound

Transcranial Doppler ultrasound (TCD) is a safe, reliable, and relatively inexpensive technology for measuring intracranial blood flow velocities. Waves with frequencies around 2 MHz are directed towards intracranial vessels using a handheld probe. The frequency shift (Doppler effect) in the reflected sound indicates the velocity of the column of moving blood.

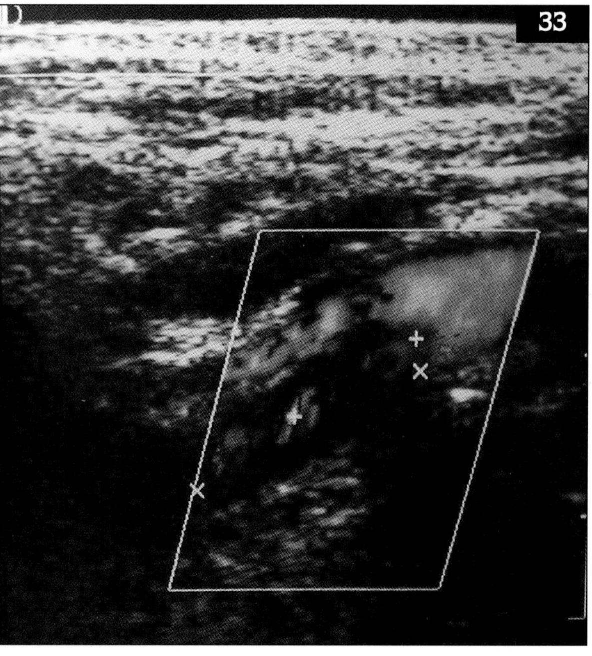

33 Carotid Doppler ultrasound showing 70% right internal carotid stenosis.

Images are reconstructed from the time-dependent intensity of the reflected sound, and vascular structures visualized. Altering transducer location and angle, and the instrument's depth setting obtains velocities from most intracranial arteries. The cranial 'windows' used are the orbit (anterior cerebral artery) and in temporal (middle cerebral artery) and suboccipital regions (basilar and posterior cerebral arteries). Age and skull thickness make insonation of vessels technically difficult. The posterior circulation is more difficult to pick up signals from than the anterior circulation. TCD is quick; 30–40 minutes is sufficient for detailed studies. The instrumentation is inexpensive and portable to the bedside. The applications of TCD are in the assessment of intracranial haemodynamics (measuring autoregulation before and after carbon dioxide inhalation or intravenous acetazolamide), detecting intracranial stenosis, spasm in subarachnoid haemorrhage, and detecting right-to-left shunts (pulmonary fistula or atrial septal defect) following the injection of intravenous agitated saline. Ultrasound may also have a therapeutic effect on clot lysis (after embolic vessel occlusion).

Neurophysiology

While imaging mainly informs on structure, the function of the brain can be assessed using various neurophysiological techniques. Mostly this involves recording spontaneous electrical activity of the brain, but also uses evoked responses, where a stimulus is provided and the brain's response to that stimulus is measured.

Electroencephalography

In electroencephalography (EEG), electrodes are placed in arrays on the scalp, equidistantly and according to an international convention (**34**). Each electrode is wired to its own channel. Electrical differences between pairs of electrodes, or one electrode and a combination of others, are recorded, and can be displayed on a screen as a series of parallel lines, each line representing one electrode. A standard EEG takes about 30 minutes to perform. Patients are usually awake, lying down with eyes closed. In addition to passive recording, provocation techniques are also routinely employed, usually hyperventilation and photic stimulation, which can sometimes induce epileptiform changes on EEG.

Normal rhythms

Detailed EEG analysis is beyond the scope of this chapter, but *Tables 7* and *8* summarize normal and abnormal electrical rhythms.

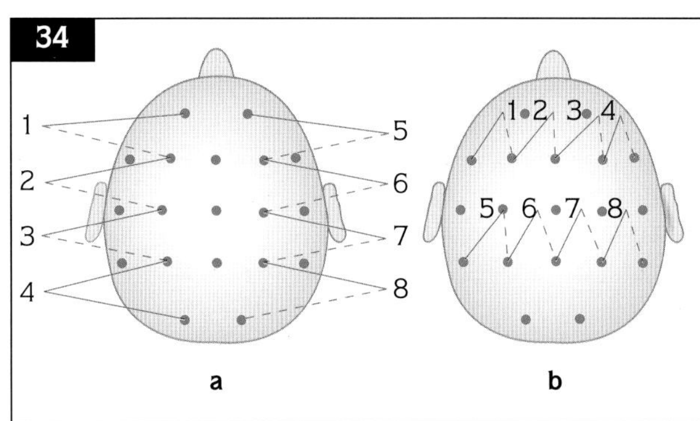

34 Diagram to show the placement of electroencephalography scalp electrodes.

Table 7 Normal electroencephalography rhythms

Alpha rhythm
- ❑ 8–13 Hz
- ❑ Symmetrical
- ❑ Seen posteriorly with eyes closed

Beta rhythm
- ❑ >13 Hz
- ❑ Symmetrical
- ❑ Present frontally, not affected by eye opening

Theta and delta rhythms
- ❑ Seen in children and young adults
- ❑ Frontal and temporal predominance
- ❑ Theta: 4–8 Hz
- ❑ Delta: <4 Hz

Table 8 Abnormal electroencephalography rhythms

Spikes or sharp waves	Epileptiform discharges
Combined spike and slow wave discharges	Commonly occur in epilepsy
Slow waves, localized	Seen over any focal lesion, e.g. tumour, encephalitis, stroke
Slow waves; generalized	Seen in metabolic or toxic coma
Periodic discharges	Seen in CJD, SSPE, metabolic encephalopathies
Absent brain waves	Severe hypoxia, hypothermia, intoxication

CJD: Creutzfeldt–Jakob disease; SSPE: subacute sclerosing panencephalitis.

Clinical use of the EEG

EEG is mainly of use in the diagnosis of altered conscious states including epilepsy. Advances in imaging have largely supplanted its use in localizing lesions. It has a niche role in diagnosis of rare cortical disorders such as Creutzfeldt–Jakob disease (CJD) and subacute sclerosing panencephalitis (SSPE), but is of little use in the differential diagnosis of dementing disorders.

Epilepsy

It must be stressed that the diagnosis of epilepsy is a clinical one. EEG is normal in 50% of patients with epilepsy, and is abnormal in 2–4% of the population who do not have epilepsy. Nevertheless, in a patient who has had a single seizure, EEG can be of some prognostic value in predicting future seizures. Even in definite seizure activity, the EEG can be of use in classification. For example, an apparent tonic–clonic seizure may indicate primary generalized epilepsy, but may also represent a focal seizure, which generalizes so rapidly that the focal onset cannot be appreciated clinically. EEG may be helpful here in differentiating between a focal (35) or generalized (36) epilepsy disorder, which has implications for the choice of anticonvulsant.

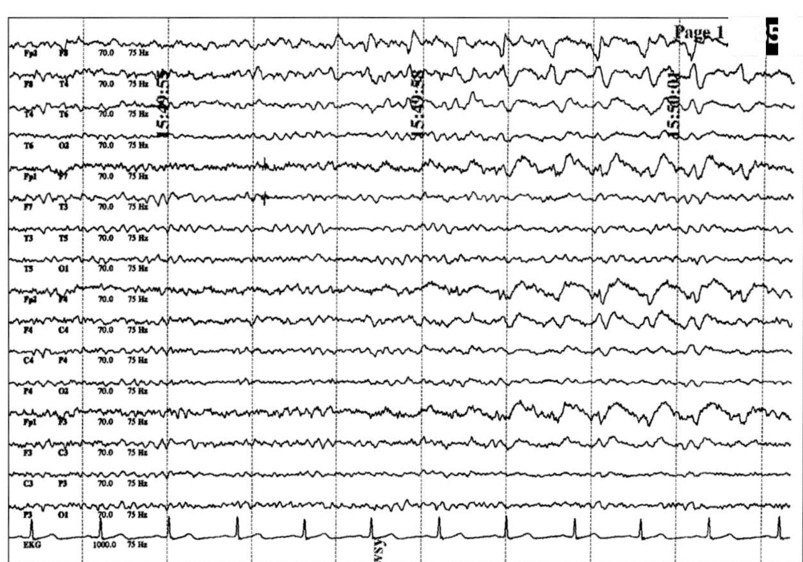

35 Electroencephalograph showing focal seizure onset (top two lines).

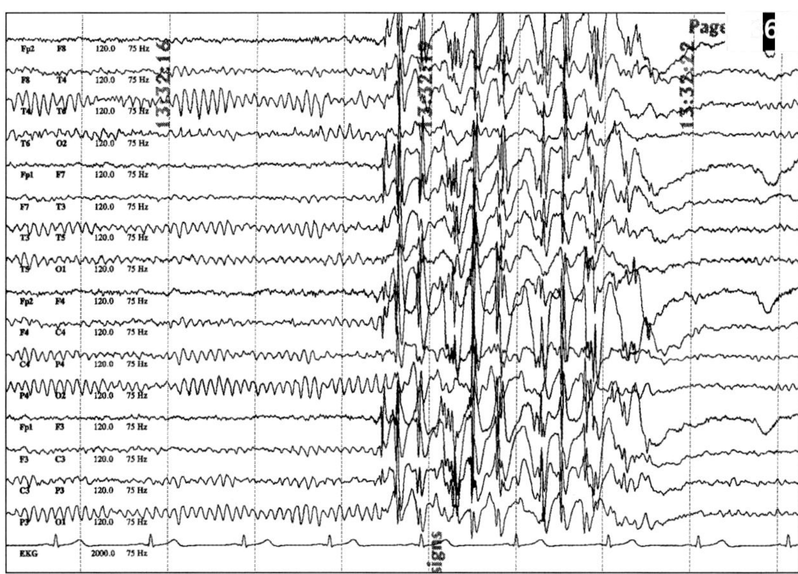

36 Electroencephalograph showing generalized seizure onset.

Other altered conscious states

EEG is particularly useful in other altered conscious states (37). It may reveal the cause of coma, and can be of use prognostically. It may also suggest neurological disorders mimicking unconsciousness such as locked-in syndrome, where the EEG will be normal.

Sleep deprived EEG

Sleep deprived EEG involves the patient remaining awake overnight, and then having EEG done first thing the following morning. Sleep can bring out epileptiform abnormalities on EEG, which may not be apparent on routine EEG. The patient tends to become drowsy quickly, or to fall asleep. Its main use is in terms of seizure classification.

Video-telemetry

As will be covered in the section on blackouts (page 64), the diagnosis of epilepsy is a clinical one, and relies on detailed questioning of the patient and relatives as to what happened during the event. There can, however, arise times when a confident clinical diagnosis cannot be made from the information available. If events are occurring sufficiently frequently, then the patient can be admitted for continuous video recording with simultaneous EEG recording. Should the patient have an event while being monitored, then careful analysis of behaviour as seen on video together with EEG data will almost always yield a diagnosis.

Short video-EEG with suggestibility

The differential diagnosis of epilepsy includes nonepileptic attacks that are of psychological origin. These turns can be induced by suggestion. On account of long waiting times for video-telemetry, it is possible to make a diagnosis of nonepileptic attacks on an outpatient basis by doing an EEG, but using suggestion techniques which increase the likelihood of a patient having an attack while being recorded.

Intracranial EEG recordings

If a patient is being considered for epilepsy surgery, the clinician must be confident of the localization of the focus of seizure activity. This is usually achieved using a combination of supporting information, including clinical semiology of the seizure, structural imaging, SPECT imaging of brain blood flow at the time of the seizure, and video-EEG. Sometimes, however, it is necessary to obtain more detailed electrophysiological data than is obtainable using surface recordings. It is then necessary to record electrical data from the brain itself. While nasopharyngeal and sphenoidal electrodes were used previously, increasing use is being made of depth electrodes, which are inserted through the brain substance. A clear hypothesis about possible sites of seizure origin must be in place, and electrodes are then placed in appropriate structures. Each electrode has several recording sites along its length. The information is then summated as a stereo-EEG (SEEG).

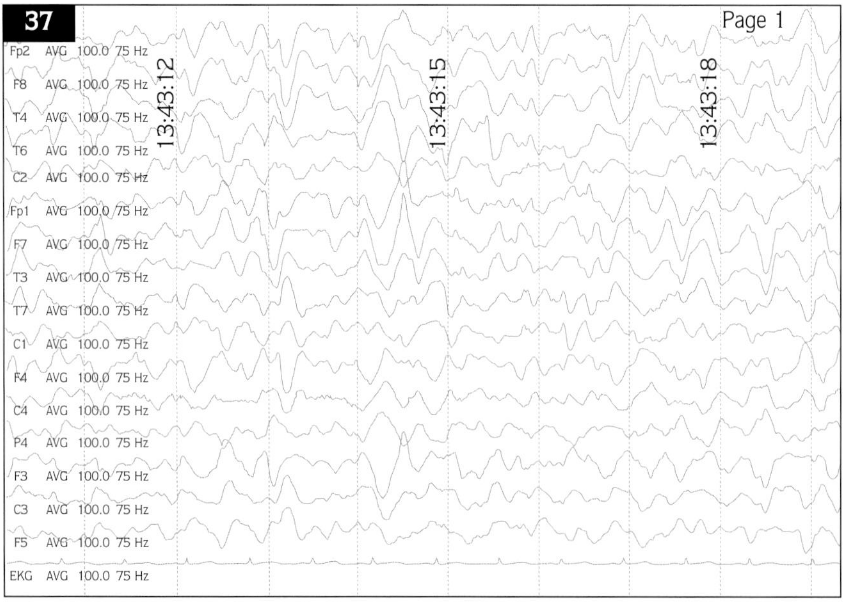

37 Electroencephalograph in encephalopathy.

In addition to recording passively from each of the electrode points, it is also possible to stimulate at each of the points along the electrode. Should stimulation at one point result in a seizure, then this makes it likely that the seizure focus is in close anatomical proximity to the electrode point.

POLYSOMNOGRAPHY

Sleep disorders are a major source of morbidity. While facilities in the UK for the investigation of respiratory causes of sleep impairment are well developed, facilities for the investigation of neurological causes of sleep disorder are relatively poor.

While some sleep disorders such as narcolepsy–cataplexy can sometimes be diagnosed with confidence in the clinic, polysomnography is the optimal technique for the investigation of sleep disorder. This involves the patient being admitted overnight, and various physiological parameters are measured during sleep. These include EEG to determine the stage of sleep, chin electromyography (EMG), electrocardiography (ECG), respiratory movements, and oxygen saturation.

EVOKED POTENTIALS

Evoked potentials are electrical signals produced by the nervous system in response to external stimuli. The stimulation may be visual, auditory, or somatosensory. Given the low voltages, it is often necessary to use computer averaging in order to discriminate the evoked potential of interest from background noise.

The main use of evoked potentials is in detecting what may be clinically silent neurological dysfunction. While they are useful for detecting abnormality in a set of brain structures, they are usually not helpful in determining the pathological cause of any such identified dysfunction.

Visual evoked potentials

In this test, the patient is asked to look at a television screen with a black and white chequer board appearance. Pattern reversal of the image is employed, and the neural signal generated is detectable with scalp electrodes over the occipital cortex as visual evoked potentials (VEPs). The clinical interpretation of the signal achieved relies primarily on the latency of the signal and whether it is delayed. Reductions in amplitude are of lesser clinical importance. Delayed visual evoked responses (VERs) indicates nervous system dysfunction somewhere between retina and occipital cortex, and can be a manifestation of subclinical demyelination (**38**).

Brainstem auditory evoked potentials

Brainstem auditory evoked potentials (BSAEPs) occur in response to an acoustic stimulus, usually a click, and arise from subcortical structures. On account of their very small size, many such stimuli must be summated in order to achieve a recordable signal.

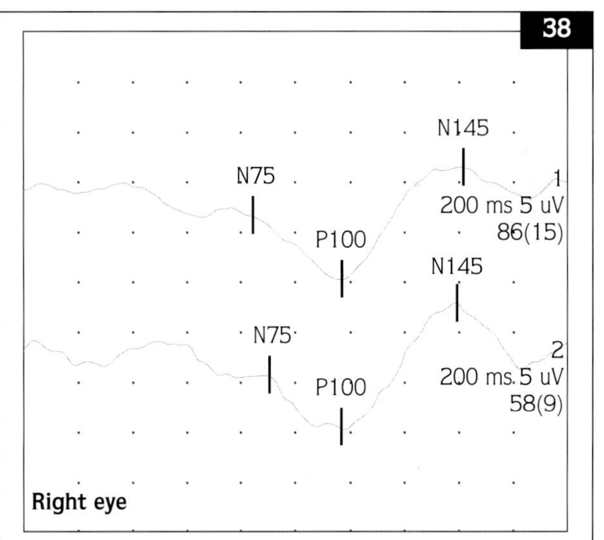

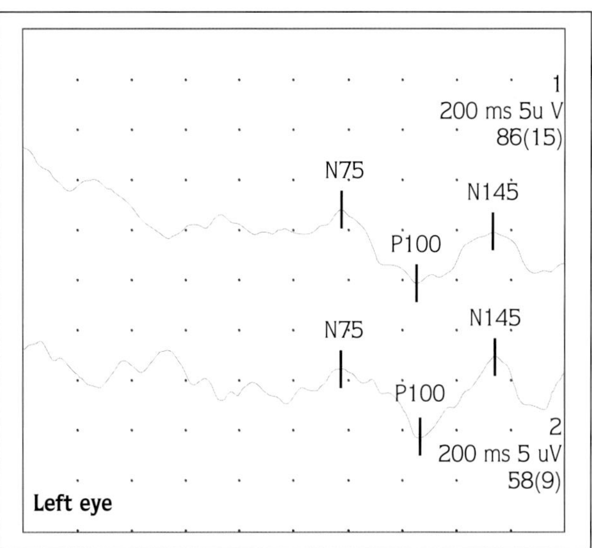

38 Visual evoked response showing delayed response on the left due to optic neuritis.

While VIIIth nerve damage may impair BSAEPs, their main use is in assessing the integrity of the brainstem. Any such pathology there, such as pontine glioma or demyelination, can result in abnormal signals.

Somatosensory evoked potentials

Using similar rationale to the above, the integrity of the somatosensory system may be assessed by stimulating sensory nerves peripherally, and measuring the time for such a signal to be recordable over the somatosensory cortex (somatosensory evoked potentials, SSEPs). Common sources of stimulation are the median nerve, common peroneal nerve, or posterior tibial nerve. Again, delayed SSEPs may occur due to disturbance anywhere in the sensory system from peripheral nerve, through spinal cord, up to cortex, and can be due to many different pathologies (**39**).

NEUROPSYCHOLOGY

Cognitive function is investigated by the clinician as part of the neurological examination, i.e. bedside cognitive testing. Due to constraints of clinic time, this allows only a brief assessment of cognition. A neuropsychologist, who has the time to fully assess cognition using standardized tests, does more detailed investigation of cognitive function.

Traditionally, neuropsychological testing employed a battery approach, where a standardized, well-validated test battery would be administered to the patient. This results in collation of much information regarding cognitive function, but is not specific to the patient's cognitive presenting complaint. An alternative approach is individualized testing, where the choice of tests is tailored to the patient. Although such tests may not be as well standardized as in the battery of tests, it does allow a dynamic, fluid approach to investigating patients. Often the neuropsychologist uses a combination of the two approaches. There are hundreds of individual neuropsychological tests, and the following only provides a brief representative sample of what is available.

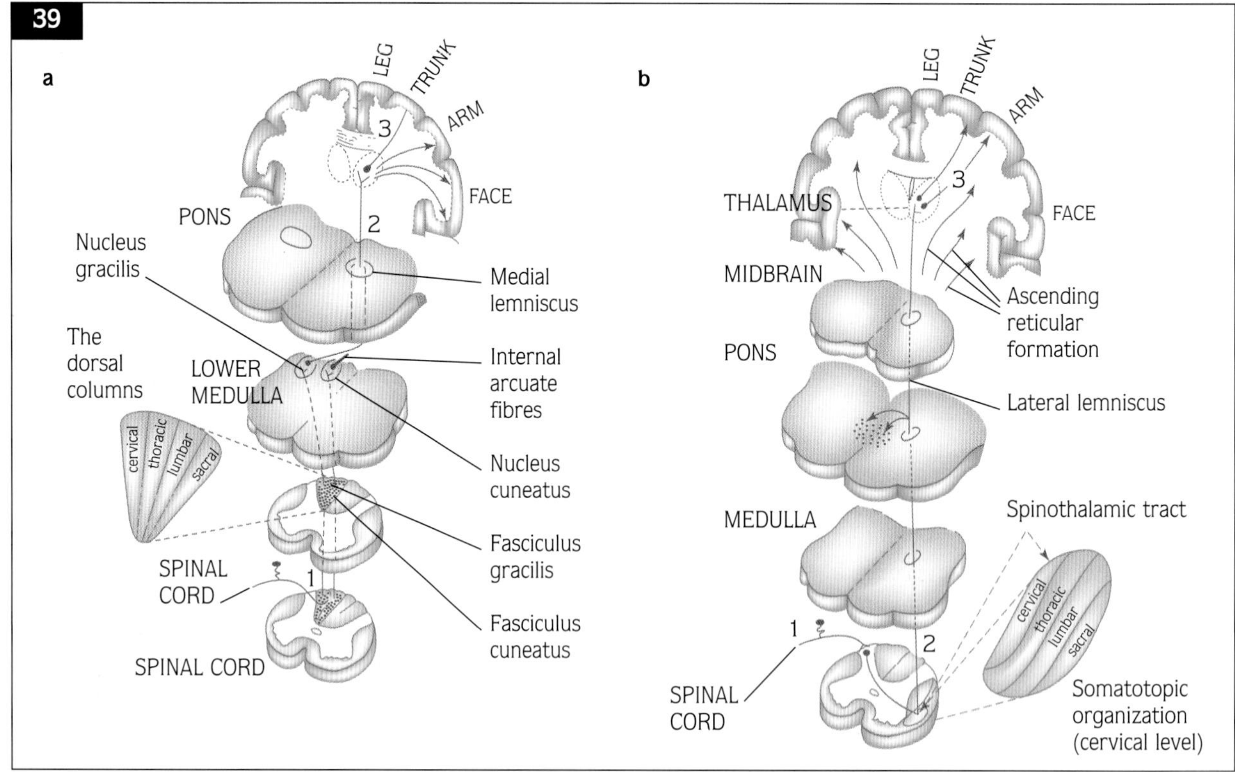

39 Diagram to show the anatomy of the sensory system. **a:** dorsal columns; **b:** spinothalamic pathway.

Orientation

This is usually assessed as part of bedside cognitive testing, where it comprises a third of the total score of the Mini-Mental State Examination (MMSE). The MMSE acts as a brief assessment of cognitive function, but is used more by the neurologist in clinic rather than by the neuropsychologist.

Attention

A simple test of attention is digit span. While this may be done forward or backward, backward digit span also involves short-term memory in addition to attention, and forward digit span is therefore the purer test of attention. The examiner simply reads out a digit sequence, each number given at one-second intervals. The length of the digit span is increased until the patient makes errors. A nonverbal equivalent of the digit span test is the Corsi Block Test, in which the subject watches the examiner touching blocks in a certain order, and must reproduce the order.

The Trail Making Test A involves connecting randomly positioned numbered circles in numeric order as quickly as possible. The Letter Cancellation Test involves cancelling selected letters from a background of nontarget letters.

Intellectual abilities

Intelligence is thought to be the ultimate expression of cognitive ability. The most widely used measure of intelligence is the Wechsler Adult Intelligence Scale-Revised (WAIS-R). This comprises various subtests. Verbal scales comprise information, digit span, vocabulary, arithmetic, comprehension, and similarities, while performance scales comprise picture completion, picture arrangement, block design, object assembly, and digit symbol. Given that a patient's current performance may reflect impairment due to neurological disease, it is also worthwhile trying to estimate premorbid IQ (intelligence quotient). One such measure is the National Adult Reading Test (NART). This utilizes the fact that IQ is correlated with the ability to pronounce irregular words, e.g. pint. It was previously thought that this ability to pronounce words is insensitive to cerebral damage, and thus provides a measure of premorbid IQ. Concerns arise, however, that semantic memory impairment (as occurs in many neurodegenerative illnesses such as Alzheimer's disease) can lead to a surface dyslexia, which results in mispronunciation of irregular words, thus leading to a false underestimate of premorbid IQ.

Reasoning, problem solving, and executive function

Executive function is complex, and involves many abilities, such as formation and planning to achieve goals, set-shifting, and searching stimuli for relevance to achieving goals. Measures of verbal reasoning include the comprehension and similarities subtests of the WAIS-R. Such tests involve questions such as 'What does '*A rolling stone gathers no moss*' mean?' or 'How are an orange and a banana alike?'

Raven's Progressive Matrices may measure nonverbal reasoning. In this test multiple designs are presented, with a final design missing. The patient has to choose from a series of alternative designs which one should occupy the missing space.

The Wisconsin Card Sorting Test involves the patient being given four target cards with designs. Probe cards are then given to the patient, who is asked to sort these according to the target card template. There are three ways of sorting, but the patient is free to sort by whichever strategy they first adopt. The only feedback to the patient is whether their sorting is correct. In this way, set shifting is also tested in addition to concept formation.

The Stroop Test comprises three parts. Firstly, the patient reads the names of colours printed in black ink. Secondly, the patient must name the colour of coloured dots as quickly as possible. Lastly, the patient must name the colour of ink of colour name words. Interference is caused by the colour name not matching the colour of the ink. The ability to inhibit this interference effect is a measure of frontal executive function.

Verbal function

An assessment of language should include spontaneous speech, naming, comprehension, repetition, reading, and writing. There exist aphasia batteries such as the Boston Diagnostic Aphasia Examination, and aphasia screening tests such as the Token Test. In this latter test, the patient is given various tokens of different shape, size, and colour. The patient is asked to point, touch, and pick up certain tokens. It is a very sensitive test to impaired language, but does not indicate which component of language is impaired. Individual language components may be tested by specific tests. An example is the Boston Naming Test, where the patient is asked to name 60 line drawings.

Memory

There are many different forms of memory, both conscious (explicit) and unconscious (implicit). Explicit memory may refer to episodic memories (i.e. learning new information, or recalling discrete episodes such as previous holidays), or semantic memory (i.e. the database of knowledge we draw on to give meaning to our conscious experience).

Practically, assessing memory as part of neuropsychological testing usually involves asking the patient to learn new information, and then testing recall after a delay. Semantic memory is also assessed, but there is considerable overlap with language.

The Wechsler Memory Scale-Revised comprises various subscales, which assess different components of memory. Verbal memory is tested using logical memory, which involves the patient reading a story paragraph, and then having to recall as much as possible. Verbal paired associates involve the presentation of pairs of words. At recall, one word is shown, and the patient must provide the other word in the pair. Nonverbal memory may be assessed in a similar fashion, but by asking for recall of sequences of taps rather than a story. Short-term verbal memory is assessed using digit span.

A further measure of nonverbal memory is the Rey–Osterrieth complex figure (**40**). This is an abstract design, which is not easily encoded verbally. The ability to copy the Rey figure is a measure of visuo-perceptual function. The ability to draw from memory after a 30-minute delay is a measure of delayed nonverbal memory.

Perception and construction abilities

While perception involves all sensory modalities, in practice the neuropsychologist is interested in visual and auditory perception.

Visual perception and construction

Object and face recognition, colour perception, and visual search activities may all be assessed neuropsychologically.

The Benton Facial Recognition Test involves the patient being shown one face, with six others on the adjacent page, one of which matches the target, and is a measure of facial recognition. The Judgement of Line Orientation Test involves a test line having to be matched for orientation with one of a series of lines arranged like a protractor. The Line Bisection Test requires the patient to put a cross halfway along several lines. It is sensitive to patients with neglect. The Clock Drawing Test is a measure of visual construction (**41**).

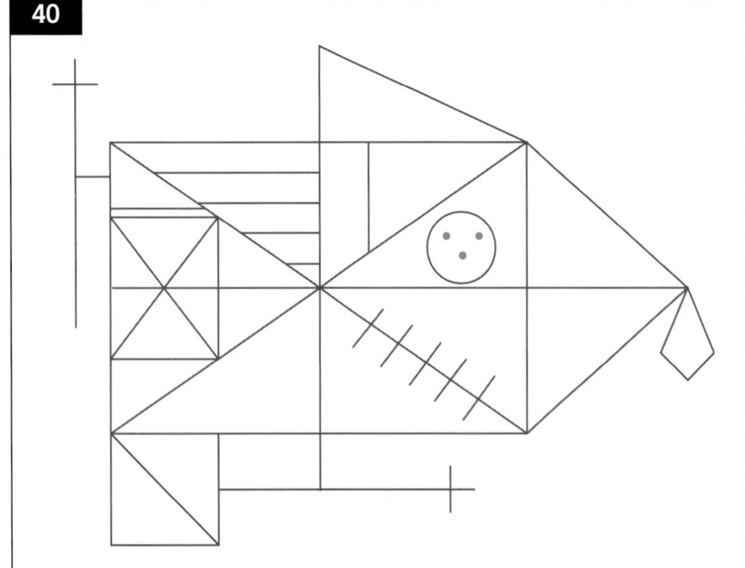

40 Diagram of the Rey–Osterrieth figure.

Specific laboratory tests

While the diagnostic sieve usually involves the above modalities to narrow down the differential diagnosis, there is a place for specific blood tests, which either confirm or refute specific diagnostic possibilities. An example of this would be dementia, where it would be appropriate to perform a blood screen to look for treatable causes of dementia, such as vitamin B_{12} deficiency and thyroid function. Depending on the clinical presentation, there may be a need to look for specific diseases. For example, if abnormal movements accompanied dementia, this would raise the possibility of Huntington's disease, and therefore genetic screening for this disorder would be necessary. In similar vein, if there were a family history of dementia, migraine, and stroke-like episodes, and if characteristic white matter lesions were seen on MRI, then it would be appropriate to test for the notch 3 mutation on chromosome 19, which would lead to a diagnosis of cerebral autosomal dominant arteriopathy with subcortical infarcts and leucoencephalopathy (CADASIL).

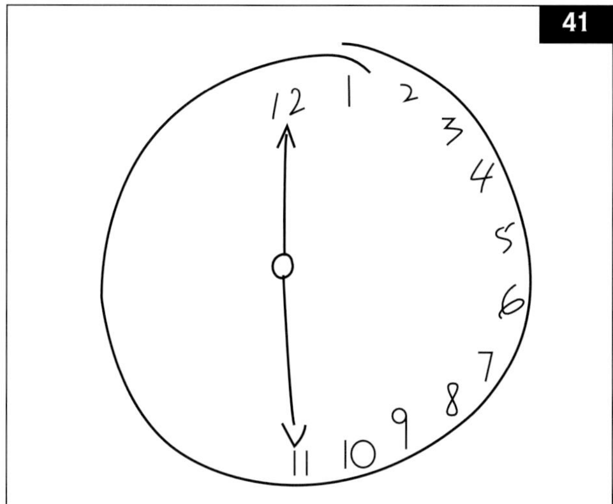

41 Clock drawing by a patient exhibiting neglect to the left hemisphere.

INVESTIGATING THE SPINAL CORD

Normal anatomy

The vertebral column comprises 7 cervical, 12 thoracic, 5 lumbar, 5 sacral, and 4 coccygeal vertebrae. The sacral bones fuse to form the sacrum and the coccygeal bones the coccyx (**42**).

With the exception of both the atlas (C1) and the axis (C2), all vertebrae share common anatomical features. Each is made up of a body, pedicles, and pairs of facets. The superior facet articulates with the inferior facet by means of the pars interarticularis (pars: part; inter: between; articularis: articulating surface). Finally, each vertebra possesses two laminae and a spinous process. The spinal cord, conus, and cauda equina lie within the vertebral canal and emerging nerve roots pass within the neural foramina. The C1 nerve root

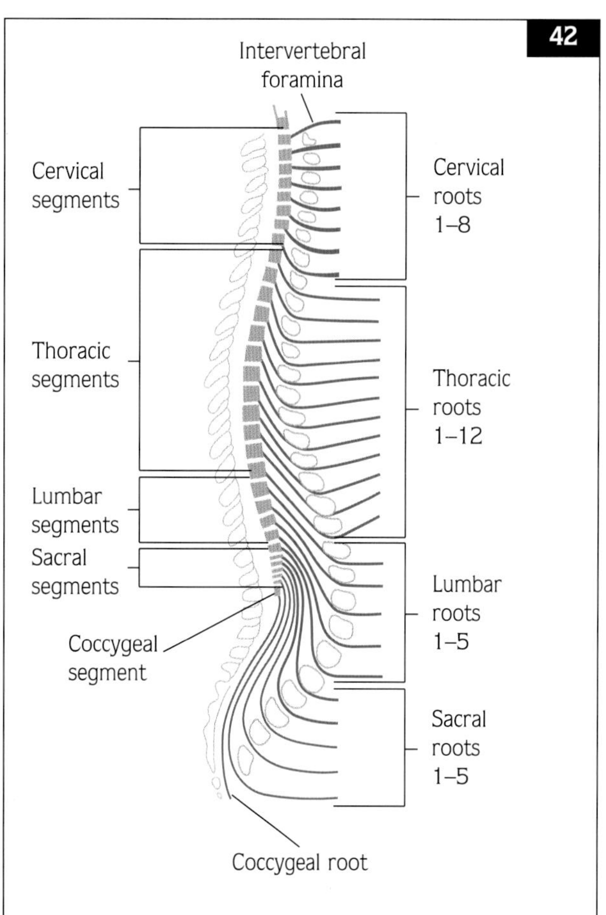

42 Sagittal diagram of the spine and spinal cord, illustrating the levels of exit for the nerve roots.

passes superiorly above the atlas, the C5 root passes above the body of C5 into the C4–5 neural foramen, the C6 root passes above C6 into the C5–6 foramen, and so on. The lowest cervical nerve root, C8, passes below the body of C7 and outwards through the neural foramen of C7–T1. The presence of the C8 root means that the T1 thoracic nerve root passes below the body of T1 through the foramen of T1–2 and all subsequent nerve roots in this manner. The last (T12) nerve root similarly passes below its vertebral body and then through the foramen of T12–L1. The first lumbar root likewise passes below L1 into the L1–2 neural foramen and the L5 root passes below the body of L5 into the L5–S1 neural foramen.

In adults, the tip of the conus lies at or above the L2–L3 intervertebral disc space. The filum terminale, a thin glial-ependymal cord, is a direct continuation of the conus terminating in the posterior aspect of the coccyx. It measures <2 mm in diameter and, if larger, is regarded as a thickened filum often associated with developmental neurological deficits (spinal dysraphism). Not infrequently, the filum contains a small amount of fat tissue, considered a normal anatomical variant of no clinical significance, though large masses, spinal lipomas, can occur.

> Understanding the relationships between the vertebral bodies and emerging nerves is indispensable for the correct correlation between the clinical examination and radiological findings.

Knowledge of spinal cord blood supply is helpful in the diagnosis of 'spinal stroke' but also in the interpretation of spinal angiography, a highly specialized infrequently performed investigation (**43**, **44**). Two paired posterior spinal arteries supply the spinal cord, arising from the posterior inferior cerebellar artery and merging to form a plexus of vessels on the posterior surface of the cord. This rich blood supply ensures protection against ischaemia and explains the relative sparing of the posterior spinal cord (dorsal columns) in spinal strokes. The arterial blood supply to the anterior two-thirds of the spinal cord is much more vulnerable, being through a single vessel. The anterior spinal artery arises by fusion of a branch from each vertebral artery. Seven to 10 unpaired radicular arteries leave it as it descends the cord. The largest, variably arising between T9–T12 levels, is called the artery of Adamkiewicz. This less efficient circulation renders the spinal cord most vulnerable to ischaemia at the 'watershed level' T8.

Radiology

The role of plain radiology in the diagnosis of spinal cord disease has become less valuable, particularly with the increasing accessibility of CT and MRI. Degenerative changes can be anticipated with increasing age and the radiological presence of cervical or lumbar spondylosis does not, in isolation, result in a clinical diagnosis. A complete radiological cervical spine assessment consists of lateral, antero-posterior (AP), open-mouth, and right and left oblique views. The thoracic spine series consists of an AP view and a lateral view, though the upper part of the thoracic spine is very difficult to visualize on the lateral view because of the overlying shoulders. A complete lumbosacral spine series consists of AP, lateral, coned-down lateral, and right and left oblique views (oblique views are useful in evaluating the pars interarticularis for spondylolysis). Guidelines on the use of plain films must be followed, thus limiting unnecessary radiation exposure.

Contrast myelography

Contrast myelography in combination with CT remains a useful investigation if MRI is contraindicated due to a pacemaker or other reason (**45**). Indeed, some neurosurgeons still rely on this investigation to visualize small disc fragments in the lateral spinal recesses. Nonionic water-soluble contrast agents are used. A history of allergy or prior contrast reaction should be enquired into (premedication with antihistamines and steroids may be necessary). Contrast is injected at the L3/4 level slowly over 1–2 minutes. Alternatively, a lateral C1–2 puncture can be performed with care to prevent intracranial flow (acute neurotoxicity). Postmyelography, patients are maintained at a 30–45° head up position to further prevent this.

Spinal CT

CT is still preferred in evaluating acute spinal trauma. Fractures are identified as lucencies without sclerotic margins, and bone impingement on the spinal canal is clearly visualized (**46**). Images are generally obtained in the axial plane with angulation of the scanning gantry where necessary. The spine is best viewed when the gantry is perpendicular to the area of interest. In the lumbar region, this necessitates considerable angulation to evaluate the lumbar discs. Images may be obtained using 1–10 mm-thick slices and sagittal reconstruction can be made; however, spinal MRI has all but ruled out the need for these. CT can provide helpful information on vertebral

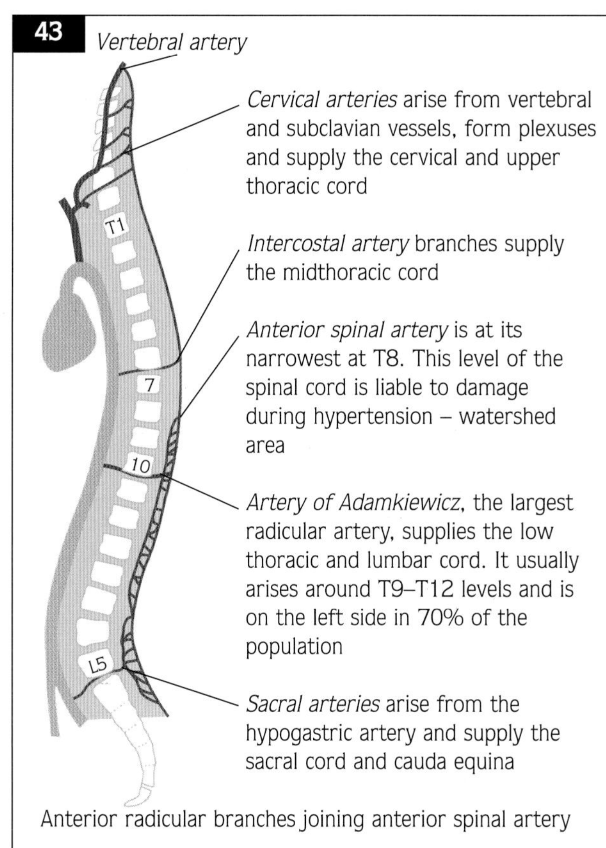

43 Sagittal diagram of the blood supply to the spinal cord.

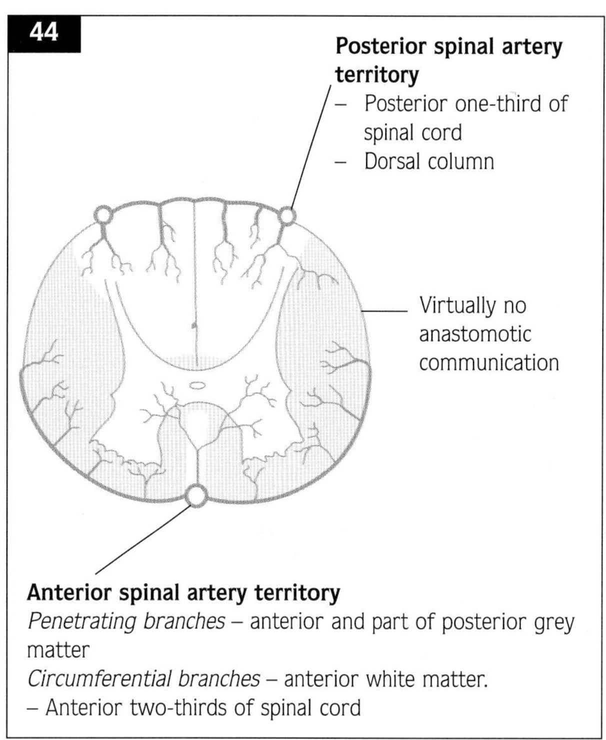

44 Axial figure of the spinal cord, illustrating anterior and posterior spinal artery territories.

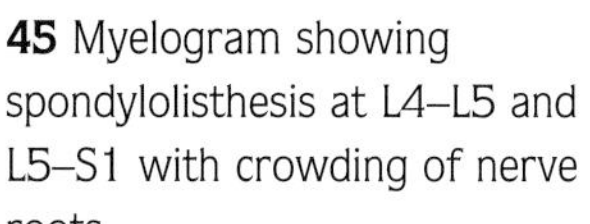

45 Myelogram showing spondylolisthesis at L4–L5 and L5–S1 with crowding of nerve roots.

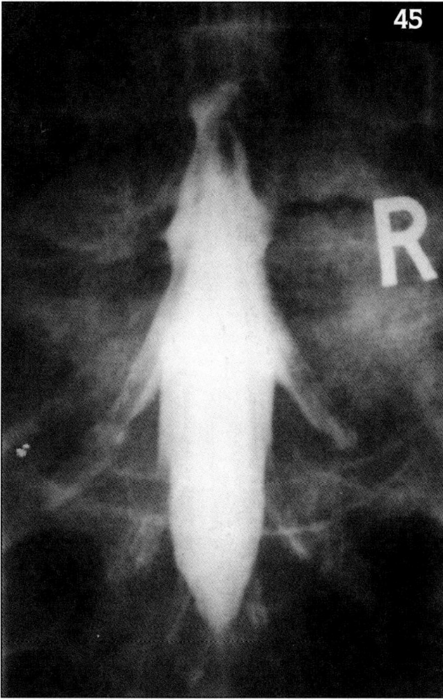

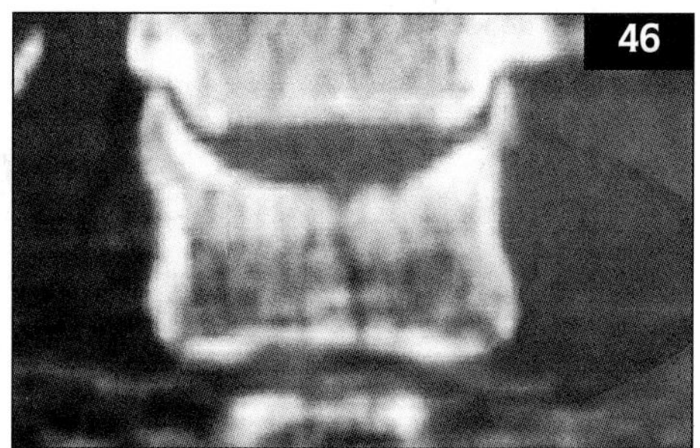

46 Coronal computed tomography scan of the spine showing a fracture at C7 not visible on plain X-rays.

body disease (tumours and infections) and may be complementary to MRI, but the latter is generally the spinal imaging modality of choice.

Spinal MRI

MRI has revolutionized the investigation of disease of the spinal cord, and recent advances have shortened data acquisition times and reduced artefacts. Its noninvasive ability to image the spinal cord and surrounding structures (CSF, dura, and ligaments) makes it indispensable in the investigative workup. Classically there are three locations for spinal neurological disease, *extradural*, *intradural/ extra-medullary*, and *intramedullary* (47). MRI has the capability to evaluate all three locations.

> A good working knowledge of basic MR imaging principles and spine anatomy is essential for understanding the imaging observations seen in various spine lesions.

For example, because of their anterior oblique orientation, the neural foramina in the cervical spine are exceedingly difficult to see on a sagittal image and are best seen on oblique sagittal or axial views. Conversely in the lumbosacral region, the neural foramina are laterally orientated and therefore are properly visualized on a sagittal T1-weighted image (48). Anatomic changes inevitably occur to the neural foramen with ageing. Posterior disk bulge, lateral herniated disk, together with vertebral body osteophytes can encroach on the neural foramen and its contents. Although MRI is poor in showing dense normal cortical bone, it shows infiltrative/infective disease well. Contrast-medium enhanced imaging can help differentiate tumours, inflammation, and active demyelinating diseases.

A common mistake is failure to order views that display the likely site(s) of the lesion. In most cases, careful history and examination will decide which of cervical, thoracic, or lumbosacral levels are to be imaged. However, this is not always possible and 'full spinal imaging' should then be requested. Some disease processes can be multilevel (multiple sclerosis [MS]) and, on occasion, the common (lumbar disc disease) and the rare (thoracic meningioma) may coexist. In any patient with a spinal cord syndrome of unknown cause, the clinician must consider the possibility of a lesion at the level of the foramen magnum, a level that is neither spinal nor cranial and consequently is often overlooked. Imaging here should pay particular attention to the possibility of malformations (Chiari malformations) and the location of the odontoid process (rheumatoid arthritis). A benign tumour of the foramen magnum such as meningioma can be confused with MS or degenerative cord diseases and, prior to correct diagnosis, progressive disability passes beyond the point of reversibility.

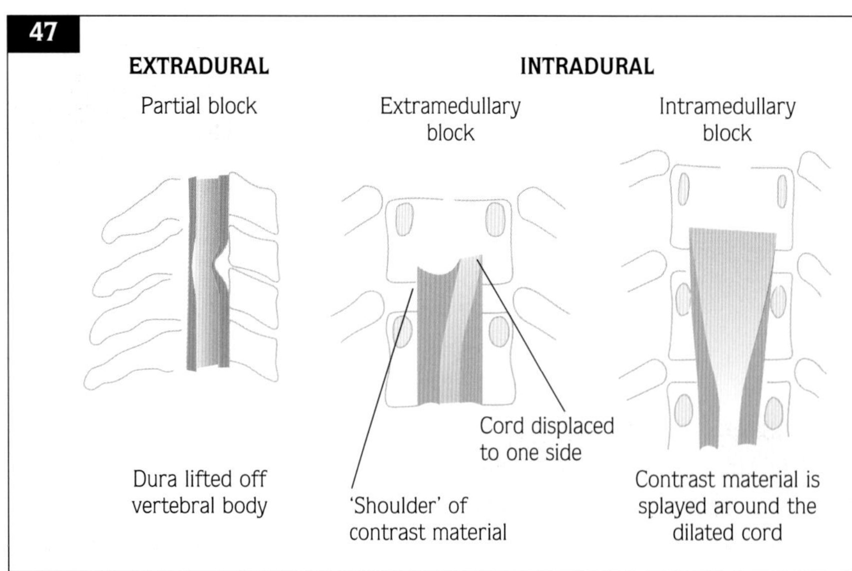

47 Illustration of extradural and intradural (extramedullary and intramedullary) spaces.

Spinal angiography

While in the head CT and MR angiography have increasingly replaced digital subtraction angiography (DSA), this is not the case with the spine. Resolution and the complexity of the spinal circulation mean that conventional angiography still remains the gold standard. However, the indications for spinal angiography are few (spinal vascular lesions such as dural fistula). This infrequently performed investigation requires considerable technical skill, and on occasion, selective cannulation of several radicular vessels may be required to demonstrate a dural fistula. CT angiography may show large dural fistulas (**49**).

Neurophysiology

Neurophysiological investigations such as EMG can be helpful in localizing the level of a lesion if this is not apparent on imaging. It is a valuable adjunct to imaging where there is uncertainty about the true significance of a compressed nerve root (cervical or lumbar radiculopathy).

Nerve conduction studies are of value in differentiating peripheral nerve from nerve root (radicular) lesions. Radicular lesions cause a segmental distribution of muscle involvement, i.e. affect muscles supplied by the same root, whereas peripheral nerve lesions may affect muscles supplied by that nerve, which may be innervated by several nerve roots. Reduction in nerve conduction velocity may indicate peripheral neuropathy. Fasciculation and fibrillations can be detected in muscles that

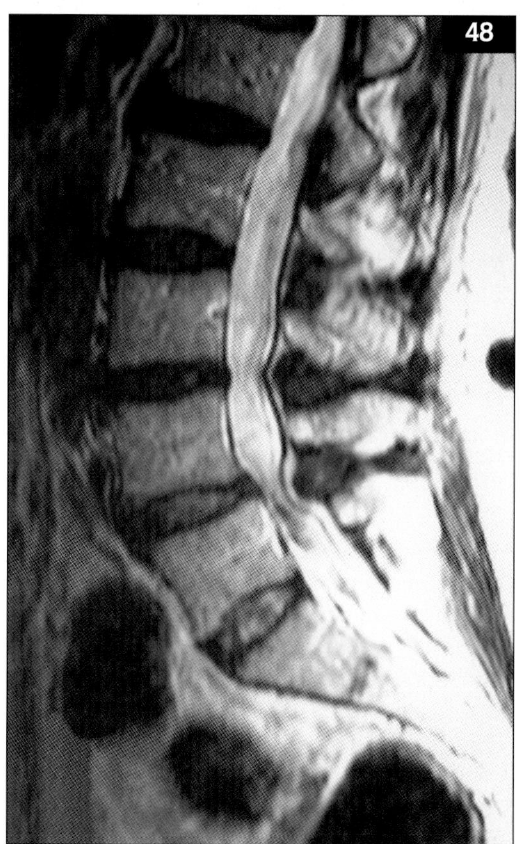

48 Magnetic resonance image of the lumbar spine showing lumbar canal stenosis.

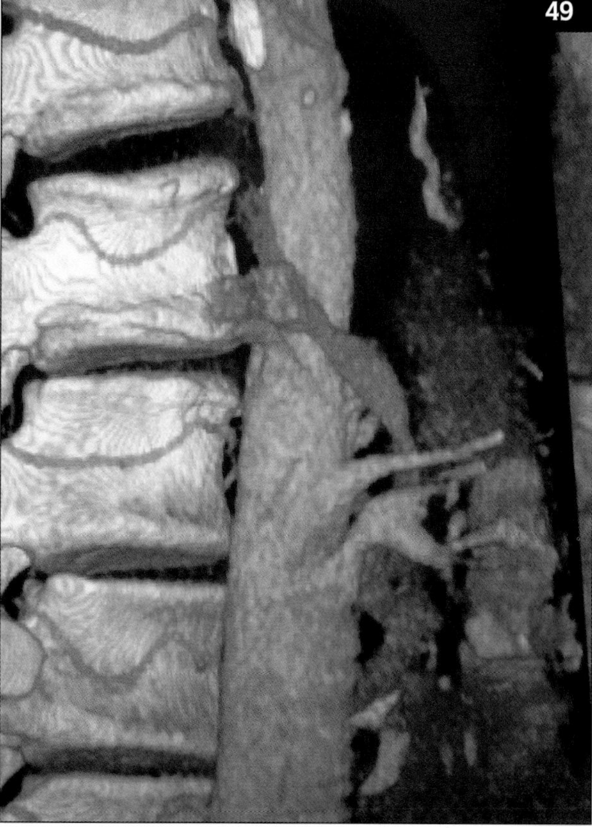

49 Computed tomography angiogram showing a dural fistula.

appear clinically not involved, e.g. certain conditions that appear purely spinal may have an anterior horn cell component (motor neurone disease/amyotrophic lateral sclerosis [MND/ALS]) and neurophysiology can be diagnostic where imaging has been normal.

Somatosensory evoked potentials

Somatosensory evoked potentials (SSEPs) test the integrity of the afferent sensory pathways, principally the large nerve fibre dorsal column–medial lemniscal pathway. They are elicited by electrical stimulation of the median and posterior tibial nerves. Evoked peaks from median nerve stimulation are detected in the brachial plexus (Erb's point), central grey matter of the cervical cord, medial lemniscus, and primary somatosensory cortex. Abnormalities of SSEPs result from single level (e.g. cervical spondylosis) or diffuse (e.g. MS) disease states. SSEPs can be used to monitor the integrity of the spinal cord during spinal surgery.

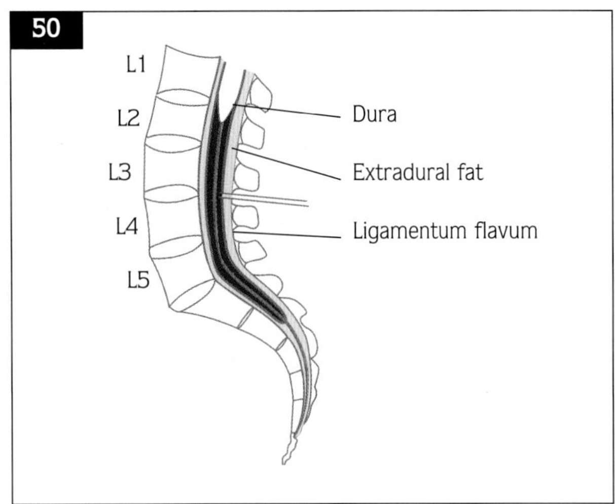

50 Sagittal diagram of lumbar spine.

Lumbar puncture

Lumbar puncture (LP) is a useful test for measuring CSF pressure and obtaining CSF samples, important in the diagnosis of inflammatory disorders (oligoclonal bands [OCBs] in MS) and infections (borreliosis, syphilis, viral infections, spinal tuberculosis) (**50**). If, however, a mass lesion is suspected, particularly if it is high in the vertebral canal, LP, without provision for prior spinal imaging and 'on-site' surgical decompression, may be contraindicated. Some patients with compressive cord lesions become abruptly worse after LP due to shifting of the cord, and they may show signs of a complete cord syndrome. If the lesion is cervical, respiratory paralysis may occur suddenly.

If spinal MRI is performed after LP, bleeding or leakage of CSF into the epidural space may result in meningeal enhancement after contrast, erroneously interpreted as part of the disease process under investigation. It is therefore normally preferable to obtain imaging prior to CSF examination.

INVESTIGATING THE PERIPHERAL NERVOUS SYSTEM (NERVE, NEUROMUSCULAR JUNCTION, AND MUSCLE)

The investigation of disorders of the peripheral nervous system relies primarily on neurophysiology, with selected use of more invasive nerve and muscle biopsy.

Neurophysiology

The use of nerve conduction studies to investigate peripheral nerve function, and EMG to investigate muscle disease, allows extensive investigation of the peripheral nervous system noninvasively.

Nerve conduction studies

By administering an electrical stimulus to a peripheral nerve, it is possible to measure signal conduction in the nerve, and thus deduce how the nerve is functioning. Motor and sensory nerves may be studied by recording the distal latency (latency from stimulus to recording electrodes), evoked response amplitude, and conduction velocity (**51**). Normal conduction velocity values vary depending on age and body temperature. Significant delay indicates impairment in nerve conduction, as is seen in demyelinating neuropathies such as Guillain–Barré syndrome or multifocal neuropathy, and in nerve entrapments.

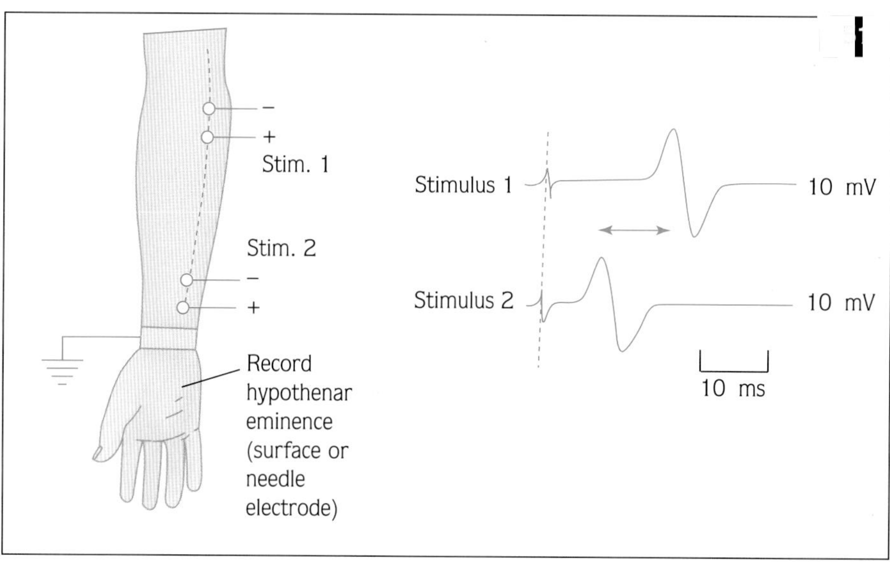

51 Diagram of nerve conduction studies.

F waves and H waves

While neurophysiology is mainly directed at disorders of nerve and muscle, it is possible to obtain indirect evidence of spinal or nerve root impairment by means of F and H waves (52). F waves require the motor nerve to be stimulated antidromically, i.e. from distal to proximal. The stimulus then travels proximally up the motor nerve axon, and then returns orthodromically (i.e. proximal to distal) back down to the initial stimulation point.

H reflexes differ in that the initial nerve stimulated is a sensory nerve. The signal in conducted proximally up to where the sensory nerve synapses with the motor nerve. The signal then returns down the motor axon and is recorded peripherally.

These F-response and H-reflex studies can be of use in peripheral neuropathies, particularly when the pathological process is too proximal to be detectable by conventional nerve conduction studies. However, in conditions such as radiculopathy, while responses may be abnormal, EMG would also be abnormal, such that F and H studies would not usually add any additional diagnostic value to EMG.

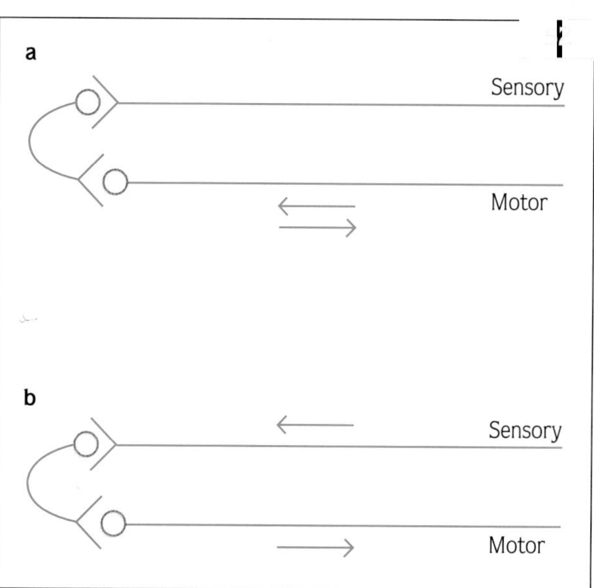

52 Diagram to show F and H reflexes in nerve conduction studies. **a:** in F waves, the signal travels from distal to proximal up the motor nerve, and then from proximal to distal down the same motor nerve; **b:** in H waves, the signal travels from distal to proximal up the sensory nerve, and then proximal to distal down the motor nerve.

Blink reflex

In this test, the supraorbital nerve is stimulated, and activity in orbicularis oculi is recorded. An abnormal blink reflex can be helpful in showing evidence of a subtle trigeminal or facial nerve lesion.

Electromyography

In EMG, a fine bore needle is inserted directly into muscle. The needle comprises a central recording electrode, and the outer casing acts as a reference. The potential difference between the two provides a measure of spontaneous muscle activity.

Normal muscle is electrically silent. When muscle is contracting normally, there appear motor unit potentials. As more of these are recruited, an interference pattern arises, which is the summation of many motor unit potentials (53). Abnormalities detected during EMG include the following: spontaneous rest activity, motor unit potential abnormalities, interference pattern abnormalities, and other phenomena, e.g. myotonia.

Spontaneous rest activity

Fibrillation potentials are due to single muscle fibres contracting, and indicate active denervation, as occurs in neurogenic disorders such as neuropathy. Sharp positive spikes may be seen in chronically denervated muscle, such as in motor neurone disease, but also occur in acute myopathy (**54**).

Motor unit potential abnormalities

In neuropathy, collateral reinnervation causes potentials of large amplitude and long duration (**55**). This is in contrast to myopathies and muscular dystrophies, where potentials are of small amplitude and short duration (**56**).

Abnormalities of the interference pattern

Neuropathy leads to a loss of motor units under voluntary control, hence a reduction in interference. By contrast, in myopathy, recruitment of motor units and the interference pattern are normal.

Special phenomena

In myotonia, voluntary movement results in high frequency repetitive discharges. The amplitude and frequency of the potentials fluctuate, resulting in the typical 'dive bomber' sound on audio monitor (**57**).

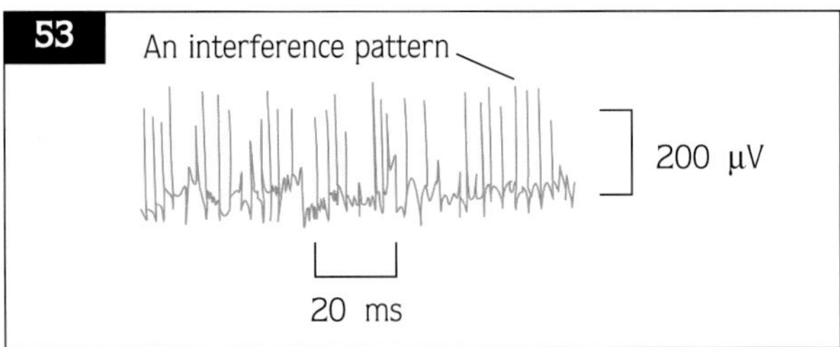

53 Diagram to show normal interference picture in nerve conduction.

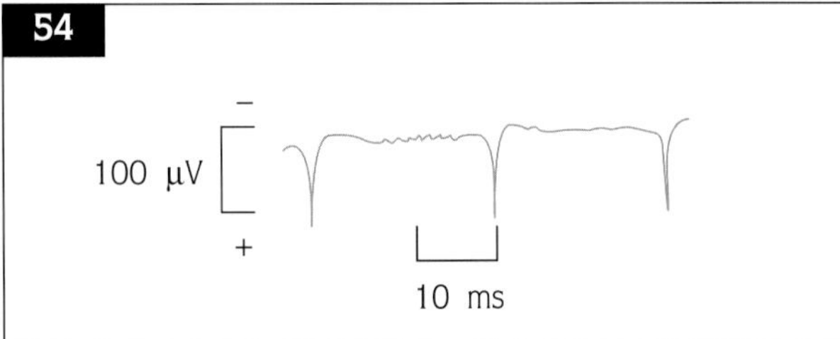

54 Diagram illustrating positive sharp waves in nerve conduction.

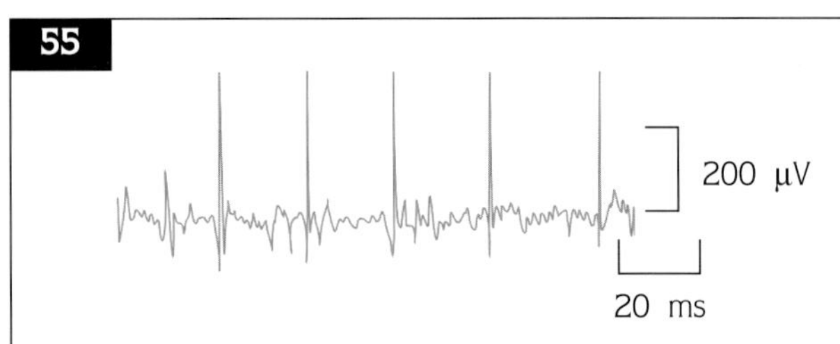

55 Diagram illustrating polyphasic, large amplitude, long duration motor unit potentials, commonly seen in neuropathy.

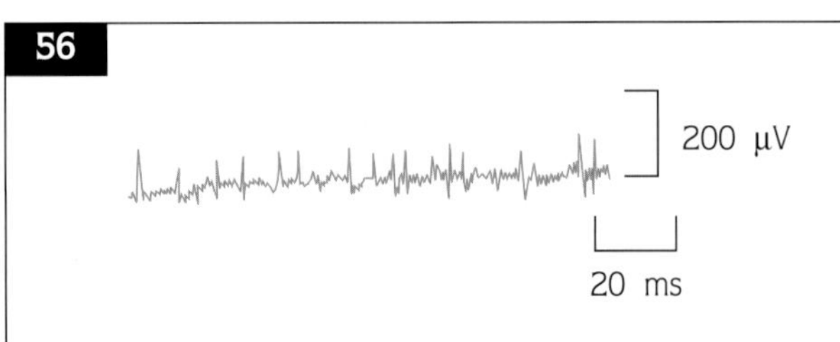

56 Diagram illustrating polyphasic, small amplitude, short duration potentials seen in myopathies and muscular dystrophies.

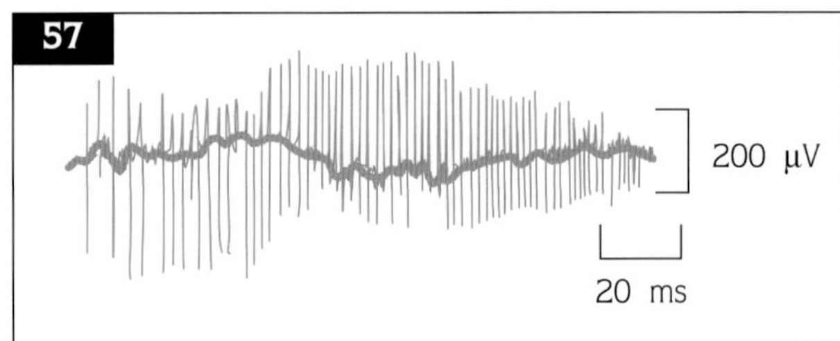

57 Diagram illustrating myotonic discharge on electromyography as seen in myotonia.

Repetitive nerve stimulation/jitter
The neuromuscular junction may be specifically investigated using these techniques. In normal subjects, repetitive stimulation of a motor nerve results in a constant muscle potential, and decrement in the amplitude only occurs when the rate of stimulation is >30 Hz. Abnormalities on repetitive stimulation indicate neuromuscular junction dysfunction. In myasthenia, there occurs a decremental response at stimulus rates as low as 3–5 Hz (**58**). In Eaton–Lambert syndrome, an incremental response occurs with rapid stimulation, i.e. at 20–50 Hz.

Single fibre EMG
A further way of investigating the neuromuscular junction is using single fibre EMG. This requires a very fine needle, which records from approximately 1–3 muscle fibres from a single motor unit, rather than the 20 or so motor units sampled when using a standard EMG needle. There is normally a degree of variability in the action potentials recorded from different muscle fibres in a single motor unit, on account of variation in neuromuscular transmission. In myasthenia, there is increased jitter due to greater variability in neuromuscular transmission (**59**). This can be helpful in supporting the diagnosis in those cases of myasthenia where repetitive stimulation may have been normal.

NEUROPATHOLOGY

Nerve biopsy

Although nerve conduction studies often give sufficient information to result in the diagnosis of a peripheral nerve disorder, it is occasionally necessary

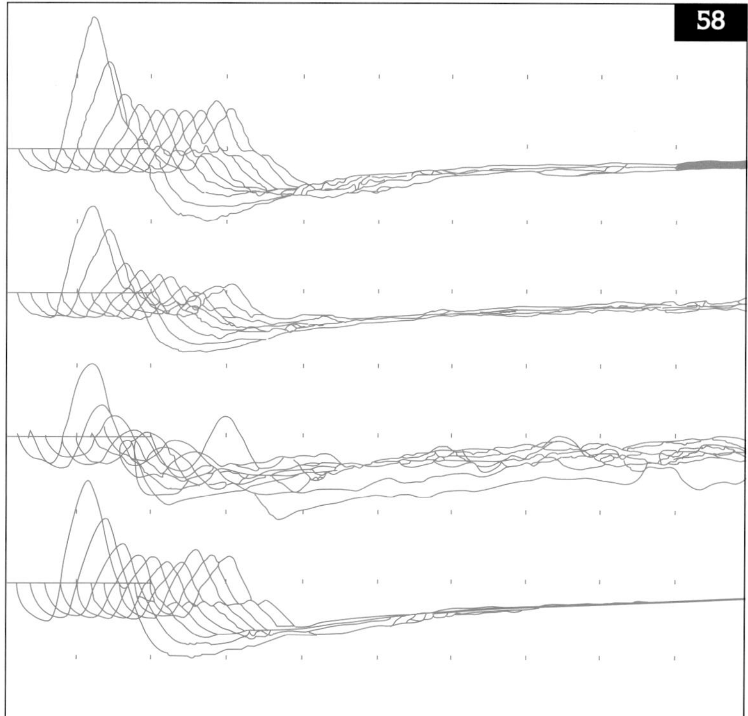

58 Electromyograph in myasthenia showing decremental response on repetitive stimulation.

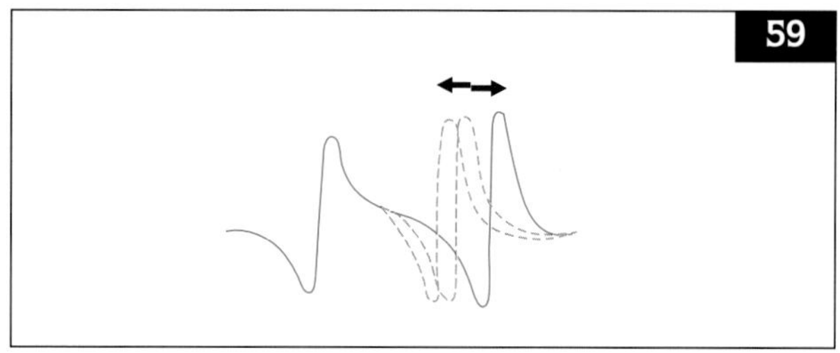

59 Diagram illustrating jitter on single fibre electromyography. The gap between the two muscle action potentials is variable, i.e. jitter.

to proceed to biopsy. It may be of use in trying to distinguish between segmental demyelination and axonal degeneration, and also in the diagnosis of a number of specific disorders such as amyloidosis, vasculitis, and sarcoidosis. The decision to biopsy must take into account the likelihood of the biopsy leading to a change in treatment, and this must be balanced against the morbidity which can be associated with this test.

Traditionally, the sural nerve was biopsied. This leads to permanent numbness affecting the lateral border of the foot. Sometimes, this can result in persistent unpleasant dysaesthesia, which can be worse than the initial symptoms. Biopsies nowadays tend to be fascicular, which at least spares a portion of the nerve, with less attendant morbidity. Normally, the specimen is analysed using light and electron microscopy, often with immunohistochemistry.

Muscle biopsy

This should only be considered after a full neurological examination, supplemented by appropriate blood tests, and often EMG. A muscle appropriate to the patient's symptoms must be chosen, and biopsy should only take place in centres where the specimen can be processed and analysed fully, i.e. histochemistry, electron microscopy, and special studies such as immunohistochemistry.

The issue of whether open or needle biopsy is better is still controversial. Open biopsies provide a larger specimen, which can be fixed at its physiological length. Needle biopsy, however, results in less scarring, and the ability to sample multiple sites. The specimen is, however, smaller and it is more difficult to orientate.

Specific laboratory tests

Antibodies

In myasthenia, the presence of acetylcholine receptor antibodies is diagnostic, although antibody-negative myasthenia may occur, especially in more restricted forms such as ocular or bulbar myasthenia. Voltage gated calcium channel antibodies are detected in 90% of patients with Eaton–Lambert syndrome, which can superficially mimic myasthenia. In certain of the hereditary motor and sensory neuropathies (HMSN some types termed Charcot– Marie–Tooth disease), it has been possible to identify the genetic mutations. Of those HMSN with a known genetic basis, HMSN types 1 and 3 have been associated with mutations in one of several genes expressed in Schwann cells, which produce myelin for the peripheral nervous system.

Mitochondrial diseases are a diverse group of conditions resulting from impairment of mitochondrial function, and leading to a wide range of clinical disorders. Some patients have symptoms that fulfil clearly delineated syndromes, such as mitochondrial encephalopathy, lactic acidosis, and stroke-like episodes (MELAS) or myoclonic epilepsy and ragged red fibres syndrome (MERRF), but most do not. Molecular genetic studies of deoxyribonucleic acid (DNA) from blood may be analysed for mitochondrial DNA mutations. Nearly all point mutations may be detected from blood, but major structural mutations, such as deletions, require skeletal muscle for analysis.

Ischaemic lactate test

This is a physiological test of muscle function. The patient is asked to grip repeatedly, with a cuff occluding the circulation. Blood is drawn at regular intervals in order to assess lactate levels. Normally, when exercise is relatively anaerobic, then anaerobic metabolism should produce lactate. In patients with deficits in the glycolytic pathway, there is no rise in lactate levels with ischaemic exercise. In contrast, in mitochondrial disease, there can be excess lactate production.

INVESTIGATING SPECIFIC SITES

Certain constellations of clinical features are of great localization value. The tempo of onset of symptoms is then of use in determining the type of pathological process responsible for these anatomically localizable syndromes.

Cranio-cervical junction

Lesions at the cranio-cervical junction may result in symptoms of poor balance (**60**). There may be a history of loss of function on one side followed by progression to signs to all four extremities. Neurological examination may reveal ataxia and cerebellar signs, together with brisk reflexes and upgoing plantars. Down-beating nystagmus, if present, points to the cranio-cervical junction. Although CT may be sufficient, the cranio-cervical junction is best imaged with MRI (**61**).

Cerebello-pontine angle

A common cause of lesions at the cerebello-pontine angle is acoustic neuroma or other tumours such as meningioma (**62, 63**). Patients with lesions here tend

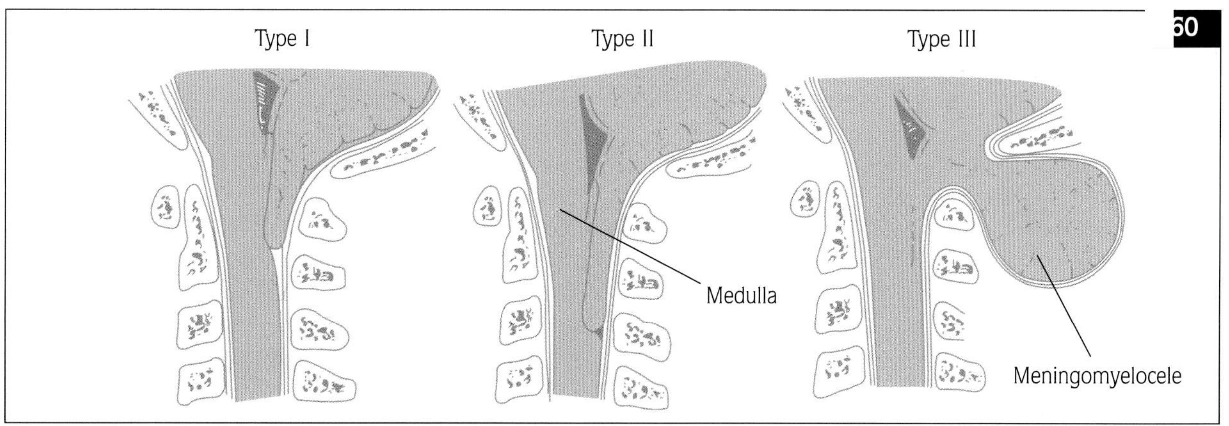

60 Diagram to show three types of Chiari malformation.

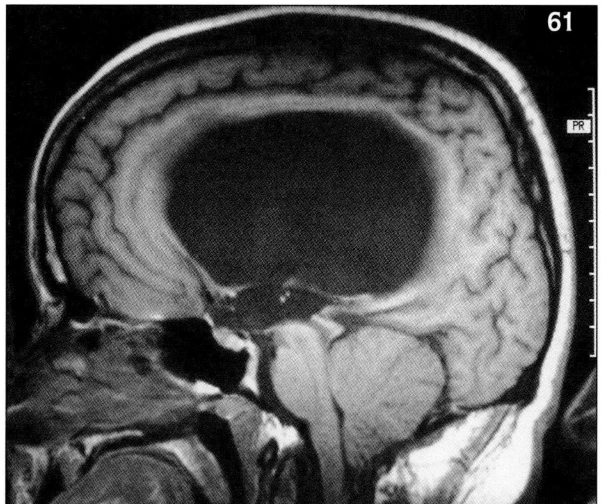

61 Magnetic resonance image showing Chiari malformation resulting in secondary hydrocephalus.

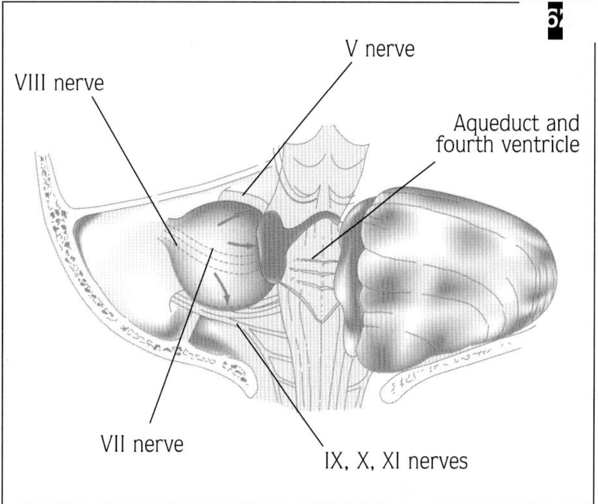

62 Diagram of a cerebello-pontine angle tumour, compressing adjacent structures.

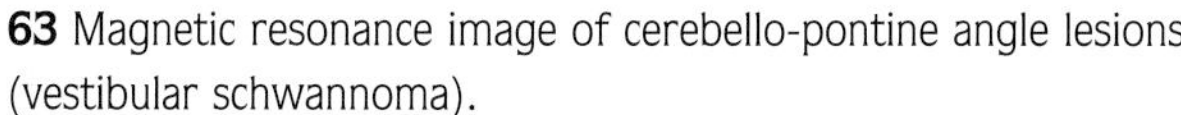

63 Magnetic resonance image of cerebello-pontine angle lesions (vestibular schwannoma).

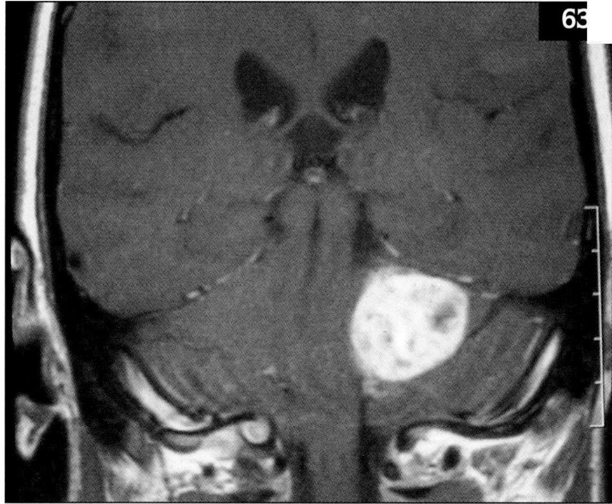

to present with mild vertigo or ataxia, and there may be accompanying ipsilateral occipital pain. Examination often reveals asymmetrical sensorineural hearing loss on examination. In the event of delayed diagnosis, as the tumour progresses there may be facial pain, numbness, and paraesthesia due to involvement of the trigeminal nerve. Depressed corneal reflex will be evident. Should the tumour result in hydrocephalus, the symptoms and signs of raised intracranial pressure will appear.

Pituitary/cavernous sinus

Lesions of the pituitary fossa may present with local space-occupying effects, or with endocrine symptoms depending on whether an active hormone is being released. Local mass effect can result in nonspecific headache. On examination, the finding of a visual field defect should raise suspicion of a pituitary lesion. Pressure on the inferior aspect of the optic chiasm results in a superior temporal quadrantanopia, but tumour progression will lead to bitemporal hemianopia. In some instances, lateral expansion will lead to compression of nerves lying in the walls of the cavernous sinus, especially the third nerve (**64, 65**).

Endocrine effects depend on whether there is hypersecretion or hyposecretion of hormones, and on which hormone is being affected. Should there be hypersecretion of growth hormone (GH), then this will result in acromegaly. This presents clinically with enlargement of face, hands, and feet, with coarsening of the skin. A tumour producing increased prolactin will result clinically in women with infertility, amenorrhoea, and galactorrhoea. In men, impotence may occur. An adrenocorticotrophic hormone-(ACTH) producing pituitary tumour will result in the features of Cushing's syndrome. This includes facial mooning, hirsutism, central obesity, and muscle weakness.

Investigation of lesions affecting the pituitary or cavernous sinus primarily involves neuroimaging and tests of endocrine function. The imaging modality of choice for investigating pituitary lesions is MRI (**66**). This gives excellent anatomical detail, and can show whether there is suprasellar extension and whether adjacent structures such as the walls of the cavernous sinus are involved. Given the close proximity of the pituitary to the optic chiasm, it is important to test visual fields as a means of monitoring involvement of visual pathways. This is best done at the bedside by assessing peripheral visual fields using a red hatpin. It may be supplemented by more detailed Goldmann perimetry, available in ophthalmology clinics.

Hypersecretion may be diagnosed by measuring blood levels of the relevant hormone. While many endocrine presentations of pituitary tumours are due to hypersecretion, it is also possible for pituitary lesions to present clinically with signs of impairment of pituitary secretion. This may present clinically as adult GH deficiency syndrome (weight gain, loss of libido, fatigue), muscle weakness and fatigue, or with the symptoms of hypothyroidism. Low levels of pituitary hormone in the presence of low target gland hormones confirm hyposecretion. This can be further

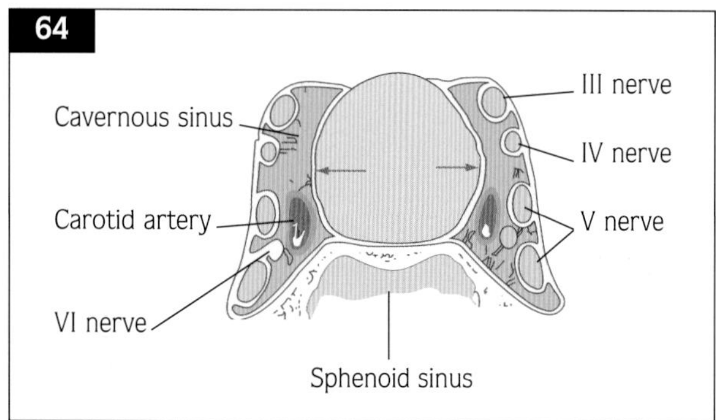

64 Diagram to show the anatomy of the cavernous sinus.

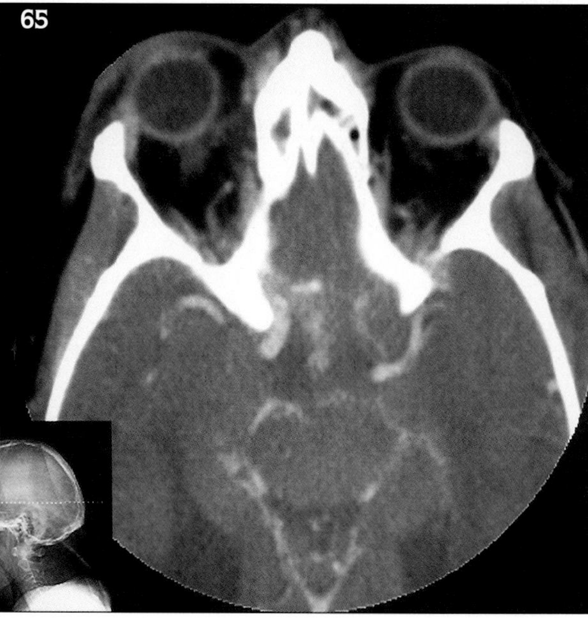

65 Computed tomography scan of cavernous sinus thrombosis.

investigated by combined pituitary function stimulation tests comprising the insulin tolerance test, also with gonadotrophin releasing hormone (GnRH) and thyrotrophin releasing hormone (TRH) injection.

DISEASE AT 'SHARED' SITES

Orbit

Orbital disorders may present to the neurologist as well as to the ophthalmologist, and it important that neurologists are aware of the appropriate investigations for this area.

Methods of visual field testing

It must be remembered that confrontation using a red pin is a relatively crude means of mapping visual fields, both for peripheral vision and for assessing the blind spot. Peripheral visual fields are better tested with a Goldmann perimeter (**67**). Here, a moving target is brought in from the periphery, and the patient must indicate as soon as he is aware of the target. It is thus possible to map out peripheral visual fields well.

While central fields may be assessed using a Goldmann perimeter, this is more accurately done using the Humphrey field analyser, which records the threshold at which a static light source is seen at various central points.

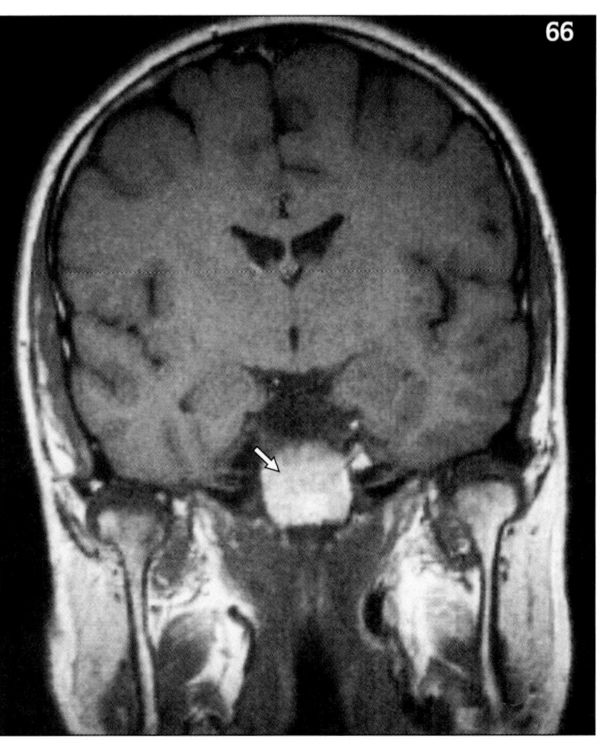

66 Magnetic resonance image of a pituitary tumour (arrow).

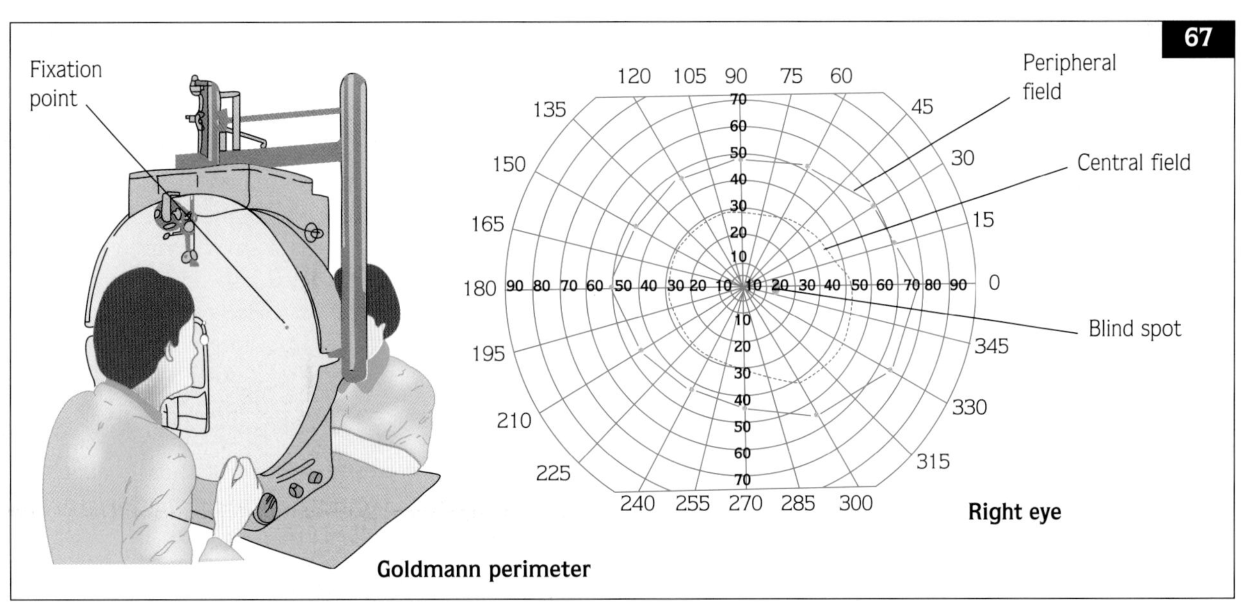

67 Diagram to demonstrate Goldmann perimetry.

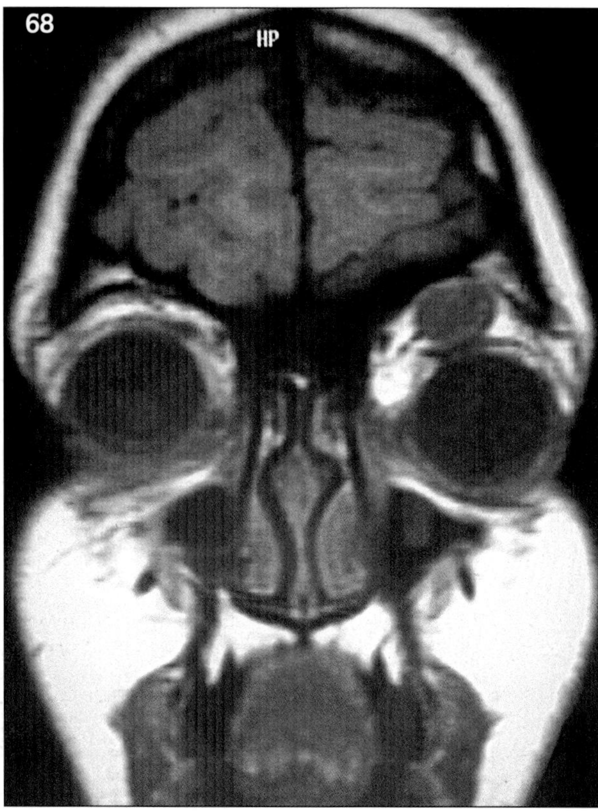

68 Magnetic resonance image showing a small tumour superior to the left eye.

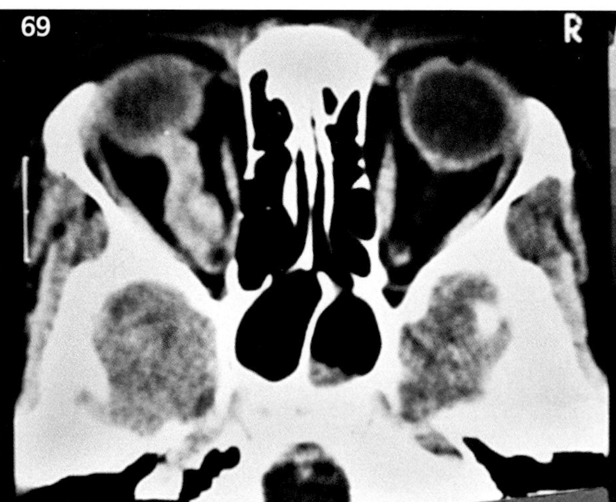

69 Computed tomography scan showing a left optic nerve meningioma. (Note Left is left on this scan.)

Imaging

Tumours of the orbit, or inflammatory conditions, are best visualised using MRI (**68**) rather than CT (**69**).

Neurophysiology

Visual evoked responses (VERs) have been described above, but are a useful means of assessing the integrity of the visual pathway from retina to occipital cortex.

Electroretinography (ERG) is a means of assessing rod and cone photoreceptor function, and is of use in assessing retinal degeneration and dystrophy.

Fluorescein angiography

This involves intravenous injection of aqueous fluorescein. A photograph of the fundus is taken before and after injection. This technique demonstrates choroidal and retinal vasculature, and can detect vascular occlusion and retinal haemorrhages. True optic disc swelling results in leakage of fluorescein, while pseudopapilloedematous discs do not leak.

The ear

Many conditions such as dizziness may present equally to a neurologist as to an ear nose and throat surgeon. One should therefore be familiar with the relevant investigations.

Auditory system

Weber's and Rinne's tests done as part of the neurological examination will usually allow classification of hearing impairment as being sensorineural or conductive, and will localize which is the impaired ear. These tests are, however, supplemented with further investigations including audiometry. Pure tone audiometry involves air conduction by means of a pure tone administered through headphones, with masking noise applied to the contralateral ear (**70**). Bone conduction is assessed by means of an electromechanical vibrator. Air-conducted sound requires a functioning ossicular system as well as cochlea and VIII nerve, while bone conduction bypasses the ossicles.

Speech audiometry uses pretaped words rather than tones, but involves the same principles as the above.

Stapedial reflex decay

Normally, a loud stimulus causes reflex contraction of stapedius, with subsequent reduced compliance of the tympanic membrane. In this test, an activating tone is applied to the ear under test, and the tympanic membrane impedance is monitored in the contralateral ear. Rapid decay of the reflex response suggests an auditory nerve lesion.

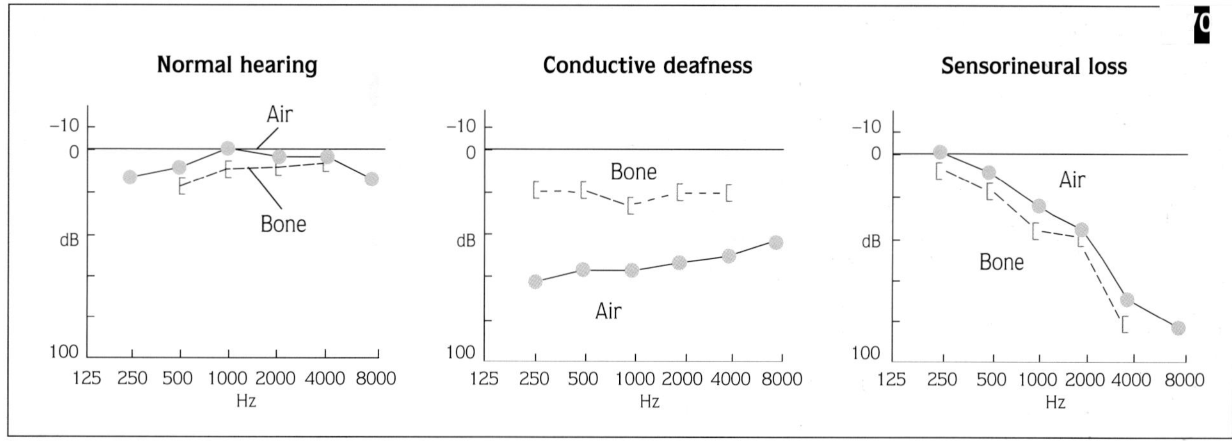

70 Audiograms of normal hearing, conductive deafness, and sensorineural loss.

Auditory brainstem evoked potential

This has been covered earlier in the chapter.

Vestibular system

Caloric testing

The vestibular system may be tested clinically using the Hallpike manoeuvre. Further investigation of the vestibular system relies on caloric testing, which utilizes the vestibulo-ocular reflex. In this test, water at 30°C (86°F) is irrigated into the ear. Nystagmus usually occurs after 20 seconds, and lasts for more than 1 minute. The test is then repeated 5 minutes later with water at 44°C (112°F). Cold water reduces vestibular output from one side, causing an imbalance and producing eye drift towards the irrigated ear, with rapid corrective movements to the opposite ear. Hot water reverses this, increases vestibular output and changes the direction of nystagmus. Time until cessation of nystagmus is plotted for each ear, at each temperature (71).

Reduced duration of nystagmus is termed canal paresis. This may be due to a peripheral or central lesion. A more prolonged duration of nystagmus in one direction than the other is called directional preponderance. It can be due to a central lesion ipsilateral to the preponderance, or from a contralateral peripheral lesion.

Combined with audiometry, these tests should differentiate peripheral from central lesions.

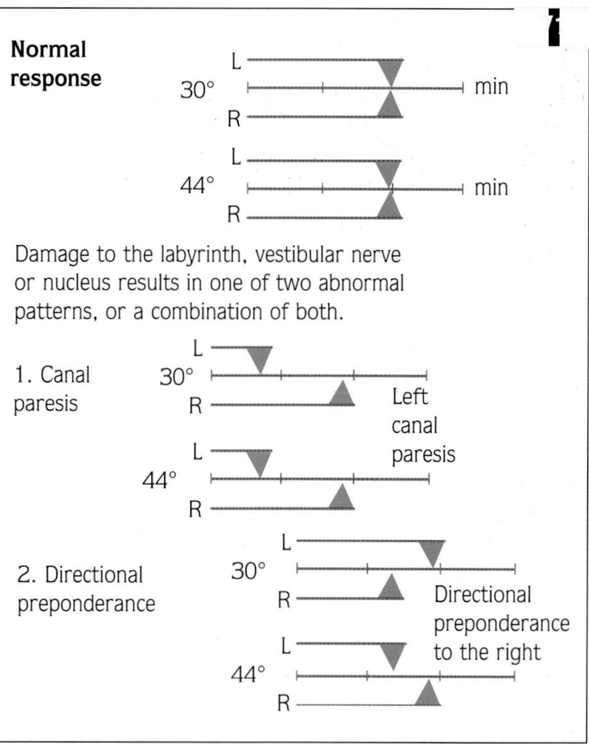

71 Caloric testing illustrating normal response, canal paresis, and directional preponderance.

Electronystagmography

Although nystagmus may be observed clinically, it is possible to assess nystagmus in a more quantitative manner by means of electronystagmography (ENG). These studies of eye movements are performed in darkness, in order to eliminate the stabilizing effects of visual fixation.

CHAPTER 3: THE PROBLEMS

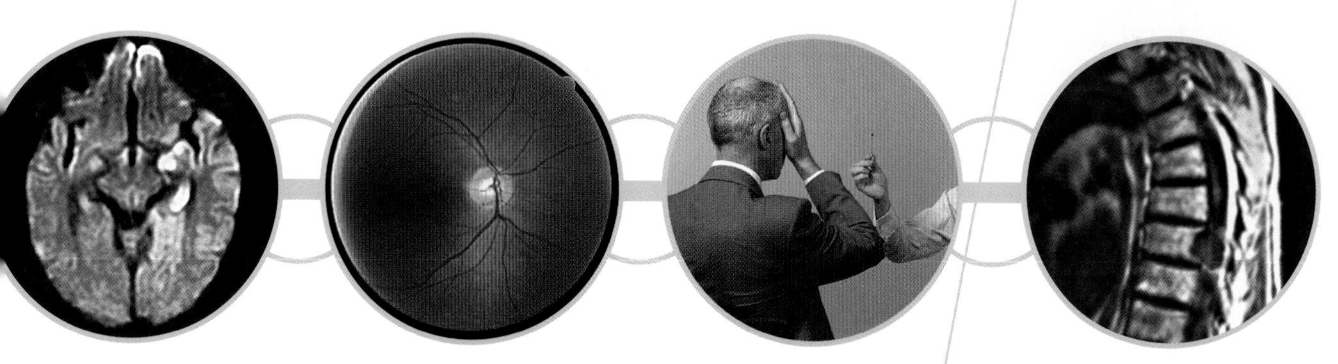

Disorders of consciousness

BLACKOUTS: EPILEPTIC SEIZURES AND OTHER EVENTS

Rod Duncan

INTRODUCTION

Clinicians in the Western world work in a diagnostic environment in which tests of one kind or another play an increasingly important diagnostic role. Disorders such as epilepsy, which manifest as recurrent, paroxysmal dysfunction of the central nervous system, continue to pose diagnostic difficulties. Why should this be?

The problem is simple to state. Between events, there are usually no abnormal examination findings, and those tests that can be applied are limited in terms of sensitivity, specificity, or both. The most accurate diagnostic tests depend on recording the disordered physiology at the time of the event (e.g. recording the changes in the electrical activity of the brain during an epileptic seizure). This type of test requires that events are frequent enough for there to be a realistic chance of capturing them, and that the resources are available to allow this. For these reasons, the use of such investigations is not practical for the majority of patients and the diagnosis of epilepsy and other disorders that come into its differential diagnosis, remains primarily a clinical one.

The differential diagnosis of epileptic seizures is wide, but this chapter will deal principally with conditions commonly considered at neurology or first seizure clinics: epilepsy, syncope, psychogenic nonepileptic seizures (PNES, previously termed 'pseudoseizures'), cardiogenic syncope, and panic or hyperventilation attacks.

The most common and important diagnostic distinction is between vasovagal syncope and epileptic seizure. It is thought that 80% of people will experience syncope at least once in the course of their lives. Epilepsy has an incidence of approximately 50 per 100,000 per year in the teenage and adult populations, with higher incidences in the paediatric and elderly populations. PNES make up 10–20% of patients who are thought to have uncontrolled epilepsy (or 2–4% of all patients thought to have epilepsy). For the nonspecialist, distinguishing PNES from epilepsy may be enormously difficult. PNES may coexist with hyperventilation or panic attacks. Cardiogenic syncope presents less commonly to neurological services, but has an importance out of proportion to its incidence, as it is potentially fatal.

CLINICAL ASSESSMENT

The diagnostic approach

The principle of the diagnostic method is that the account of the patient and that of the eyewitness allow the clinician to put together a 'video' in his or her mind of what happens to the patient during the event. This virtual video can then be compared with the clinical features of different types of event in order to try to make a match. An understanding of the pathophysiology of disorders such as epilepsy and syncope, and how that pathophysiology produces signs and symptoms, can also provide a framework for diagnosis from first principles. This can especially help where events are atypical. In this chapter, pathophysiology will, as far as possible, be related to the clinical features (sometimes called the *clinical semiology*) of events.

In taking the history of an event, it is important to be systematic. The account from the patient should include the circumstances of the event (i.e. what the patient was doing at the time of onset of the event, and for a few minutes before), the patient's experience of the onset of the event, the patient's experience of the event itself (if any), and the patient's symptoms after the event, up to the point where the patient feels back to normal. It is important that the duration of each stage is established as accurately as possible. In taking the history from the eyewitness, it is important to begin at the point when the eyewitness first realized something was amiss, and again to take the witness stage by stage through the event, once more taking care to establish durations. It is important to establish whether all the events are the same. A distinction must be made between events that vary in severity, and events that are completely different in kind. If there are both mild and severe events, it must be established whether the severe events lead on from mild ones, or occur independently.

While this chapter will deal mainly with the clinical features of the events themselves, the overall history of the disorder, and more specifically the distribution in time of the events may be diagnostically useful to some degree. Triggering of events may be seen in a number of disorders, and is crucial to the diagnosis of vasovagal syncope. In contrast, information relating to the background of the patient should not be given inappropriate diagnostic weight. A teenage patient with one first-degree relative with epilepsy, for example, has an increased risk of having epilepsy, but the absolute risk is of the order of a few percent, and syncope remains the most common diagnosis in this population. Where several first-degree relatives are affected, the increased risk becomes more significant, and more weight may be given to family history. Similarly, a history of mild head injury is associated only with a small increase in liability to develop epilepsy, and should probably not be given significant diagnostic weight (the more so as >50% of patients with PNES give a history of mild head injury prior to the onset of the disorder). If, however, the head injury involved a depressed fracture with craniotomy, the risk of epilepsy is substantial.

The role of clinical examination

Neurological signs suggestive of a cortical lesion indicate a potential cause for epileptic seizures, but should not be given undue weight in deciding whether events are seizures or not. Cardiovascular examination can, however, be important, and is dealt with under the relevant disorders.

Mechanisms of altered consciousness

Mechanisms in the brainstem are thought to determine consciousness, but it is not clear how this applies to disorders such as syncope and epilepsy. In syncope, the whole brain is ischaemic and therefore dysfunctional. In seizures, the whole brain may be involved (the cortex being responsible for generating the seizure discharge, which is then conducted down subcortical pathways, presumably including the brainstem reticular formation), or specific parts of the brain may be involved. In the latter case, the history may well fail to determine whether the patient is amnesic for a period of time, or has been unconscious. Unresponsiveness may be misleading: patients not infrequently remember some of their jerking movements. The author is aware of one case where a patient claimed to be aware during his tonic–clonic seizure and to remember this after the event, and indeed could recount information presented to him during generalized seizures. The seizures presumably only appeared to be generalized, in reality affecting only the motor strips bilaterally, causing unresponsiveness.

Syncopal attacks

Vasovagal syncope can be provoked by a number of stressors, physiological and psychological:

- Postural change.
- Medical procedures.
- Physical trauma.
- Psychological trauma (sight of blood, bad news).
- Micturition.
- Defecation.
- Eating.
- Swallowing.

More than one factor may operate: for example, postural change may provoke vasovagal syncope in combination with predisposing factors such as heat, stress, or alcohol. Some medications such as antidepressant and antihypertensive drugs predispose to syncope. If a predisposing factor such as heat is present, then maintaining the upright posture for a prolonged period may result in spontaneous syncope. Postural syncope may be one of several symptoms that might suggest disordered autonomic function. Triggering is crucial to the diagnosis of syncope. Without establishing the existence of a credible trigger for each attack, the diagnosis cannot be made with confidence.

Postural dizziness and 'presyncope'

A change in posture to the standing position causes a rise in the orthostatic pressure in the veins. The veins passively dilate, accommodating a greater volume of blood so that circulating volume to the rest of the body falls. Cardiac output and perfusion pressure to the head and brain therefore fall also. The brain has effectively no metabolic reserve, so that symptomatic dysfunction occurs within seconds. Where syncope is triggered by a 'noxious stimulus' such as the sight of blood, the pathophysiological sequence begins with vagal overactivity, leading to bradycardia and reduced blood pressure.

The initial symptoms (prodrome) of loss of perfusion pressure to the head are also crucial to the diagnosis of syncope. The retina is as sensitive to loss of perfusion pressure as the brain, so visual symptoms are common. Usually, these consist of blurring, dark spots, or darkening of the visual image. However, a wide variety of effects may occur, and the author has encountered almost every elemental visual modification imaginable: bright spots, coloured spots, darkening from the periphery inward, from the top down, and so on. Dizziness is usual (the word may be the patient's interpretation of unsteadiness, disorientation, a feeling of unreality, or other sensations). Auditory effects may occur, a buzzing noise being the most common. Reduced perfusion pressure in the carotid arteries activates the carotid baroceptors. Signals are sent to the heart, to increase cardiac output, and to the peripheral veins to increase tone in their walls. In normal circumstances, this will restore perfusion pressure to the head and any symptoms will resolve. Symptoms may also resolve if the patient sits with the head between the legs (sitting upright is usually not sufficient) or lies down.

Postural dizziness provides a useful tool in the diagnosis of syncope. Almost everybody experiences postural dizziness at some point in their lives, and therefore knows what it feels like. When a patient presents with an episode of loss of consciousness with a prodrome, the patient can be asked to compare the prodrome with the feeling they get if they 'stand up too quickly'. Clearly, the duration and severity of the feelings can vary, but if the patient identifies them as qualitatively the same, then the clinician can be clinically confident that the patient has lost consciousness because of lack of perfusion pressure to the brain. During presyncope, an eyewitness may not notice anything at all, or may note that the patient looks dazed or confused.

Vasovagal syncope

In some circumstances, the above sequence of events may either be insufficient to restore cerebral perfusion, or may trigger vagal overactivity, resulting in loss of consciousness and fall. In elderly patients and those with neuropathy involving loss of control of blood pressure, a change to the upright position may directly cause loss of perfusion pressure to the head, and the onset of syncope may be rapid, with no remembered prodromal symptoms. However, it is more usual, especially when the trigger is postural change, for the process to take some time. Thus, if a person gets up from a chair to leave the room, the onset of symptoms may be delayed for a few steps, and loss of consciousness typically does not occur until the patient has reached the next room. It is therefore important in taking the history to be sure to go back to precisely what the patient was doing and what his or her posture was at least 1 minute or so before the onset of symptoms.

When loss of consciousness occurs, the patient normally falls. The orthostatic pressure differential between the head and the legs is then lost, perfusion pressure to the brain is restored, and the patient recovers. Typically, therefore, the duration of unconsciousness in syncope is short. However, if for some reason a fall is prevented or if the patient is propped up in the sitting position, then perfusion pressure to the brain may not be restored, and the patient may not regain consciousness for some time.

During syncope, brain ischaemia may be sufficient to cause seizure-like manifestations, such as brief stiffening and a few jerks. If the patient does not fall or if hypotension is severe, then these manifestations may be quite marked. The accurate identification of this situation as an effect of syncope depends crucially on obtaining a clinical history of the triggering factor, and of the prodromal symptoms typical of syncope.

Cardiogenic syncope

In cardiogenic syncope, the patient loses consciousness when perfusion pressure to the brain is lost due to arrhythmia or cardiac outflow obstruction. However, because perfusion pressure tends to be lost much more quickly, there may be no prodrome. If loss of perfusion pressure is severe then stiffness may occur, but a simple fall to the ground with no convulsive movements is usual.

Cardiogenic syncope should be suspected in the following situations:

- ❑ If the eyewitness account suggests syncope, but no history of triggers can be elicited.
- ❑ If there is a history of cardiac disease.
- ❑ If there are additional cardiac symptoms.
- ❑ If there is a family history of sudden unexplained death.
- ❑ If loss of consciousness is provoked by exercise (very important).

Cardiogenic syncope presents relatively uncommonly to neurology clinics; long QT syndrome usually presents in childhood (72). It may be misdiagnosed as epilepsy and subsequently present as longstanding epilepsy in an adult, probably because of its tendency to cause loss of consciousness with a tonic phase. It is important to identify, as it is associated with attacks of ventricular fibrillation and death.

Carotid sinus hypersensitivity may cause episodes of loss of consciousness. An exaggerated response to physical stimulation of the carotid sinus, in some cases provoked even by turning the head, may cause sinus arrest. It occurs mainly in the elderly. The patient often has no warning, is aware of a gap in their awareness, and then of coming round with rapid return to normality. An eyewitness seeing such a collapse notes the patient lying still, without convulsive movements, for a short period. Sometimes the patient notes an association with head turning, or a particular position of the neck.

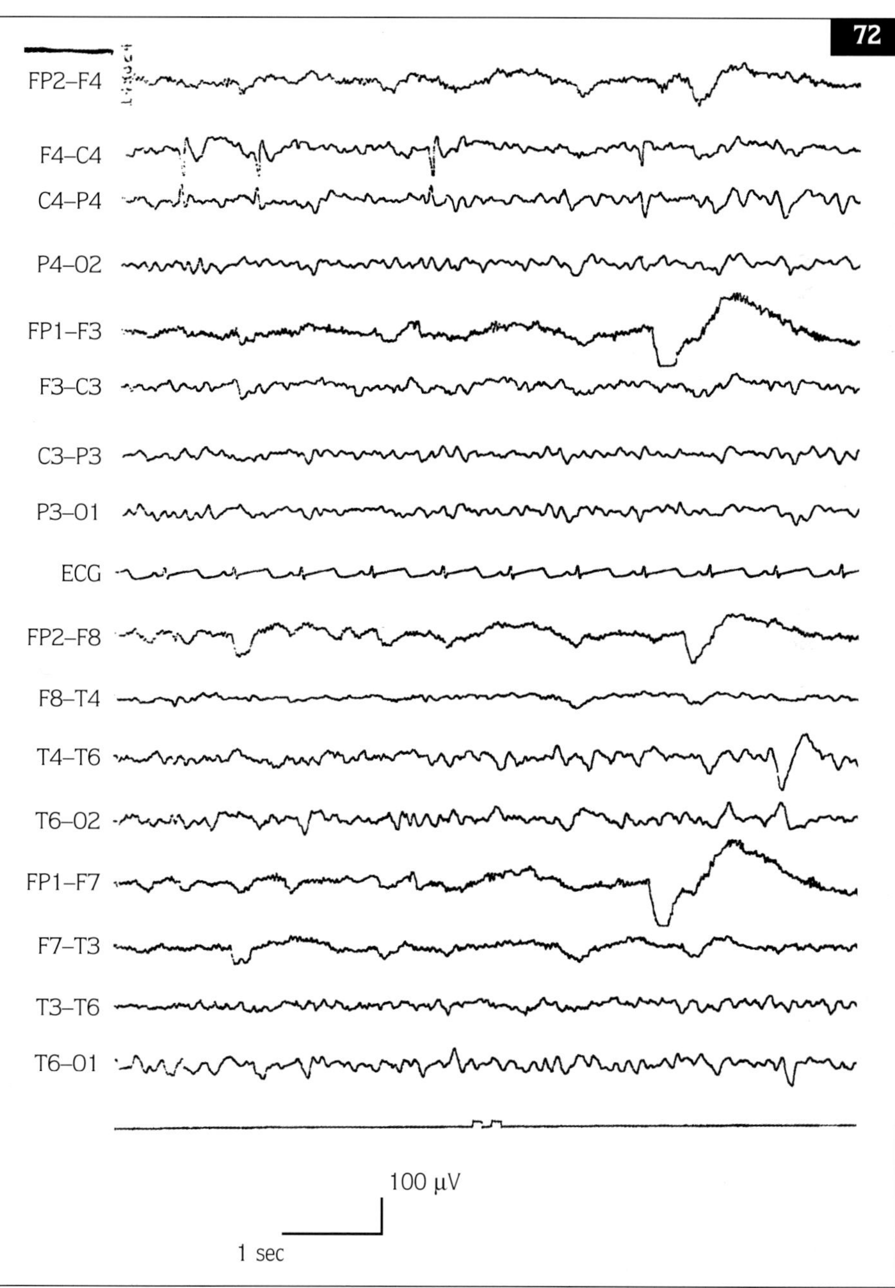

72 Interictal encephalographic recording in a boy aged 11 years, showing focal frontal spikes on the right (second and third channels from the top). The electrocardiographic recording (9th channel from the top) shows normal sinus rhythm but a prolonged QT interval of 0.52 seconds (upper limit of normal is 0.46 seconds). The spikes were thought to be incidental as the patient had never been witnessed to have had an epileptic seizure. He had documented episodes of cardiac arrest (ventricular fibrillation, 'torsades de pointe' pattern), manifesting as loss of consciousness with stiffness and cyanosis. The diagnosis was long QT syndrome.

EPILEPTIC SEIZURES

Classification of seizures

Epilepsy is usually defined as a tendency to have recurrent epileptic seizures (ESs). It follows from this that to diagnose epilepsy the patient's events must be identified as being epileptic seizures, and more than one has to have occurred. The classification of the epilepsy depends on identifying the type(s) of seizures the patient suffers from. *Table 9* identifies common seizure types.

The relationship between the pathophysiology of seizures and their clinical manifestations is most easily illustrated by considering focal motor seizures. A 'spike' refers to a phenomenon seen on electroencephalographic (EEG) recording, and is the basic 'unit' of seizure activity. It is a sudden and brief increase in the measured voltage at an electrode or electrodes. It is due to an aggregate of neurones firing simultaneously, or nearly so. The voltage and current produced are much higher than those which occur during normal brain function. If the current is produced in a given part of the brain (for example that part of the right motor cortex which corresponds to the left hand), then it is conducted down pathways which impulses from that cortex would normally be conducted down. In the case of the motor cortex, the impulse is conducted through the relevant parts of the internal capsule, basal ganglia, brainstem, spinal cord, brachial plexus, and peripheral nerves to the muscles. The result is a jerk (a movement with a fast contraction phase and a slower relaxation phase [clonus or a clonic movement]) (73).

If the discharge takes the form of a series of spikes very close together, the jerks will occur too frequently for the muscle to relax between, and the result will be a sustained contraction (stiffness, or tonus). If the discharge consists of repetitive spikes (of whatever frequency), then areas of cortex adjacent to that originally involved may begin to be 'recruited'. In this way, as a discharge spreads (or propagates) along the motor strip, the jerks or tonus correspondingly spread to the parts of the body served by the cortex. For

Table 9 Common types of seizure

Seizure type	Description	EEG discharge	Type of epilepsy
Primary generalized tonic–clonic	Tonic–clonic seizure (vocalization, stiffness followed by generalized jerks, with postictal stupor and confusion). No focal onset	Generalized from onset, spike, spike/wave	Primary generalized
Primary generalized absence	Also called petit mal: short interruption of activity and contact	Generalized 3/sec spike and wave	Primary generalized
Myoclonic	Jerk, usually of 1 or more limbs	Generalized or focal spike	Primary generalized or focal
Atonic	Abrupt loss of muscle tone and drop to the ground	Variable. May be generalized or focal spike	Primary generalized or focal
Simple partial	Focal seizure with no disturbance of consciousness (usually clonic movements of limbs or sensory symptoms)	May have no detectable surface EEG change. May show focal change (spike, slow wave)	Focal
Complex partial	Focal seizures with disturbance of consciousness (usually arrest of activity, loss of contact with automatic movements)	Focal onset, usually with bilateral spread	Focal
Secondary generalized tonic–clonic	Simple or complex partial seizure evolving to clonic	Focal onset then generalized	Focal

example, if a seizure discharge begins in that part of the motor cortex serving the hand, as it spreads upward and downward through the cortex, the jerks (or stiffness if the spikes are frequent enough) will gradually spread to involve the rest of the arm, the face, and the leg. This phenomenon is called the 'Jacksonian March'. The discharge may then go on to involve the whole brain, producing a generalized seizure. In this event, the spikes are synchronous throughout the motor cortex, are conducted down motor pathways, and reach the muscles simultaneously, producing a jerk that is synchronous in all four limbs.

These are the basic processes by which the positive elements of clinical seizure semiology are produced. They are translatable pretty much directly to other primary cortices (sensory and visual principally). In cortices with complex integrative functions, 'simple' epileptic discharges feed in to networks, producing complex effects that may mimic or parody normal brain function. These complex effects may consist of organized automatic movements, complex hallucinations, or other effects and behaviours.

Seizure discharges produce not only positive phenomena (e.g. jerks) but also negative phenomena, as they will prevent normal function. Dysfunction may also occur in the postictal phase, thought to be due to neuronal exhaustion. If a focal motor seizure involves one arm, for example, then the arm may be weak for a period postictally. If the seizure activity involves Broca's area, then the postictal deficit is likely to be dysphasia. Seizures may be followed by widespread brain dysfunction, causing effects such as confusion and drowsiness.

Seizure discharge and the clinical manifestations of tonic–clonic seizures

During a tonic–clonic seizure, the EEG shows an initial discharge of high frequency generalized spikes, which then gradually breaks up into frequent discrete spikes, slowing as the seizure progresses. Once the spikes have stopped, there is absence of, then slowing of, cerebral rhythms. The clinical correlate of this is direct. The fast discharge of spikes coincides with the tonic phase of the seizure. As the fast discharge begins to break up into discrete spikes, the tonic phase gives way to persisting stiffness but with a superimposed fine jerky tremor. The tremor and stiffness gradually break up further into discrete jerks, which slow down as the seizure progresses. The absence or slowing of rhythms in the postictal period reflects cortical dysfunction, which is clinically associated with confusion, drowsiness, and headache. In the aftermath of the seizure, the patient may report incontinence and having bitten the side of the tongue or the cheek. The next day, the patient may complain of myalgia.

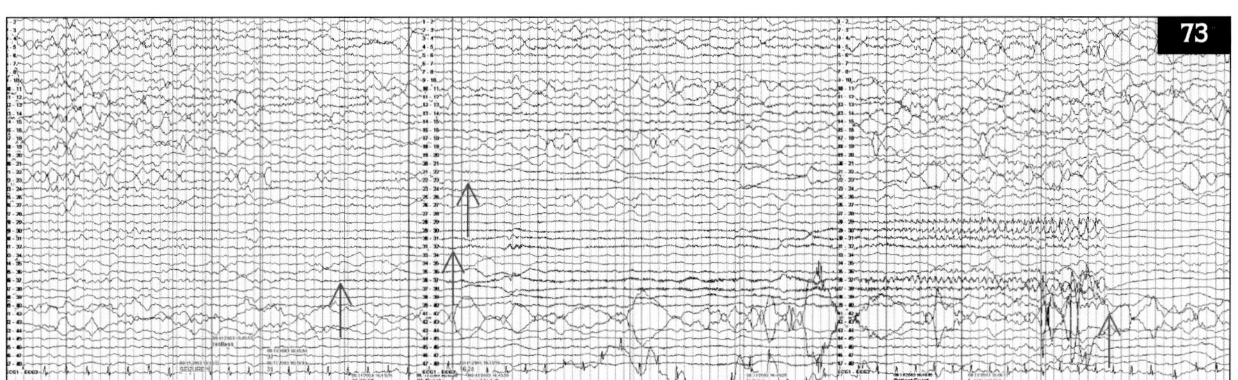

73 Recording from a subdural grid of electrodes placed over the lateral frontal cortex just anterior to the motor strip. The electrical manifestations of the seizure begin in channels 35–36, 36–37, and 37–38 as a high frequency spike discharge (arrow). As the seizure progresses, the discharge spreads to adjacent cortical areas (arrows). The discharge evolves into a slower spike-wave form and terminates (last arrow) with postictal flattening of the trace most severe in the channels most affected by the seizure discharge (28–29, 29–30, 30–31, 31–32, 36–37, 37–38, 38–39). Clinically, the fast spike discharge was associated with stiffening of the contralateral upper limb, and the spike-wave discharge with jerks. The postictal flattening represents neuronal dysfunction, and was associated with weakness (i.e. Todd's palsy).

An understanding of this pathophysiological sequence has an important clinical implication. A generalized spike produces a jerk that is necessarily synchronous in all four limbs, and is not capable of producing alternating movements of limbs or side-to-side movements of the head. If an event appears to be a generalized seizure but the movements are alternating, then the event is likely to be a PNES (*Table 10*). It should nevertheless be remembered that complex movements might occur during complex partial seizures or during postictal confusion, again illustrating the importance of having an eyewitness account of the whole event.

Classification of the epilepsies

The International League against Epilepsy (ILAE) classification of epilepsies includes a large number of syndromes. However, many are relevant primarily to epilepsies presenting in childhood, and in adolescents and adults by far the most important classification issue is whether the epilepsy is primary generalized or focal. The importance of making this distinction lies in the fact that primary generalized epilepsies respond only to certain anticonvulsant drugs, tend not to remit, and tend to relapse on withdrawal of current treatment.

Primary generalized epilepsies make up 10% of adult epilepsies as a whole, but up to 50% of epilepsies presenting in the late teens. The most common phenotype is juvenile myoclonic epilepsy (JME). This presents with tonic–clonic convulsions in combination with myoclonic jerks, which usually occur in the morning. Some patients have a photoconvulsive response (**74**), which may manifest as a tendency to have seizures in response to flashes of certain frequencies. A minority of patients also have true petit mal absence seizures; these consist of arrest of activity and loss of contact lasting several seconds (**75**). In some patients, seizures occur in the context of sleep deprivation, or following alcohol excess. Other phenotypes, such as early morning tonic–clonic seizures in adolescence, may be encountered. It is rare for primary generalized epilepsies to present after the age of 25 years.

Auras

The aura of a seizure is a subjective feeling that the patient associates with the beginning of the seizure. It is in fact the very beginning of the seizure, reflecting the effects of the seizure discharge while it remains very localized, and therefore is usually a feature of focal or secondary generalized seizures. Auras are

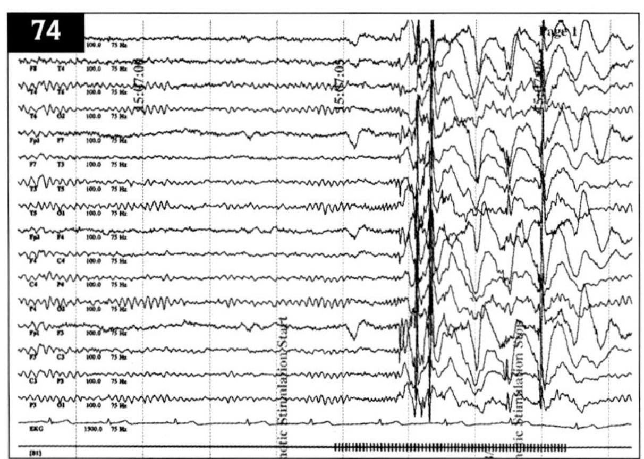

74 Interictal electroencephalographic recording with photic stimulation at 19/second (flashes are marked on the trace at the bottom of the picture). Photic stimulation induces a generalized spike-wave discharge, typical of a primary generalized epilepsy such as juvenile myoclonic epilepsy.

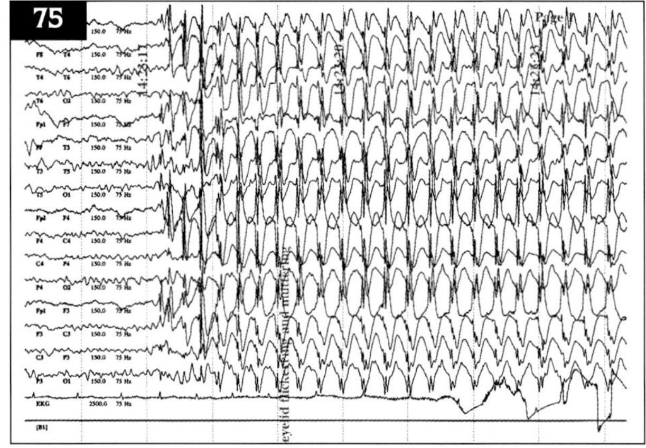

75 Electroencephalographic recording during a generalized 'petit mal' seizure, showing generalized 3/second spike and wave discharges.

particularly common where the seizure originates in cortex with sensory or associative functions. If a seizure originates in the sensory cortex, the aura is likely to be one of tingling, the tingling being felt in that part of the body served by the part of the sensory cortex that is affected. If a seizure originates in the primary visual cortex, then the aura is likely to consist of an elementary visual hallucination, seen in the contralateral visual field. In temporal lobe seizures, a number of auras may occur, the most common being a feeling of déjà vu and an abdominal sensation of butterflies rising up through the chest. Auras consisting of smells and sounds may occur.

Complex partial seizures

Complex partial seizures may originate from any part of the cortex, but most commonly originate in the temporal lobe. From the eyewitness point of view, there is an interruption of activity and a loss of contact. The patient tends to stare into space, and may remain motionless. Automatic activity may occur. This most commonly consists of chewing or lip smacking movements of the mouth, or fiddling movements of the hands, whereby the patient will pluck at his clothing or fiddle with some object near him. The seizure typically lasts 30–90 seconds, with a variable phase of postictal confusion, drowsiness, or sometimes headache.

Table 10 Factors which may lead to a clinical suspicion of PNES

- ❏ 'Fall down, lie still' type attacks lasting >2 minutes*
- ❏ Recurrent attacks in medical situations (in scanner, clinics)
- ❏ Many major attacks in the day with no morbidity
- ❏ Alternating movements
- ❏ Side-to-side head movements
- ❏ Emotional outburst associated with attack
- ❏ Situational response
- ❏ Eyes closed during attack

*If shorter may be syncope or cardiac syncope.

Frontal lobe complex partial seizures may be associated with bizarre automatisms, causing them to be mistaken for PNES, or may simply consist of short periods of immobility.

Panic and hyperventilation attacks

Hyperventilation is a common reaction to anxiety. Hyperventilation decreases carbon dioxide levels in the plasma and induces respiratory alkalosis. This causes instability of excitable membranes and results in a number of symptoms, including light-headedness, or a sensation of unreality. Excitability of peripheral nerves causes peripheral paraesthesiae. Where hyperventilation is marked, spasm of some muscles may occur, particularly those of the hands and occasionally the eyes. Rubefaction may be marked. Hyperventilation may induce vasovagal syncope, confusing the diagnostic picture. If it is remembered that it is often not possible to obtain a clear history of a precipitating situation, the history is usually fairly clear. While there is no diagnostic test as such, the patient can be asked to hyperventilate under observation, and the effects then compared to those of the events complained of by the patient.

Psychogenic nonepileptic seizures

Confirmation of the diagnosis of PNES is the function of the specialist, but it is important that all clinicians coming in contact with epilepsy and similar disorders know when to suspect PNES (*Table 10*).

Most patients with PNES are young and most (75%) are female. Only 10–15% have epilepsy. A significant proportion (probably approximately 50%) has a background of sexual or physical abuse, and psychopathology is common. While useful in understanding the condition, these factors should be used with care in diagnosing PNES, as their discriminatory value is poor.

While the occurrence of social triggering is a useful pointer to PNES, its absence should not allay diagnostic suspicion; in many patients with PNES there is no discernible social triggering. There is a distinct tendency for PNES to occur in medical situations, and the diagnosis should be considered in patients who have a history of events during scans, hospital outpatient visits and so on. Patients with PNES may well have events in response to photic stimulation.

The clinical semiology of PNES

PNES are usually frequent. Two types of event are particularly common. They may be labelled 'convulsive', where patients have variable movements of limbs, head, and trunk, and 'swoon' where patients fall down and lie still. PNES tend to be longer than epileptic seizures, though the ranges overlap. Where there are 'convulsive' movements, the observation of alternating limb movements and side-to-side head movements, especially with coordinated alternating agonist and antagonist activity (effectively a tremor) or thrashing movements, are highly suggestive of PNES. Jerking movements do occasionally occur, but are asynchronous. Forward pelvic thrusting is seen in a variable proportion of patients. Signs of emotional distress during or after the event suggest PNES.

'False friends'

Some clinical features widely thought to indicate epilepsy do in fact occur in PNES, in particular urinary incontinence and injury (with the exception of thermal burns). PNES are often said not to be stereotyped, but a number of studies have shown this not to be true. Patients may have PNES while appearing to be asleep, and a history of events arising during sleep should not be taken as conclusive evidence for ES.

INVESTIGATIONS

Routine (interictal) EEG should be used with care in the diagnosis of epilepsy. A single recording has a false-negative rate of at least 50%. The test is therefore of absolutely no use at all in excluding a diagnosis of epilepsy, and should not be requested for this purpose. Nonspecific abnormalities are common, especially in certain patient groups (e.g. the elderly, history of brain trauma) and should not be regarded as relevant to the diagnosis of epilepsy. Epileptiform abnormalities (**76**) occur rarely (1%) in the young, healthy, nonepileptic population, although they are less specific for epilepsy in the elderly and in patients with a history of brain trauma.

EEG should be used as a diagnostic test when the patient history and eyewitness account are suggestive of epilepsy, but the clinician is not quite sure. Where the history indicates some other type of event (e.g. faint), then the prevalence of epilepsy in this population will be low: few positives will be obtained, and a high proportion of them will be false positives. The test should not be carried out in this circumstance.

> There is no point in carrying out an EEG recording for diagnostic purposes in a patient who has an unequivocal history of seizure. Neither a positive nor a negative result will change the diagnosis.

In patients in whom the diagnosis of seizure is made, however, EEG may usefully be carried out for three indications other than diagnosis. It may aid the classification of the epilepsy where that is clinically uncertain. It can detect a photoconvulsive response,

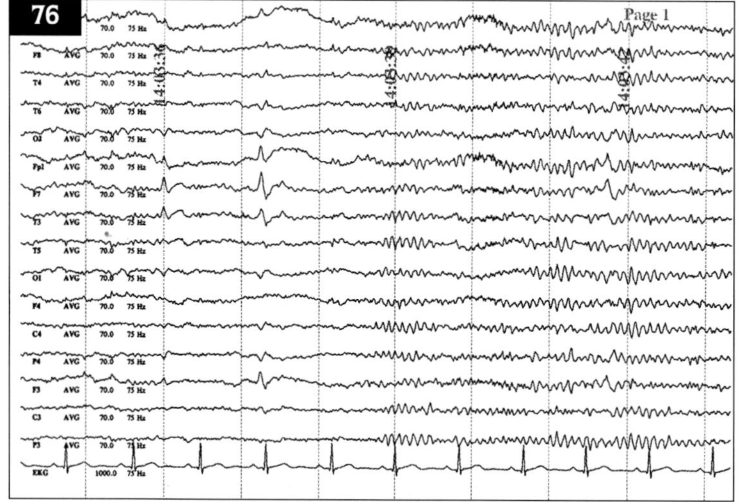

76 Interictal electroencephalographic recording showing left fronto-temporal spikes, maximal in channel T3, typical of interictal discharge seen in mesial temporal lobe epilepsies.

allowing the patient to be advised to avoid certain situations. If carried out soon after a first seizure, the finding of epileptiform abnormalities indicates an increased probability of recurrence.

In patients presenting diagnostic difficulties, simultaneous video and EEG recording of events is usually diagnostic. Events do, however, have to be reasonably frequent for this to be practicable. Ambulatory EEG recording may also be used, and in some circumstances simple video recording may be useful. Electrocardiography (ECG) should be carried out in any patient whose attacks include loss of consciousness. If the clinical picture indicates a significant possibility of cardiogenic syncope (see below), then ambulatory ECG monitoring may be indicated. Referral to a cardiologist should be considered. Patients who have had a seizure should have cranial imaging, to exclude a structural cause that may require treatment. MRI is recommended, in view of its greater sensitivity, though CT is more generally performed.

SUMMARY

- ❑ The diagnosis of epilepsy is normally made on clinical grounds alone.
- ❑ Knowledge of and the ability to diagnose other common attack disorders are required.
- ❑ Vasovagal syncope may present features suggestive of epilepsy; the key to diagnosis is to identify triggering factors and the aura.
- ❑ Cardiac syncope should be suspected when attacks are provoked by exercise or when there is a family history of sudden unexplained death.
- ❑ Psychogenic nonepileptic seizures are common among patients who are thought to have intractable epilepsy. It is important to know what factors should trigger referral for reassessment of diagnosis.
- ❑ Standard EEG can be useful in diagnosis and classification, but should never be used to 'exclude' epilepsy.

CLINICAL SCENARIOS

CASE 1

A 35-year-old male had an episode of loss of consciousness. The general practitioner obtained an account of the event from the man's wife. She said that he had been sitting on the couch the previous evening, had lost consciousness, slumping to one side. He went stiff, and had had a few jerks, and gradually came round, feeling groggy for a few minutes.

At this point, the diagnosis is one of epileptic seizure. However, it is important to be clear on the circumstances of any attack, so further questioning is indicated.

The general practitioner had not unreasonably diagnosed epileptic seizure. At the clinic, however, the patient was asked how he had been feeling that night. He said that he had a cold. He had been sitting on the couch in front of a warm fire, drinking a glass of whisky. He had got up to refill his glass, and approximately half way to the living room had felt unwell.

There were three factors that might predispose to syncope. Firstly, the patient had a cold. Secondly, he had consumed a small amount of alcohol. Thirdly, he was in a warm environment. A change in posture interacted with three predisposing factors to produce syncope. The initial history placed the onset of the event on the couch. In reality, the onset was after the patient had got up and walked a few steps, and it was necessary to go back a few minutes in time to elicit the history of postural change.

He turned round, and went back and sat on the couch. There was then a gap in his awareness until he came round. He was asked in what way he had felt unwell just after he got up from the couch. He said that he felt dizzy, and that his vision had become blurred. He identified this feeling as being similar to the one he had on standing up too quickly, a feeling of dizziness accompanied by blurring and darkening of the vision.

The patient fainted in the sitting position, preventing an immediate fall, and preventing restoration of perfusion to the brain. Unconsciousness and recovery were longer than usual, and the patient had stiffness and jerks.

Case 2

A 27-year-old female presented with a history of episodes of loss of consciousness. These had started when she was 6 years old and had originally been infrequent, at one or two per year. Over the preceding year, the frequency had increased to the point where she was having three or four per week.

At this point the disorder appears like worsening intractable epilepsy, but a change in the behaviour of epilepsy should prompt a reassessment.

She herself had no warning of the attacks. Following them, she felt drained, but had no specific postictal symptoms. Her husband gave a description. She would become agitated, with a progressively severe tremulous movement involving both arms. This would increase over several minutes, and spread to the point where she had violent alternating movements of all four limbs, with side-to-side movements of the head. This would go on for several minutes, occasionally for longer. There was no cyanosis, tongue biting, or incontinence.

This description is not compatible with tonic–clonic seizures, and suggests PNES, possibly of recent onset on the background of a longstanding seizure disorder.

She was admitted for video EEG recording, and several attacks were recorded in the first 3 days. All corresponded to the husband's description, and all were PNES. Enquiry discovered a background of childhood sexual abuse. No interictal EEG abnormalities were detected.

The diagnosis of PNES is established, but the possibility of a background epilepsy remains. Onset of PNES aged 6 years is not usual, and the events were infrequent for many years, suggesting another cause.

Her medication was gradually withdrawn after her discharge from hospital. On review at 1 month, her husband said that the attacks had greatly reduced, but said that he now realized there had been two types of attack, the more recent, frequent attacks being different from the original ones. A detailed description of the more recent attacks was obtained. The patient would fall abruptly to the ground, initially floppy, then stiff. She would then go blue. After 30 seconds or so, she would recover her colour, then relax and gradually recover consciousness, with a short phase of confusion.

When different attacks are occurring eyewitnesses may find it difficult to distinguish between them. In this case, it was only when the frequent type of event ceased that the husband could give a clear description of the less frequent type. In this case it was not possible to establish the diagnosis definitively, but the eyewitness description of the recent attacks is highly suggestive of cardiac arrest. The fact that the patient had a history of sexual abuse illustrates the diagnostic limitations of background factors.

An ECG was performed urgently, and showed a prolonged QT interval.

There is a good argument for performing routine ECG in all patients presenting with attacks of loss of consciousness.

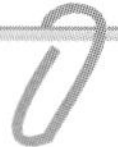

Case 3

A 55-year-old female presented to the neurology clinic complaining of memory difficulties over the previous few months. On taking a detailed history, it became clear that her problem was intermittent. She was actually complaining of short gaps in her memory, at intervals of every few hours or so, though sometimes with gaps of a few days. The gaps in memory were brief, lasting 2 or 3 minutes at most. According to her own account, she behaved completely normally during these gaps, and appeared to carry on normal activity. She felt completely normal before the attacks and after.

While the initial complaint was of poor memory suggesting a cognitive problem, a paroxysmal disturbance of memory over a time of seconds or minutes should always arouse suspicion of seizures.

The eyewitness account was obtained. It transpired that most of the gaps in memory passed without an eyewitness being aware of anything amiss. However, on one occasion she had a gap in her memory while driving. The eyewitness reported that she had become disoriented, and seemed unaware of where she was. She continued to drive, but could not carry on a sensible conversation for 30 seconds or so.

This illustrates the tendency for focal epileptic seizures to vary in severity (reflecting a variation in the extent of the propagation of the discharge). In this case, it was only when a more severe seizure occurred that it became evident that the functional disturbance extended beyond memory.

A standard EEG was normal. Ambulatory EEG monitoring was carried out. This showed frequent spike discharges over the left temporal region, which correlated with periods of loss of memory.

Revision questions

1 Vasovagal syncope:
- a Presents with lateralized visual aura.
- b Causes biting of the tip of the tongue.
- c Is usually infrequent.
- d May cause myoclonic jerks.
- e May be provoked by exercise.

2 True petit mal seizures:
- a Are associated with a generalized spike-wave discharge.
- b Usually last 30–60 seconds.
- c Usually originate in the temporal lobe.
- d May occur many times per day.
- e May occur in juvenile myoclonic epilepsy.

3 Psychogenic nonepileptic seizures:
- a Are usually frequent.
- b May cause injury.
- c Are not stereotyped.
- d Are associated with synchronous clonic movements.
- e Are associated with head injury.

Answers

1
- a False. Lateralized visual aura suggests epileptic seizure.
- b True. In tonic–clonic seizures, tongue biting is usually lateral, or the inside of the cheek is bitten.
- c True.
- d True.
- e False. Provocation by exercise should suggest cardiogenic syncope.

2
- a True.
- b False. Seizures last several seconds at most.
- c False. They are generalized seizures.
- d True.
- e True.

3
- a True.
- b True, though in a minority of patients.
- c False.
- d False. Movements are normally alternating or tremulous. Asynchronous jerks may occasionally occur.
- e True. A history of minor head injury is elicited in approximately 50% of patients.

ACUTE CONFUSIONAL STATES

Myfanwy Thomas

INTRODUCTION

About 20% of acute medical admissions come under the broad heading of neurology, though not necessarily due to a precise and easily defined primary neurological condition. Alerted arousal (coma) and disturbed content of consciousness (e.g. confusional states) are encountered on a daily basis in the acute medical wards. Many patients, particularly the elderly, have comorbid illnesses that cross medical disciplines. This is particularly true of the acute confusional state, which can be produced by a systemic illness and disorders remote from the central nervous system; in practice, more than half of elderly patients with a confusional state have a non-neurological disease underlying it. However, the same is not true of younger persons where primary neurological disease must be the prime suspect.

Definition of the acute confusional state

Confusional states are behavioural syndromes, which can be caused by a number of physical illnesses. Confusion results in the patient being unable to formulate thoughts coherently; concentration is impaired, attention cannot be maintained or is constantly shifting, and thought processes are slowed and disorganized. Orientation for time, place, and person is disturbed. The immediate world becomes a bewildering place as patients cease to comprehend and register what is happening around them, put this in context, draw inferences from such happenings, and plan appropriately taking account of changing circumstances. Sometimes, this is accompanied by visual or auditory hallucinations. The sleep–wake cycle is disturbed and there is either increased (agitated) or decreased (hypoactive) psychomotor activity. The onset is almost always acute or subacute. Once the underlying physical cause is treated, confusion rarely lasts more than 1 week. The prognosis depends on causation, but if the underlying cause is eradicated then recovery can be expected to be complete.

Some diseases which lead to stupor or coma have as part of their evolution an acute confusional state. Confusion is a characteristic feature in dementia, but dementia is a chronic disorder and does not form part of this chapter. Finally, it is worth remembering that intense emotion may interfere with coherence of thought.

Sometimes there is a practical difficulty in deciding between confusion and dysphasia (see page 94). However, features central to discriminating between the confused and the dysphasic are retention of concentration and the speed of attempting a reply. The examiner should ask 'are they able to listen attentively to what is being asked?'; 'Do they struggle to reply while concentrating?' If so, they are dysphasic rather than confused.

Anatomy of attention

The ascending reticular activating system (ARAS) in the upper brainstem and the polymodal association areas of the cortex must be intact for normal attention (77). The function of the ARAS in this context is to prime the cortex for stimulus reception. However, a lesion of the ARAS produces sleep or coma rather than impaired attention or a confusional state. Once primed, the polymodal association cortex focuses this arousal energy for attention, and lesions in these cortical areas will affect selective attention. Other areas feed into these polymodal areas; the prefrontal cortex is particularly involved in

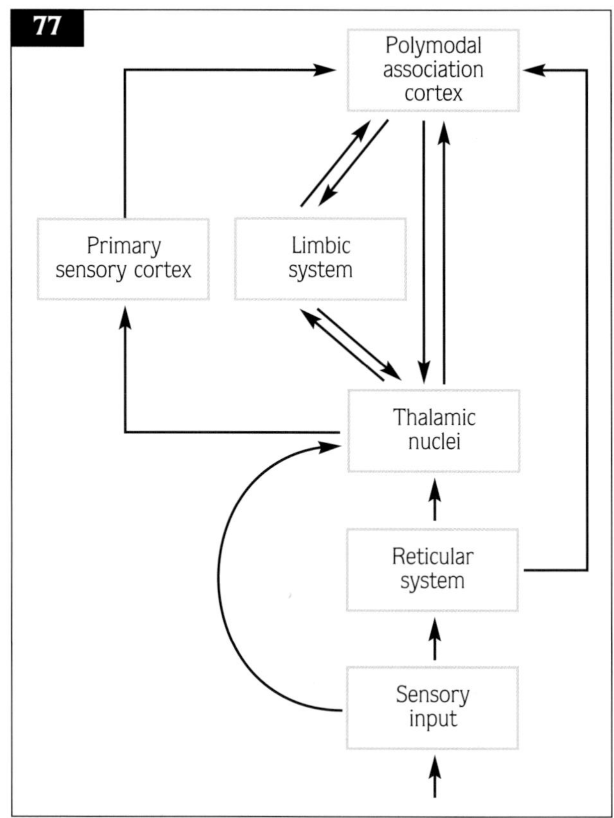

77 Diagram to show the parameters of attention.

maintaining attention. The limbic system and the primary sensory cortex also feed into these polymodal areas. It is thought that the limbic system has quite a major role in delirium because of its connections with the temporal lobe polymodal areas.

As well as maintaining attention to the subject in hand, the attention system must also monitor the environment to detect any new or changing factors to which the brain must respond, must decide which need a response and which can be ignored, and then must be able to shift attention to any of these new stimuli. Blood flow studies have shown that the polymodal cortical areas are the regions of monitoring and shifting. Specifically, the posterior parietal cortex and other polymodal areas feed back to the reticular nucleus of the thalamus, which itself modulates sensory input to the cortex from the thalamus.

In summary, sensory input arrives in the thalamus, which relays it to the primary sensory cortex from where it is relayed to the polymodal association areas (prefrontal cortex and posterior parietal cortex) where selective attention takes place. Additional input arrives directly from the reticular system and the limbic system.

Pathophysiology

Theoretically, a structural lesion in the attention system (though never in the ARAS) may cause a confusional state, but the vast majority of cases are due to a diffuse metabolic or infective cause. The pathological changes found at postmortem are minimal and entirely nonspecific. The diffuse causes and the fact that there is a universal susceptibility to developing acute confusional states (it can happen to all of us) suggest that there is biochemical or enzymatic impairment to a common metabolic pathway in neurones. A diffuse metabolic cause can interrupt neurotransmitters such as acetylcholine and noradrenaline. These two neurotransmitters are perhaps particularly significant, since acetylcholine increases the responsivity of cortical neurones to other inputs. Noradrenaline increases postsynaptic evoked responses. Anticholinergic drugs, which were widely used to treat Parkinson's disease, are particularly likely to induce confusion, suggesting that perhaps cholinergic function is the key dysfunctional neurotransmitter in the acute confusional state. Furthermore, the pathways involving the ARAS and the polymodal cortex may be especially vulnerable, since these two areas have the most polysynaptic chains.

Anatomy and pathophysiology

There is no one single abnormal finding in the confused state; the pathology depends on the underlying cause. For example, in a patient who is confused as part of an evolving brain disorder such as a metabolic disturbance or a severe systemic infection such as pneumonia, there may be few or no pathological changes in the brain. The electro-encephalogram (EEG), however, may show marked slowing, with the predominant rhythm being in the slow theta (4–8 Hz) or, not uncommonly, the delta range (<4 Hz). The student should remember that confusion forms a consistent part of the postseizure state, so primary pathological changes in the brain may be at a molecular cellular level.

Clinical assessment

Clinical characteristics

The development of a confusional state occurs over hours or days. The state consists of two subtypes: the lethargic and the delirious. These two subtypes are distinguished by psychomotor activity. In the former, there is psychomotor retardation with obtundation. In delirium, there is a heightened state of arousal, patients are hyperalert and over-react to stimuli with agitation, tremulousness, and excitement, are distracted by irrelevant stimuli, and cannot sustain attention. Sometimes, this is coupled with wild delusions and terrifying fantasies and insomnia. It should be noted that even though the two subtypes may seem superficially distinct, they often overlap and indeed may occur alternately in the same patient as well as have the same cause. Both types are characterized by acute mental changes with accompanying attentional deficits.

Attention and memory

Poor attention span is the cardinal feature: these patients can be distracted, and they cannot sustain attention to external stimuli, e.g easily lose the thread of a conversation. Trivial stimuli may gain inappropriate attention and important stimuli be ignored. Patients cannot shift their attention or manipulate material and concentrate on a task.

When looking for an attentional deficit in a patient, the patient is asked to recite the days of the week or the months of the year in reverse order. Digit span is tested by asking the patient to subtract serial 7s from 100. All these require sustained concentration and the ability to manipulate material. Another good test for attention is to ask the patient to produce words beginning with a certain letter or from specific semantic categories, e.g. animals. Patients with impaired attention can produce few examples, and may return to a previous category or perseverate.

Disorientation for time is always present at some point in acute confusion and is usually an early feature. There is invariably a disturbed appreciation of the passage of time. As the confusional state worsens, there is disorientation for place, and later for person.

The memory disturbance is mainly due to poor attention. New material or incoming stimuli are not appropriately registered. Therefore, immediate repetition of a name and address will be poorly performed and the clinician may need to repeat the information several times before the patient can correctly or even approximately repeat. Long-term memory is intact; the problem is to access it in the presence of impaired attention. Sometimes confabulation (a wildly inaccurate account of events) occurs as part of a confusional state.

Fluctuations

During the confusional state there are sometimes marked swings in attention and arousal. These may occur unpredictably and irregularly during the day and worsen at night. 'Sundowning' with restlessness and confusion at night is frequent. Sometimes a confusional state is only apparent at night when the sleep–wake cycle is disturbed, with drowsiness occurring during the day and wandering at night. Once the patient has recovered from the acute state, there is a dense amnesia for the period of the illness, though if the illness has been marked by fluctuations there may be islands of memory remaining.

Thought and speech

The organization and content of thought are disturbed. In the lethargic subtype, the stream of thought is slowed. In delirium, the stream of thought may be accelerated but, in both subtypes, there is difficulty in ordering thoughts to carry out a sequenced activity and goal-directed behaviour. Even mildly confused patients will have problems formulating a complex idea and sustaining a logical train of thought. Confusion can be understood as an inability to maintain a stream of thought with the usual coherence, clarity, and speed. The patient has problems with concept-formation and tends towards a rather concrete type of thinking. Asking the patient to explain a proverb such as 'a rolling stone gathers no moss' can test this. The clinician can test to see whether the patient can detect differences and similarities between classes of object (similarity judgement), and whether they can define single words.

Sometimes, the thought content has a dream-like quality and it may be dominated by the patient's concerns, beliefs, and desires. There are often brief, poorly elaborated, and inconsistent delusions which have a paranoid content, such as that their life is in danger or that relatives have been killed.

The patient's speech may reflect this muddled thinking, in that it is imprecise, shifting from subject to subject, is usually circumlocutory and goes off at a tangent. There are hesitations, repetitions, and perseverations. Often the rate is abnormal and hurried with a dysarthria.

Perceptual deficits

Perception refers to the ability to extract appropriate information from the environment and one's own body and to integrate this information so that it can be useful and is meaningful. Clearly an attention deficit accounts for many of the perceptual disturbances; the most common disturbance is decreased perception: the patients are missing things going on around them. However, there may be disturbances of vision and hearing, visual hallucinations occurring particularly in the younger patient. These are vivid and coloured. Sounds may be distorted or accentuated. Body image may be affected with a perceived alteration of size or shape. Feelings of unreality and depersonalization are common, but psychotic auditory hallucinations with voices commenting on behaviour do not generally occur in the acute confusional state. Generally, patients with delirium rather than the lethargic subtype develop hallucinations and those patients who are alcohol- or benzodiazepine- dependent and have been withdrawn from them are particularly likely to hallucinate.

There are some additional perceptual phenomena worth mentioning: an altered time sense when nonrelated events are juxtaposed. Sometimes the unfamiliar is mistaken for the familiar. Bizarre reduplicative phenomena may occur, when a patient perceives a person with two heads but one body. Similarly, reduplicative paramnesia, or the replacement of persons or places, occurs because of an inability to integrate recent observations with past memories.

Emotion and behaviour

Emotional disturbances are common: there is emotional lability with swings from agitation and fearfulness to apathy or depression. Generally, the impression is of someone who is rather perplexed, but this can suddenly change to a frightened, angry, and aggressive patient. The mood changes occur with delusions and impaired perception. It has been suggested that these are a direct result of a confusional state on the limbic system and its regulation of emotions.

As described earlier in this chapter, behavioural changes are always present with two contrasting patterns. These patterns are not fixed and patients commonly alternate between them. The first pattern is the hyperalert state: this is the excitable patient whose gaze and attention are constantly shifting. These are the patients who develop vivid hallucinations. Any stimulus will receive an immediate and excessive response with pressure of speech and abnormal and excess emotion such as crying or laughing inappropriately. This is accompanied by increased physical activity and repetitive and purposeless behaviour such as plucking at the bedclothes repeatedly. Attempts to restrain the patient if they try to get out of bed produce an aggressive outburst. Coupled with this is evidence of autonomic hyperactivity such as pupillary dilatation and tachycardia. The lethargic subtype is quite different: these patients drift in and out of sleep if not stimulated and lie quietly. Their replies are slow and their speech is often incoherent. Although they may be hypoalert, such patients can be experiencing delusions.

Causes of the acute confusional state

The easiest way to classify causes and formulate an investigative approach is to subdivide causes into four groups (*Table 11*).

Infectious non-neurological illness

Confusion can be an accompaniment to an infectious non-neurological illness, particularly pneumonia or a urinary infection in the elderly. Confusion often accompanies a septicaemia and forms part of the postoperative state. It is also worth remembering that an acute confusional state in a child can be due to a lobar pneumonia. Focal or localizing neurological signs do not accompany this type of acute confusional state.

Neurological disease

Neurological diseases producing focal or lateralizing signs on neurological examination can cause confusion. Vascular disease, particularly the so-called 'top of the brainstem' syndrome, often due to small infarcts involving the posterior circulation, where the basilar artery divides to form the two posterior cerebral arteries, is an example. There are small end-arteries, the mesencephalic arteries that supply the posterior part of the thalamus. Infarction of these presents with a confusional state. Almost any infarction or haemorrhage of the temporal or parietal lobes (but particularly involving the right parietal lobe) can present with confusion, as can lesions of the upper brainstem. As this is 'site-sensitive' rather than 'pathology-sensitive', any pathology, be it vascular, neoplastic, or infective in this area may cause confusion. Cerebral trauma with concussion can produce acute confusion with disorientation.

Acute bacterial meningitis presents with headache and increasing confusion. Tuberculous meningitis has a rather more gradual onset than does bacterial or purulent meningitis, and often presents with fatigue, apathy, lethargy, and somatic symptoms, sometimes

Table 11 Causes of acute confusional states

Acute non-neurological illness:
- ❑ Commoner in the elderly
- ❑ No focal neurological signs

Neurological disease:
- ❑ Focal or lateralizing signs
- ❑ Vascular disease
- ❑ Trauma
- ❑ Meningitis
- ❑ Encephalitis
- ❑ Subarachnoid haemorrhage
- ❑ Drugs and alcohol
- ❑ Postictal confusion

Chronic confusion with lethargy or retardation:
- ❑ Metabolic disease
- ❑ Hypoxia
- ❑ Severe infectious disease
- ❑ Post-operatively

Drug intoxication

over days or even weeks. The somatic symptoms (headache, neck stiffness, and vomiting) tend to be predominant in bacterial meningitis, particularly in younger patients, whereas confusion may outweigh the somatic symptoms in the elderly, but this is not an absolute rule.

Herpes simplex virus (HSV) encephalitis usually begins with a seizure and lateralizing signs but other viral causes may not, e.g. the encephalitis associated with infectious mononucleosis or measles.

In subarachnoid haemorrhage, the accompanying neurological signs should be apparent, but it is worth remembering that in a young person rupture of a small aneurysm along the course of the middle cerebral artery as it winds along the Sylvian fissure may produce no or very little neck stiffness. This is because the reactive swelling of the brain surrounding the aneurysm presses on the aneurysm and prevents much blood leaking into the subarachnoid space. Postictal confusion is usually short and should be self-limiting.

Drugs and alcohol

More correctly, this should really be 'withdrawal from drugs and alcohol'. In the chronically habituated or addicted patient, the withdrawal from alcohol will produce an acutely delirious state, delirium tremens, as described earlier. (Although benzodiazepine withdrawal does not produce an acute confusional state remember that acute withdrawal in a chronically dependent patient can produce seizures.) The use of barbiturates is now rare. Acute withdrawal produces an initial improvement for 8–12 hours. This is rapidly followed by tremor, nervousness, and insomnia, but the initial improvement may last up to 2 or even 3 days in the chronically addicted patient. These symptoms can be associated with generalized seizures and these may be followed by a state very similar to delirium tremens. This though is variable and some patients have seizures without delirium while others develop delirium without seizures. Acute psychosis should make the clinician consider the possibility of drug abuse. Opiates in large doses can produce a clouded, agitated state of consciousness. Some of the drugs previously commonly prescribed for Parkinson's disease, such as the anticholinergics, can cause confusion. Also, unfortunately some of the drugs which are currently used, such as L-dopa preparations and dopamine agonists, have similar side-effects.

Confusion with lethargy or retardation

Confusion can occur with an underlying medical or surgical disorder and can occur with any of the metabolic disorders such as hepatic encephalopathy, uraemia, or hypoglycaemia. It can arise as a part of the hypoxic state following resuscitation after cardiac arrest, or indeed in hypoxia of any cause such as congestive cardiac failure. Equally, confusion may occur in CO_2 retention. This type of confusion can occur as part of severe infectious diseases (the list of potential infections is vast but rare 'opportunistic infections' need to be considered in the immunosuppressed).

> Postoperatively, particularly in the elderly or frail patient, confusion may be seen. The pathophysiological basis for this is commonly a mixture of drug (sedatives/analgesics) intoxication and (possibly) a degree of hypoxia.

Summary

- ❑ In an elderly patient who has become confused, consider an underlying infection.
- ❑ If there is no infection, look at the drugs they may have been taking.
- ❑ In a young patient, consider a neurological cause.
- ❑ Remember that an acute confusional state can present either with agitation and tremulousness or with lethargy.
- ❑ There are no typical postmortem features in the acute confusional state; any pathological changes are minimal and nonspecific.
- ❑ Remember that Wernicke's encephalopathy does not just occur in the alcoholic patient but can occur in the context of repeated vomiting and poor nutritional intake.

CLINICAL SCENARIOS

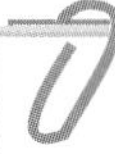

CASE 1

A 77-year-old right-handed male was admitted to the Acute Medical Receiving Unit in his local hospital from home. He was unable to give any information himself but was accompanied by his son and daughter-in-law. They said that he was normally an independent man, looking after himself and, since being widowed, living on his own. His health was good for a man of his age.

This is therefore a sudden change and not someone who has slowly deteriorated over a period of weeks or months. There is no suggestion that he has a dementing illness nor is there any suggestion of an acute deterioration in a chronic disease.

He had telephoned them complaining of chest pain and when they arrived at his house, found he had vomited and he said he had been off his food. His relatives were alarmed that he could give them no other information and he did not seem able to answer their questions at all so they brought him to the local hospital.

His symptoms suggest an acute physical cause plus some other factor.

When he was admitted to the ward he was conscious, but made no spontaneous complaints. When asked directly whether he had any chest pain, or whether he had been sick, he gazed around him and eventually replied 'yes' to the questions but was quite unable to add further details. When pressed for further information he could not supply any, tending to ignore the questions and gaze around the ward (an old-fashioned Nightingale ward) which seemed to surprise him. It became clear that he was vague and distracted. Attempts at a formal neurological examination were fruitless as he either ignored requests (e.g. to follow a moving finger) or turned towards some other stimulus such as a noise outside the curtain. Intermittently, he would make a brief effort to concentrate, only to be distracted by a fresh stimulus. However, when asked whether he drank a lot, he indignantly denied this and his relatives equally indignantly denied this.

This man is not dysphasic. In spite of being distracted, it is clear that he comprehends and is capable of a response, although intermittently. His distractedness, his vagueness and, most importantly, the testimony of close relatives that this is quite unlike his usual behaviour, suggest that this is an acute confusional state.

An attempt was made to carry out some tests of higher cortical function. When asked to name the days of the week, he gazed around before settling himself back on the pillow. He did not seem to understand when asked to name five animals and became irritated when pressed to try. When asked where he thought he was, he said 'the market' (he had been an auctioneer). He then started giving a rambling and confused story about something being found in his garage but he could not elaborate on this. When his son tried to assure his father that everything there was safe, the patient became agitated and accused him of stealing something, it was not clear what, and he tried to get out of bed. At this point he started accusing the admitting clinician and became more restless and difficult to manage. Further attempts at formal examination were fruitless.

This is now quite clearly an acute confusional state. Formal examination is often difficult, in fact sometimes impossible. But we still have no clue as to why it has occurred. Earlier in the history he had mentioned chest pain, when he phoned his relatives. It is possible he may have had a myocardial infarct (MI), perhaps with hypotension.

At this point, noticing that he had Dupuytren's contractures, he was asked whether he would like a drink. He brightened up immediately and said yes. On examination of his respiratory system, he was found to have coarse crepitations bilaterally but particularly at the left base. Abdominal examination showed his abdomen to be soft and his liver was not enlarged.

This seems to be an elderly man who drank regularly. Some of the clinical picture may be alcohol withdrawal, perhaps combined with chest infection, although a MI has not been ruled out.

(Continued overleaf)

Case 1 *(continued)*

An MI screen was negative. However, 48 hours after admission, he became agitated and confused. His relatives admitted at that point that he consumed alcohol on a regular basis; they thought this might be as much as half a bottle of whisky per day and he was therefore treated as having alcohol withdrawal. However, on the following day when it was realized that his liver function tests were normal, neurological review was requested. On the assumption that his confusion was due to alcohol withdrawal, he had been given a benzodiazepine and had become very drowsy, making assessment difficult.

On examination, he was an elderly rather plethoric man who said that he had no complaints about his health. When asked, he said that he had worked as an auctioneer for many years but gave no other details about himself although pressed to do so. His cerebration was slow and he tended to perseverate. He had recurrence of all primitive reflexes (pout, glabellar tap, and palmo-mental responses). His fundi were normal with rather attenuated arteriosclerotic vessels and he had a full range of ocular movements. However, he had neglect of his left visual field. There was no objective weakness of his limbs. Sensory testing was carried out and it was not possible to say whether or not he had neglect, because by that stage of the examination the patient was not able or willing to cooperate. His reflexes were all very sluggish apart from his ankle jerks, which were absent. His plantar responses were abnormal in that his left plantar response was extensor, the right equivocal.

Sensory testing is often considered the most difficult part of the neurological examination, as the patient must first comprehend what is being done, must be able to cooperate with the examination, and be able to formulate an appropriate reply, clearly not possible in a confused patient. The focal signs, with visual neglect, hint of a right parietal lesion in an elderly man with a previous history of steady alcohol intake and signs of a chest infection. His chest X-ray and his computed tomography scan (78) confirmed this.

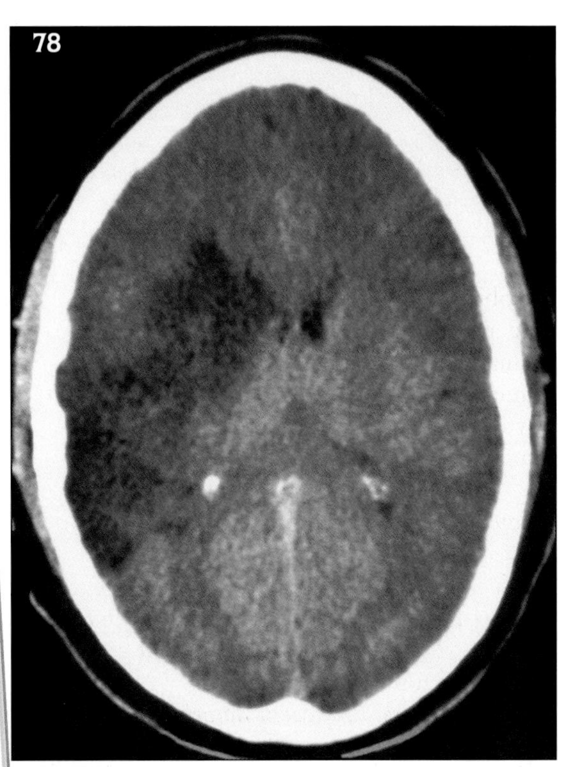

78 Computed tomography scan of right parietal stroke.

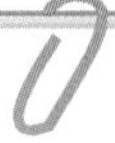

Case 2

A 54-year-old female with long-standing anxiety and depression was admitted to the Medical Unit at her general practitioner's (GP) request. Her husband provided all information on admission.

This is unusual for a woman of 54 years and immediately alerts the clinician to a new situation. Whether it is an organic change or a functional change is as yet unknown.

He said that over the previous 6 months his wife had slowed down and she had started to shuffle. Her mobility had deteriorated quite dramatically over 3 days and, because she had fallen many times at home, he asked the GP for a home visit. He added that although her walking and her behaviour had been unusual in the past, he had never seen his wife like this. Over 48 hours she had become confused and then mute. The patient herself made no complaints of any sort but sat gazing in front of her. She could not or would not answer any questions. In reply to a series of standard questions, her husband said that she had not vomited, nor had she complained of headache and had never had a seizure.

This is a subacute situation. It is clear that this patient has been deteriorating gradually until the 3 days before admission, when matters had accelerated. This is not the history of a bacterial or a viral infection, but could be due to trauma. Her GP thought that for some reason her chronic psychotic state had decompensated, although he also wondered about a hysterical fugue state. Both these are good suggestions, but the question is then, why should her psychotic state have decompensated?

Her husband was adamant that although she had fallen many times, she had not hit her head and had never been unconscious.

Therefore, the recent deterioration is not due to trauma and there is no explanation for her symptoms over the past few months. It is possible that due to her long history of anxiety and depression, drug therapy may be relevant. Or the possibility of some superadded infection?

Her husband said that she had been taking phenelzine (45 mg) each day, zopiclone (15 mg) every night, and one tablet of diazepam (5 mg) and one of prochlorperazine (5 mg) each three times a day. On checking the referring letter from her GP, it emerged that she was also taking tramadol (50 mg), MST Continus (15 mg), a cox-2 inhibitor, and beclomethasone and seretide inhalers.

Finally, the possibility of an inherited disorder should be pursued; this patient had no family history of any neurological disease. There is now a good history, and an account of a gradual deterioration with a more rapid change over the past few days. Trauma has been ruled out, and the history does not sound like infection.

On examination, she was conscious, agitated, groaning, and sweating profusely, with a tachycardia of 128 per minute. Her temperature was 37.7°C (99.9°F). Her eyes were open and her pupils reacted to light directly and indirectly. Her neck, trunk, and limbs were rigid with clonus in both legs and a generalized hyperreflexia with extensor plantar responses. She moved around the bed spontaneously. There was no facial weakness. There was a pout reflex but no other primitive reflexes. There was no rash, although livedo reticularis was noted over the abdomen. Heart sounds were normal and her chest was clear. There was no lymphadenopathy and no abdominal masses. Although the patient was conscious, she made no verbal response to either questions or commands. Her concentration was limited and she was easily distracted, repeatedly trying to sit up.

It was thought that infection was a possibility and so following a CT scan, which showed some atrophy, her cerebrospinal fluid (CSF) was examined, and a range of blood tests were requested. Clinically, the picture looked like the neuroleptic malignant syndrome, although the drugs and doses the patient had taken did not wholly support this diagnosis.

(Continued overleaf)

Case 2 *(continued)*

Initial investigations:

WCC:	*$13.3 \times 10^9/l$*	*ALP:*	*306 IU/l*
ESR:	*3.2 mm/h*	*AST:*	*167 IU/l*
CRP:	*21 mg/l*	*CK:*	*9499 IU/l*
Bilirubin:	*30 μmol/l*		

WCC: *white cell count;* ESR: *erythrocyte sedimentation rate;* CRP: *C-reactive protein;* ALP: *alkaline phosphatase;* AST: *aspartate aminotransferase;* CK: *creatine kinase.*

Although the initial diagnosis clinically was thought to be a septicaemic illness, the very high CK level suggested the neuroleptic malignant syndrome. The prochlorperazine was stopped and she was given supportive treatment with a rapid improvement in her clinical state from admission, to being symptom-free, apart from her depression.

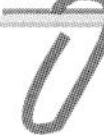

Case 3

A 55-year-old female presented to a District General Hospital with a week's history of a flu-like illness. During the first 3 days she had been very lethargic and rather drowsy, but brightened up on the fourth day and so returned to work the following day. At work she had had a seizure; eyewitnesses said she had become very pale, her eyes rolled up, and she fell, becoming rigid. The seizure lasted about 1 minute and an ambulance was called and she was brought to the Accident and Emergency Department. The information was given by her daughter, the patient herself being very drowsy. The patient had no history of epilepsy, had not had a head injury and her general health was excellent. She had not vomited and her complaints during the previous few days had been of feeling 'shivery' and aching all over, including a headache.

This is not just a postictal state, though part of the confusion may be related to the seizure. This patient has never had a seizure before and it was preceded by a febrile illness with an alteration in her alertness. No medical help was sought initially as her family assumed she had the flu until she had the seizure.

On examination, she was confused and drifted into sleep unless stimulated. She answered questions slowly but appeared to have little understanding. Her temperature was 37.7°C (99.9°F). There was no neck stiffness; Kernig's sign was negative. Her fundi were normal and there were no focal neurological signs.

There is the hint of a subacute confusional state; there is no clinical evidence of meningitis.

Over the next few hours there was no improvement in the patient's clinical state, she remained drowsy and confused, and her initial blood tests were normal apart from a gamma-glutamyl transferase (GT) of 87 IU/l. Over the next few hours her temperature rose slightly to 38°C (100.4°F) and later that day to 39°C (102.2°F).

These results provide further confirmation that this is not a postictal confusion, but there is an additional illness, which does not clinically look like acute meningitis, although this has to be considered. There is no history of head injury or of any drug ingestion. The course and tempo of the illness suggest an encephalitic illness.

A CT scan shortly after admission was normal and lumbar puncture was carried out. The CSF had a mild increase in protein of 0.77g and WCC of $457 \times 10^9/l$, 99% of these were lymphocytes. Staining and culture for bacteria were negative.

(Continued on page 85)

CASE 3 *(continued)*

This is very suggestive of encephalitis, with a mildly raised protein and a lymphocytosis. Could this be tuberculous meningitis, which in reality is a meningoencephalitis and often has a subacute or even a gradual onset? This is unlikely given the short history and the clinical examination gave no hint of any meningitic features. Moreover, tuberculous meningitis is predominantly basal meningitis with a high CSF protein and cranial nerve signs. Positive HSV polymerase chain reaction (a sensitive and specific test for herpes simplex) and a magnetic resonance image (79) showing swelling of the right temporal lobe confirmed the clinical suspicion of herpes simplex encephalitis. Her EEG showed the classical periodic slow wave and sharp wave discharges over the right temporal region.

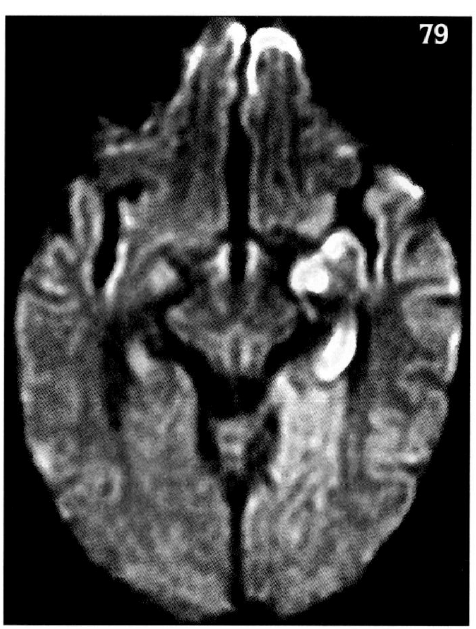

79 Diffusion-weighted magnetic resonance image of herpes simplex virus encephalitis, showing temporal lobe involvement.

REVISION QUESTIONS

1 In an acute confusional state the stream of thought can be either slowed or accelerated.
2 A lesion of the ascending reticular activating system may cause a confusional state.
3 Fluctuations in a confusional state may occur by day and by night, but are more marked by night.
4 In an acute confusional state, remote memory is intact.
5 There is no universal susceptibility to developing an acute confusional state.
6 The predominant EEG rhythm in an acute confusional state is fast theta or alpha rhythm.
7 Autonomic hyperactivity, e.g. a tachycardia, is usually present.
8 The acute confusional state is always accompanied by increased psychomotor activity.
9 Visual hallucinations are rarely seen in the acute confusional state.
10 In an acute confusional state there is disorientation for time before that for place or person.
11 The two subtypes of a confusional state never coexist in the same patient.
12 Following recovery from an acute confusional state, the patient has an amnesia for the period of confusion.
13 There are specific features found at postmortem following the acute confusional state.
14 Emotional lability is a frequent accompaniment to the acute confusional state.
15 The acute confusional state lasts <24 hours.

Answers

1 True.
2 False.
3 True.
4 True.
5 False.
6 False.
7 True.
8 False.
9 False.
10 True.
11 False.
12 True.
13 False.
14 True.
15 False.

Disorders of cognition

MEMORY DISORDERS

John Greene

INTRODUCTION

Perhaps the commonest cognitive complaint presenting in the clinic is gradually worsening memory. Symptoms of forgetfulness may simply be due to mild depression, but equally can be the harbinger of neurodegenerative illness such as Alzheimer's disease. In order to exploit fully the clinical examination in making the diagnosis, it is essential for the clinician to have a detailed understanding of the anatomy, physiology, and pathology of memory. There are many different types of memory, e.g. learning a name and address, recalling a previous holiday, knowing the capital of France. These different types of memory rely on different brain structures. Disease affecting different areas of the brain can therefore result in different types of memory impairment.

MEMORY AND ITS DIVISIONS

The taxonomy of memory is complex, but the broadest distinction is between explicit and implicit memory (80). Explicit memory refers to memories which can reach consciousness. By contrast, implicit memory refers to unconscious learned responses, including conditioning and motor skills, which rely on cerebellum and basal ganglia.

> Knowledge of the neural substrates underlying the above subcomponents of memory allows the clinician detecting a memory deficit to know which brain structures are affected.

Explicit memory is divided into short-term (or working) and long-term memory. Strictly speaking, short-term memory refers to a system that retains information for seconds at most, while long-term memory refers to memories held even for as short as a few minutes. These terms are widely misused by clinicians, who use short-term memory to mean events of a few weeks' or months' standing, and long-term memory to refer to memories of years' standing. The terms will be used here as correctly defined by neuropsychologists.

Short-term memory can be tested by digit span or by asking a patient to immediately repeat a name and address. Working memory requires the frontal lobes, language areas for verbal material such as digit span,

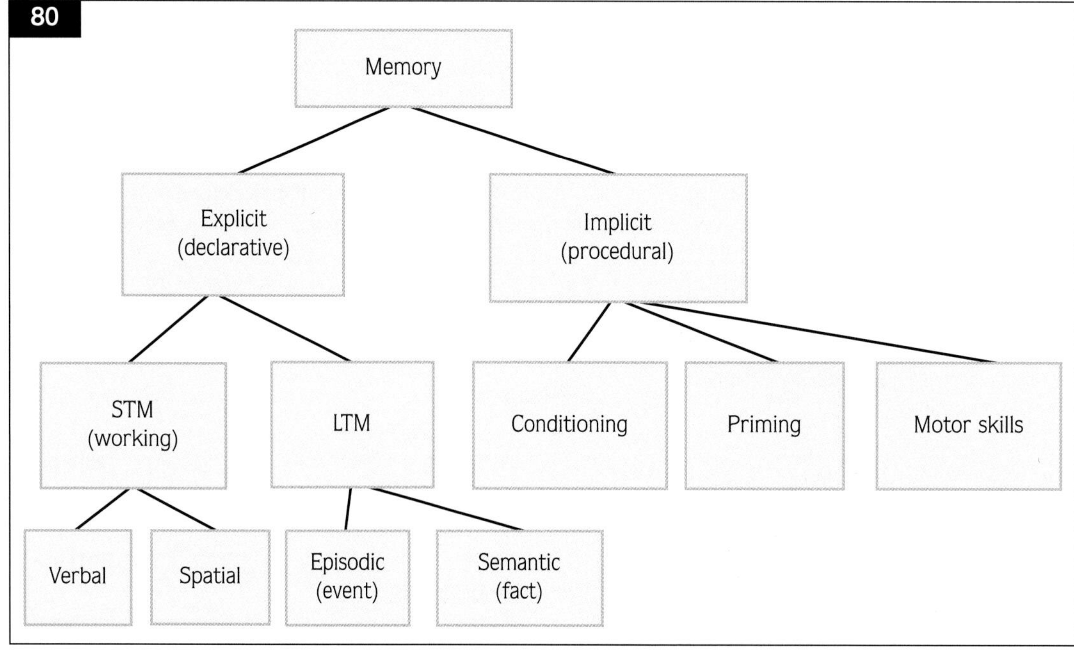

80 Diagram to show the components of memory. LTM: long-term memory; STM: short-term memory.

and nondominant hemisphere for visual material. Asking a patient to recall a name and address given 10 minutes previously, or anything longer tests long-term memory. Long-term memory is further subdivided into episodic and semantic memory: episodic memory refers to personally experienced events (e.g. recalling a conversation earlier in the day or a previous holiday), while semantic memory refers to facts, concepts, and words and their meaning (e.g. boiling point of water, capital of France). Episodic memory and semantic memory require different brain regions. While semantic memory utilizes mainly dominant temporal neocortex, the structures crucial for establishing and retrieving episodic memories appear to be components of the limbic system (**81**).

The limbic system comprises the hippocampus, the thalamus and mamillary bodies, and the basal forebrain. Although all limbic structures are involved in episodic memory, different components have differing roles (*Table 12*). The hippocampus is primarily involved with laying down new memories, and consolidating recently acquired ones. Hippocampal pathology can cause difficulty encoding new ongoing memories (i.e. an anterograde amnesia) and impaired consolidation of those very recently acquired, before injury (i.e. a temporally-limited retrograde amnesia). The thalamus, by contrast, is involved not only in laying down new memories, but also in retrieving previously acquired memories. Thalamic pathology (e.g. Korsakoff's syndrome, thalamic infarction) will manifest clinically as an anterograde amnesia with a temporally extensive retrograde amnesia, i.e. patients have difficulty in recalling events which occurred years or decades before the onset of the pathology.

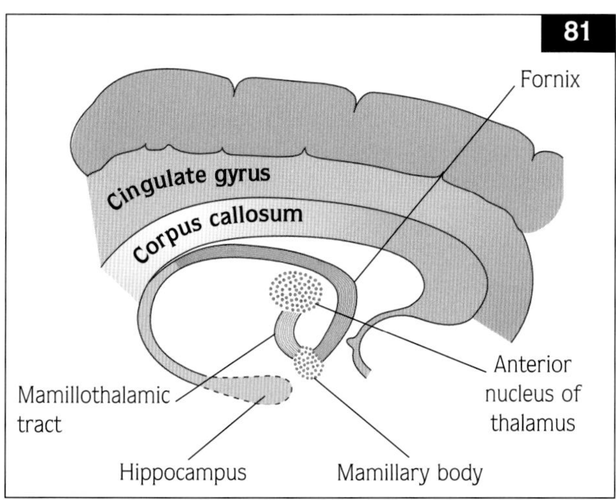

81 Diagram illustrating the anatomy of the limbic system.

Table 12 Divisions within long-term memory

Type	Role	Neural substrate
Episodic	New learning, retrieval of autobiographical events	Limbic system
Semantic	Knowledge of the world	Temporal neocortex
Implicit	Motor skills, e.g. playing a musical instrument	Basal ganglia, cerebellum

Memory disorders

The practical relevance of knowing the above anatomy is that identifying a specific type of memory disorder will allow the clinician to localize the site of the pathology. Accepting the above subdivisions, it should be noted that there are many different types of memory disorder, the commonest of which will be described here. Memory disorders may be pure (i.e. amnesias) or mixed (with additional cognitive deficits, i.e. confusion if acute, dementia if chronic). *Table 13* presents the causes of memory impairment.

Table 13 Causes of memory impairment

Type	Pure amnesia	Mixed
Transient	Transient global amnesia	Delirium
	Transient epileptic amnesia	
	Drugs	
	Psychogenic amnesia	
Persistent		Dementia
	Hippocampal	
	❑ Early Alzheimer's disease	
	❑ HSV encephalitis	
	Diencephalic	
	❑ Korsakoff's syndrome	

HSV: herpes simplex virus.

Acute transient disorders of episodic memory

Many pathological conditions are responsible for transient impairment of episodic memory. Any disorder that transiently impairs medial temporal function will result in a reversible episodic memory deficit.

Transient global amnesia is a disorder in which the patient becomes acutely amnesic for several hours, usually with a cycle of repetitive questions. It is benign, tends not to recur, and is thought to have a migrainous basis. *Psychogenic amnesia* results in loss of previous autobiographical memory and may result in loss of personal identity, which almost never occurs in organic disease. There is usually a major precipitating life event, and usually a psychiatric background. The condition may last for up to months. *Epilepsy* can occasionally present as transient episodes of pure amnesia, but this usually occurs in the context of more obvious seizures.

Chronic disorders of episodic memory – the amnesic syndrome

Here, there is inability to learn new information, but there can also be a retrograde amnesia of variable duration. It is broadly divided into hippocampal and diencephalic amnesia. Hippocampal damage results in dense anterograde amnesia with temporally limited retrograde amnesia, while parahippocampal pathology can cause a more extensive retrograde amnesia. Hippocampal pathology may arise as a result of conditions as varied as herpes simplex virus (HSV) encephalitis, hypoxia, or early Alzheimer's disease.

In diencephalic amnesia, in addition to anterograde amnesia, there is an extensive retrograde amnesia with a temporal gradient (i.e. relative preservation of distant memories). A classic example of this is Korsakoff's syndrome, in which acute thiamine deficiency results in damage to the mamillary bodies. Bilateral thalamic infarcts or third ventricle tumours may also damage the diencephalon.

Disorders of semantic memory

Damage to temporal neocortex classically occurs in semantic dementia (temporal variant fronto-temporal dementia) (**82**). The pathology affects the temporal neocortex and tends to spare the hippocampus, resulting in profound semantic memory impairment with relative sparing of episodic memory. On occasion, HSV encephalitis or stroke may selectively impair semantic memory.

Mixed disorders of episodic and semantic memory

The above discrete syndromes are useful for delineating the functional neuroanatomy of memory. In practice, mixed episodic and semantic memory disorders are more common, such as occur in neurodegenerative disease such as Alzheimer's disease.

CLINICAL ASSESSMENT

History taking from the patient and relative is crucial to the diagnostic process for memory disorders. In assessing a patient complaining of memory impairment, the following questions need to be addressed:

- Is there a memory problem?
- If yes, what aspect(s) of memory is/are affected?
- What is the neuroanatomical substrate?
- Is the memory problem transient or chronic?
- Is it a pure amnesia or a mixed picture (i.e. is it purely a memory problem, or are others aspects of cognition such as language or visuo-perceptual function also impaired)?
- Are the memory complaints organic?
- Does the tempo of the illness suggest the likely pathological process?
- If the clinical picture suggests dementia, is the pathology likely to be cortical or subcortical?
- Which disease is causing the dementia?

The patient interview

Patients with memory complaints are often aware that the possibility of dementia is being considered. Initial questions regarding background (occupation, family circumstances) will establish rapport, and establish whether history taking from the patients themselves will be informative. It is helpful to establish whether the patient knows why they have been referred to the clinic. Further open-ended questions regarding how symptoms began, what current difficulties there are, and the effect this has had on activities are worth recording, as they illustrate the extent of the problem.

It is imperative to know what is meant by 'poor memory'. This can be used to mean forgetting the names of things or people (semantic memory), forgetting new information or past events (episodic memory), or forgetting what one has gone into a room to get (attention). A further useful distinction is between memories acquired before and after onset of pathology (i.e. anterograde and retrograde). It is, however, not always easy to determine the date of onset of pathology, especially in early dementia, whereas this is straightforward in the case of head injury or acute stroke. Specific probing questions can elucidate which aspects of cognition are impaired. With regard to the subdivisions within memory, the most important issue is whether the patient can learn new information, as impaired anterograde episodic memory is the first manifestation of Alzheimer's disease. This can be assessed by whether the patient can recall conversations, describe current affairs, or current TV programmes. Has the patient started to make lists, become repetitive, or started frequently to lose things at home? Retrograde memory can be assessed by asking autobiographical questions (e.g. holidays, previous houses) or asking about old news events, which occurred before the onset of symptoms.

Semantic memory can be assessed by testing general factual knowledge (e.g. capitals of countries, names of people, places, and things). Is there a recent history of word-finding and naming problems, or loss of meaning of less common words? The patient's employment, education, and premorbid intelligence quotient (IQ) must be taken into account in assessing a patient's cognitive status, especially when testing semantic memory. Specific difficulties indicating a language disorder include word-finding problems, word errors, grammatical mistakes, difficulty understanding words and grammar, or problems with reading and writing. Ability to dress and route finding are a measure of visuo-spatial function. It is always worth enquiring about mood, energy, sleeping and eating patterns, as depressive pseudodementia can superficially resemble early dementia.

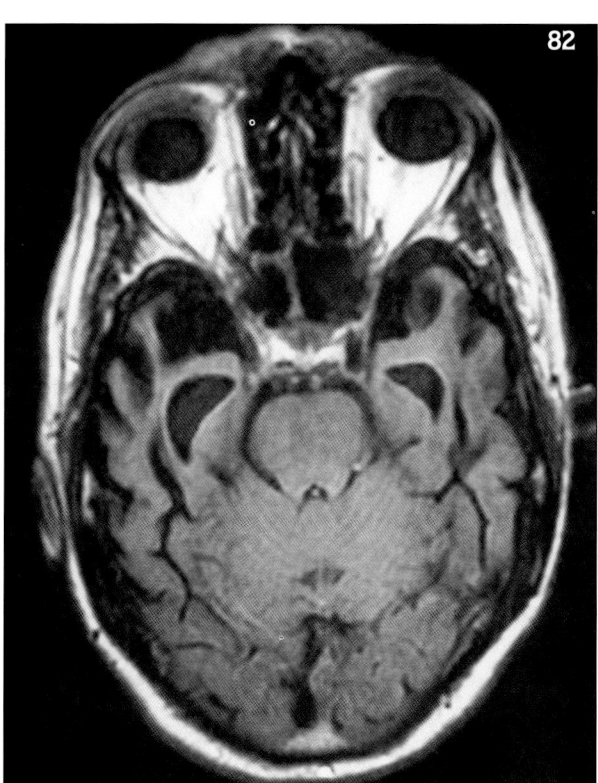

82 Magnetic resonance image showing anterior temporal lobe atrophy in semantic dementia, i.e. temporal variant fronto-temporal dementia.

The informant interview

Relatives can often identify when symptoms were first noted, and what the initial symptom was. This is of diagnostic use as different dementias present specifically, while latterly they merge. The suddenness of onset and rate of progression are again diagnostically useful. How symptoms sequentially have affected activities of daily living is also informative.

Other history

Past medical history should pay particular attention to previous head trauma, epilepsy, meningitis, or psychiatric illness. Drug history is important, as is family history. Alcohol and other drug consumption is also relevant.

Clinical examination

In addition to the general and neurological examinations, the bedside cognitive examination is crucial in the patient with memory disorder. While it is important to assess all aspects of cognition (e.g. language, visuo-spatial function) to see if the memory complaint is part of a more widespread dementing illness, the following will focus on memory in particular.

The Mini-Mental State Examination (MMSE) is a widely used test, initially developed as a screening tool for dementia. Due to its brevity it has several limitations. In terms of this chapter, it has deficiencies in assessing memory. The ability to learn and retain new information is very important in bedside cognitive testing of memory, as impaired delayed recall is often the first indication of early Alzheimer's disease. In the MMSE, the patient is asked to remember three items. The ability to subtract 7 from 100 repeatedly is then tested, and then the patient is asked to recall the three items. This is not properly delayed recall, as insufficient time is allowed to pass before testing recall. An intelligent patient may do serial 7s very quickly, and may in fact have been holding the three items in working memory during this task, so that recall of three items is not in fact testing true delayed episodic memory.

In an effort to improve on this, the Addenbrooke's Cognitive Examination (ACE) significantly expands on bedside testing of memory. In addition to the MMSE, the patient is also given a name and address to remember. To ensure that they have had a chance to register the new information, the address is given three times. Secondly, delayed recall is not tested until towards the end of the ACE, with many intervening items having been given in the interim. It is thus a proper test of delayed recall.

The ACE also assesses semantic memory through category fluency (as many animal names in 1 minute), and in more rigorous testing of object naming. It is brief enough to use in a busy outpatient setting. It is clearly shorter than a full neuropsychological assessment but serves to screen those patients who might require more detailed neuropsychology.

Bedside cognitive function comprises tests of orientation, attention, frontal executive function, memory, language, calculation, and praxis and right hemisphere function. Given that this chapter refers to forgetfulness, comment is restricted to those components that assess memory.

Working (or short-term memory) may be assessed using digit span, with items presented at one per second. The patient should be able to repeat at least five digits. For practical purposes, the most important part of memory testing is whether the patient can learn and retain new information. This is best done by giving a name and address three times, testing immediate registration after each presentation, and then testing recall after an interval of not less than 5 minutes. True hippocampal pathology, such as early Alzheimer's disease, should result in a patient scoring 7/7 on each of the trials of immediate recall, yet scoring 0/7 on delayed recall. By contrast, subcortical pathology, such as depressive pseudodementia, results in impaired immediate registration, e.g. 1, 3, 5/7, yet the proportion retained after an interval is above baseline, e.g. 3/7. This distinction is by no means absolute, but is a useful clinical pointer. Quizzing the patient about previous conversations and so on may also test anterograde memory.

Should a patient fail to recall a name and address, this may be due to either impaired encoding of this information, or failure to retrieve it. By then giving a choice of three items, should the patient tend to choose correctly, then a retrieval defect seems likely. If, however, they score at no more than chance, then it is likely that information was not encoded in the first place. More detailed assessments of anterograde verbal memory include story recall and word-list learning.

Anterograde nonverbal memory impairment usually parallels that of verbal memory disturbance. Damage to nondominant hippocampus can cause anterograde nonverbal memory impairment, but there is no easy bedside test of this. Walking a route outside the clinic and asking the patient to repeat it can suffice. Delayed recall of the Rey figure (an abstract design, see **40**), also tests nonverbal memory. Remote memory may also be assessed, e.g. previous major news events, but also autobiographical memory. This is necessarily more subjective and there is significant variation in individuals' knowledge of famous events. Autobiographical memory also requires cross-verification with relatives to ensure that plausible responses are not merely confabulation. Semantic memory may be assessed by category fluency, asking for the names of as many exemplars as possible in 1 minute, e.g. animals. Object naming also taps semantic memory.

Summary

- ❑ The clinician cannot accept a complaint of 'poor memory' at face value, but must further clarify what this means.
- ❑ Different areas of the brain subserve different aspects of memory.
- ❑ It is often best to interview the patient and informant separately for part of the examination, as the presence of the patient can inhibit the informant from relaying a clear account of the symptoms.
- ❑ It is necessary to ascertain whether the cognitive deficit is restricted to memory, or whether other areas of cognition are involved.
- ❑ Inability to recall a name and address given 10 minutes previously is a useful screening test, which can be of some use in detecting patients with early Alzheimer's disease.

CLINICAL SCENARIOS

CASE 1

A 66-year-old male presents to the Memory and Cognitive Disorders Clinic complaining that his memory is failing. He has been troubled with this for a few months. He has been failing to keep appointments and finds it difficult to follow weekly TV series from one week to the next. He has started using lists for the first time. He denies low mood. His wife has noted forgetfulness for over a year. It was of insidious onset, and is progressing. He has become repetitive, and does not learn new information. He appears otherwise unchanged, with no alteration of personality.

Insidious progressive forgetfulness is very suggestive of early dementia. Examples of his memory problems are of failing to keep appointments or to remember TV programmes from one week to the next, i.e. true episodic memory deficit. The patient denies low mood, making depressive pseudodementia less likely. No early change in personality makes a frontal dementia unlikely.

On bedside cognitive examination, he was oriented except for the date. Cognitive deficits were restricted to memory. While immediate registration of name and address was normal, delayed recall was poor at 0.

Normal bedside cognitive testing with very poor delayed recall demonstrates a specific deficit of episodic memory. As definitions of dementia require impairment in at least two areas of cognition, he is not by definition demented. However, the very early changes of Alzheimer's disease affect the perihippocampal areas, resulting in a pure amnesia initially. He thus is not demented, but his progressive amnesia is likely to be due to Alzheimer's disease.

Magnetic resonance imaging (MRI) showed bilateral hippocampal atrophy (83), while single photon emission computed tomography revealed bilateral temporo-parietal hypoperfusion (84). He was commenced on anticholinesterases.

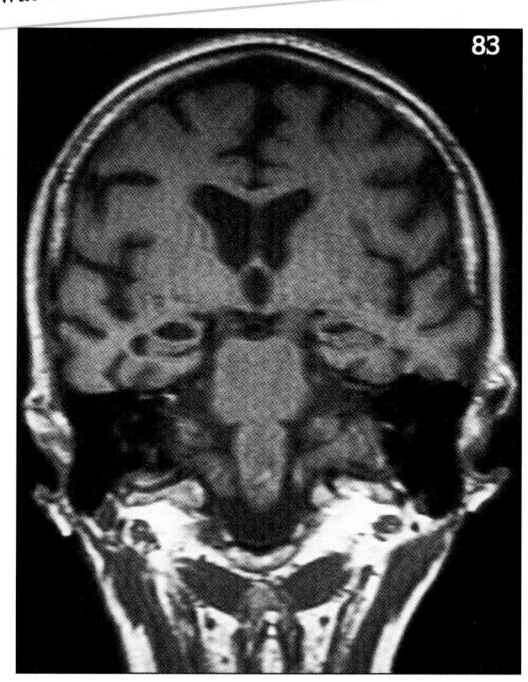

83 Magnetic resonance image showing medial temporal atrophy in Alzheimer's disease.

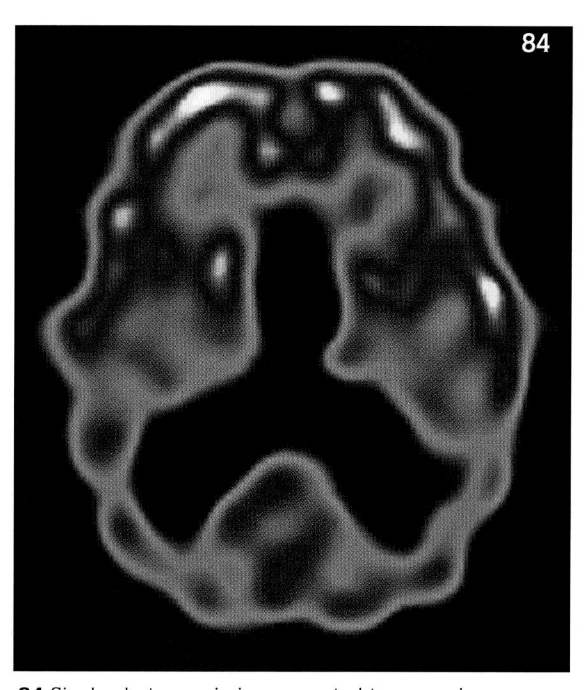

84 Single photon emission computed tomography scan showing temporo-parietal hypoperfusion in Alzheimer's disease.

Case 2

A 55-year-old female presented complaining of poor memory and concentration. This had come on fairly suddenly 6 months previously. She admitted to early morning wakening and poor appetite. She felt low, but was adamant that this was a consequence of her poor memory. She was worried she had the beginnings of dementia. Her family described her as having become very apathetic and no longer attending to much around her. She had also become more irritable.

Subacute onset of symptoms is not in keeping with early dementia. She has some somatic markers of depression, as well as low mood. Apathy and irritability are in keeping with depression.

On cognitive assessment, she was poorly oriented for time. She had difficulty with serial 7s, could not spell WORLD backwards and digit span was reduced to four. Category and letter fluency were both reduced. Anterograde memory was impaired: she had great difficulty with immediate registration of name and address. She had a tendency to answer, 'I don't know' to many questions.

She has problems with tests of attention and concentration. The tendency to say, 'I don't know' or to give up easily is suggestive of depressive pseudodementia. In organic pathology such as dementia, the patient will usually try to do the test, even if they subsequently fail. This is typical of depressive pseudodementia. Imaging was normal, and she responded well to antidepressants.

Case 3

A 60-year-old male was admitted with acute confusion under the influence of alcohol. He was found to be dehydrated, and was given intravenous dextrose infusion. On recovery, it was noted that he tended to ask nursing staff the same questions repeatedly. He also insisted that he was 25 years old, and needed to go back to his army base.

Repeated questioning suggests that he is amnesic. His insistence that he is 25 indicates that the amnesia also has a significant retrograde component. The sudden onset of his symptoms precipitated by alcohol raises the possibility of Wernicke's encephalopathy followed by Korsakoff's psychosis.

His sister commented that he was sure it was the 1960s, and he appeared to have no knowledge of his personal life events since then. He was unable to learn new information about the family, which she had told him. He had been living alone on an inadequate diet, and had been drinking heavily before admission.

Inability to learn new information shows that he has anterograde amnesia. His lack of knowledge of personal events since the 1960s demonstrates retrograde amnesia. The inadequate diet suggests that he may have thiamine deficiency. Administration of intravenous dextrose in hospital can precipitate Wernicke–Korsakoff syndrome.

On general examination, he had evidence of a mild peripheral neuropathy, but also had a broad based gait, and was unable to tandem gait. On bedside cognitive examination, he was disoriented for time, thinking it was 1968. Letter fluency was reduced with perseverations. On testing memory, he registered name and address, but delayed recall was 0. He had an extensive retrograde memory deficit, and could not describe public or autobiographical events more recent than the 1960s. Language and visuo-spatial function were normal.

(Continued on page 93)

CASE 3 *(continued)*

His cognitive deficit is restricted to memory. Absent delayed recall confirms anterograde amnesia. This is acute onset anterograde amnesia. There is also a significant retrograde amnesia, extending back 40 years. MRI showed altered signal in the periaqueductal grey matter of the midbrain (85). It transpired that when presenting to the Accident and Emergency Department, he had been given IV dextrose but no thiamine cover, and this had precipitated acute Wernicke's encephalopathy with subsequent Korsakoff's syndrome. Ataxia and peripheral neuropathy also occur in this condition.

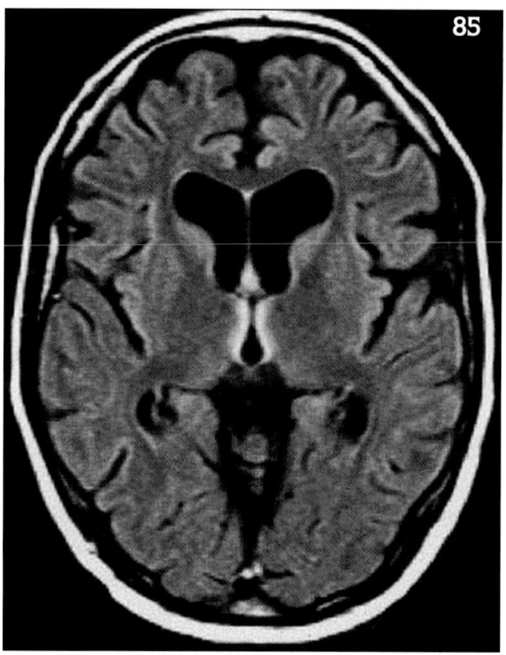

85 Magnetic resonance image showing increased signal in periaqueductal grey matter of the midbrain, consistent with Korsakoff's syndrome.

REVISION QUESTIONS

1 All memories reach conscious awareness.
2 Remembering last month's holiday is short-term memory.
3 Premorbid intelligence does not affect bedside cognitive performance.
4 It is easy to determine the time of onset of neurodegenerative disease.
5 A normal Mini-Mental State Examination score excludes Alzheimer's disease.
6 Digit span is a useful bedside test of short-term memory.
7 Korsakoff's syndrome results in a significant retrograde amnesia.
8 With memory impairment, loss of personal identity usually indicates a nonorganic cause.
9 Herpes encephalitis may selectively impair either episodic or semantic memory.
10 Insight may be retained early in Alzheimer's disease.
11 Depression can superficially resemble early dementia.
12 Hippocampal pathology primarily results in an anterograde rather than retrograde amnesia.
13 Short-term memory relies on the frontal lobes.
14 Retrograde memory can be tested by asking about autobiographical memories, and also by asking about famous public events.
15 Semantic memory can become impaired only if there is also episodic memory impairment.

Answers

1 False.
2 False.
3 False.
4 False.
5 False.
6 True.
7 True.
8 True.
9 True.
10 True.
11 True.
12 True.
13 True.
14 True.
15 False.

SPEECH AND LANGUAGE DISORDERS

John Greene

INTRODUCTION

Speech and language are crucially important for everyday life. The student must therefore have a good grasp of the anatomy and physiology of language, how the process may be upset by disease, and how to assess the patient with a possible speech or language problem. The role of clinical examination in neurological diagnosis involves two stages. The first is to know what level in the nervous system is responsible for the symptoms. This can be at the level of brain, spinal cord, peripheral nerve, neuromuscular junction, or muscle. The second stage is to ascertain the nature of the pathology responsible for the symptoms. The tempo of onset of the symptoms is of use here in that sudden onset symptoms may well have a vascular basis, while insidious onset of progressive symptoms may be due to tumour or neurodegenerative disease.

> In order to be able to deduce from the nature of a language disorder where in the nervous system the symptoms are arising from, the student must first study normal language.

Anatomy and physiology of language

It is important firstly to distinguish between language and speech. Language refers to the entire system used for communication, including understanding others' speech, reading, speech output and writing, as well as other forms of expression such as gesticulation and sign language. Speech simply refers to the oral production (the mechanics) of language.

The understanding and production of language utilize brain regions specializing in language working in unison with the motor system responsible for the articulation and expression of speech. The language centres are located in the left hemisphere in nearly all right-handers, and in about 60% of left-handers. The following account of language is necessarily simplistic. In truth, the brain does not work through a linear set of actions, but functions through multiple parallel streams of processing (parallel distributed processing). Having said that, the following remains a clinically useful teaching aid.

The comprehension of language will be described first. The heard word is initially processed by auditory cortex in the temporal lobes. The signal is then sent upstream to Wernicke's area in the superior temporal gyrus. This area allows comprehension of language and initiation of speech output. This is then passed forward to Broca's area (inferior frontal gyrus), which is responsible for supervising the production of language (86). Adjacent motor cortex then prepares the motor act of speech, and signals are sent down cortico-bulbar fibres to the muscles controlling speech. These descending fibres are modulated by the cerebellum and basal ganglia and terminate on motor nuclei of cranial nerves controlling tongue and larynx. The appropriate muscle action results in desired articulation and speech (87).

Reading and writing

Reading differs from listening in that the occipital cortex processes language visually. Information is then passed forward to Wernicke's area for understanding of what is being read. Normal processing of written material involves two processes. One is a superficial system in which words are read and pronounced simply on the basis of the letter strings, e.g. MINT is pronounced as one would expect from the component letters. For the other (deep) system, correct pronunciation is intimately tied up with meaning, e.g. PINT can only be correctly pronounced if the patient knows the meaning of the word. With a regular word such as MINT, there is no disparity between the superficial and deep systems. With irregular words such as PINT, there is a disparity in pronunciation between the surface and

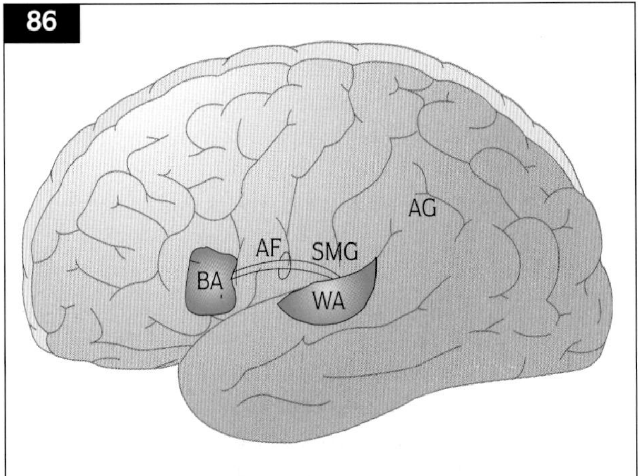

86 Diagram illustrating the principal language areas of the brain. AF: arcuate fasciculus; AG: angular gyrus; BA: Broca's area; SMG: supra marginal gyrus; WA: Wernicke's area.

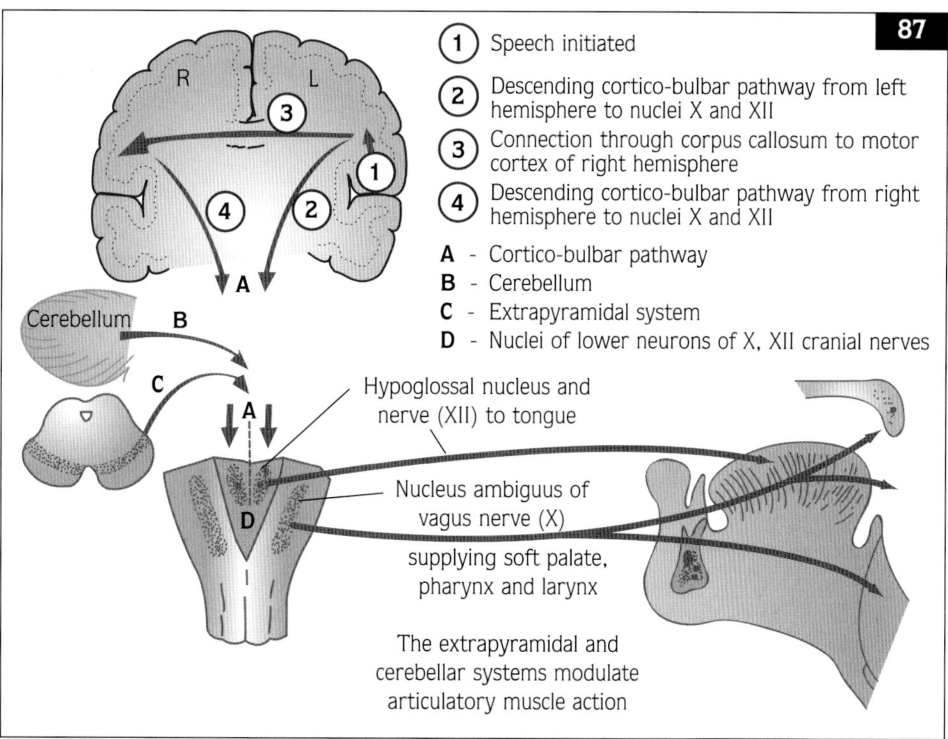

87 Diagram to illustrate the anatomy of articulation.

deep systems, but the deep system overrules, and the word is pronounced correctly (88). Should reading aloud be required, Broca's area is activated, and the above cascade occurs. Writing requires motor areas controlling hand movements to be involved in the production of written symbols.

Pathology of language and speech

In caring for a patient with an apparent disorder of speech or language, the clinician must first establish whether there is a true language impairment (i.e. a dysphasia), or whether the deficit is due to more peripheral damage. If there is an apparent deficit in comprehension of language, it is important to establish whether basic hearing and vision are sufficient to allow the heard or seen word to be passed upstream to become accessible to language, or whether it is a true language deficit. Similarly, in terms of speech output, it is again important to establish whether there is a true language output disorder (i.e. expressive dysphasia), or whether the problem is more peripheral (i.e. impaired motor control of facial and vocal musculature to allow speech expression). Dysphasia refers to a loss of comprehension, production, or both of spoken (and/or written) language. Dysarthria refers to poor articulation of speech yet with language intact.

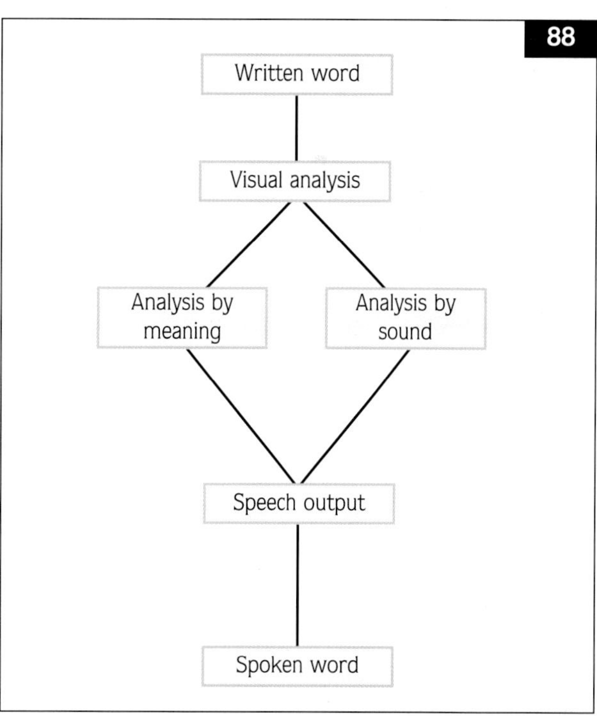

88 Diagram to illustrate the dual route hypothesis of reading.

Dysphonia refers to impaired vocal cord control, which affects speech. Pathology affecting any individual part of this extensive system can result in specific language or speech impairment. The nature of the language deficit varies depending on the site of pathology. Thus clinical examination can help the clinician to localize what level in the neuraxis is responsible for the impairment.

DISORDERS OF LANGUAGE

Classification of aphasias

Given the understanding of the systems involved in language, it is possible to address how selective lesions to the language and speech regions result in specific aphasia syndromes. The prime factors to be assessed in determining the type of aphasias are: fluency, repetition, comprehension, and naming (89).

Fluent speech is of normal rate and normal phrase length. Damage to anterior language areas results in nonfluent (or expressive) aphasia, in which speech is slow, and said to resemble 'telegraphic' communication. Fluency is impaired in Broca's aphasia, but is spared in Wernicke's aphasia.

Impaired repetition indicates pathology in the perisylvian language areas. An isolated impairment of repetition is called *conduction aphasia*, while selective sparing of repetition occurs in the *transcortical aphasias*.

Comprehension is impaired in Wernicke's aphasia, and relatively spared in Broca's aphasia. While naming is impaired in all the aphasias, the nature of the naming defect can provide clues as to the type of aphasia, e.g. phonemic paraphasias in Broca's aphasia.

Neuroanatomy of the aphasias

Wernicke's aphasia

Lesions to Wernicke's area produce problems with decoding of spoken and written language (fluent dysphasia). Here, speech is fluent and there is little effort in speaking. Paraphasias (i.e. word errors) occur. These may be semantic paraphasias (e.g. APPLE for ORANGE), or new words (neologisms) may occur in the acute stage. The disorder is sometimes described as jargon aphasia (or a word salad). Syntax (correct use of grammar and nonsubstantive words) is relatively preserved. Auditory comprehension is always impaired and repetition is impaired. For instance: 'We redo, er, the place, em, near the nettek, thing with wheels', instead of 'We went to the seaside by car'.

Transcortical sensory aphasia

Transcortical sensory aphasia is identical to Wernicke's aphasia, except repetition is preserved. The pathology usually involves cortical or deep white matter damage at the periphery of the perisylvian language areas.

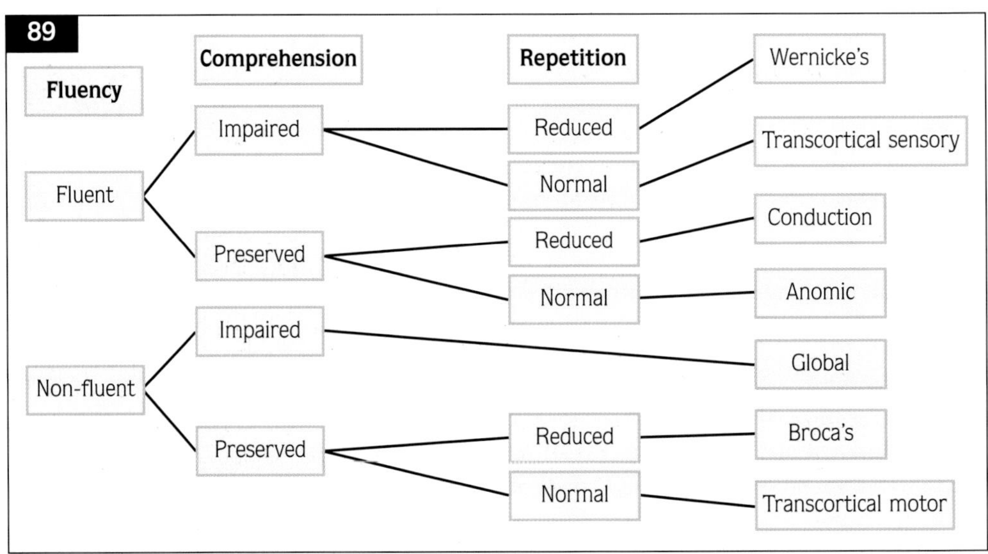

89 Diagram to show the classification tree of aphasias.

Conduction aphasia

Speech is fluent but paraphasic, with significant impairment of repetition, and is due to perisylvian pathology. Asking the patient to repeat 'No, ifs, ands or buts' can test this.

Broca's aphasia

Broca's aphasia is nonfluent, with distorted language output and disturbed syntax. Speech is slow and laboured, often described as telegraphic speech, with phonemic paraphasias (e.g. SITTER for SISTER). Broca's aphasia occurs due to damage to the fronto-parietal region in general, rather than specifically isolated damage to Broca's area. For instance: 'The tea in, um, cup. Put on tagle.' instead of 'Put the cup of tea on the table'.

Transcortical motor aphasia

This is similar to Broca's aphasia except that repetition is preserved.

Anomic aphasia

Anomia is a poor localizing sign, and is present in all aphasias. For instance: 'It's a, er, the thing you put water in to, a cup' instead of 'It's a glass'.

Disorders of reading, writing, and speech

The dyslexias

Ability to read is one of the most sensitive markers of language dysfunction, and in aphasia there is nearly always some impairment of reading aloud or comprehension of text.

There are several different types of reading disturbances (dyslexias). Analysis of the type of reading deficit allows classification of the dyslexia, aiding anatomical localization. Broadly speaking, dyslexia may be peripheral (i.e. due to impaired visual decoding of the written word) or central (due to a breakdown in true language resulting in deviation from the normal meaning of words).

Peripheral dyslexias

Alexia without agraphia

In this disorder, written material cannot be understood, yet the patient can recognize words spelt aloud. Writing is preserved, but patients cannot read what they have written. It is usually due to disease (usually infarction) of the medial aspect of the left occipital lobe and splenium of the corpus callosum, and there is normally an accompanying right homonymous hemianopia (see page 104). Due to the left occipital insult, visual information is only relayed to the right occipital cortex (**90**). The signal cannot be conveyed from there to Wernicke's area, thus the patient cannot read. Pathways from right occipital cortex can, however, reach more anterior language and motor areas, and the patient is therefore able to write down what is being seen.

Neglect dyslexia

Here, the patient does not attend correctly to left hemispace, and the inability to read the left side of words is therefore part of the more general phenomenon of neglect.

Central dyslexia

It is possible to understand subtypes of central dyslexia, by referring to the above dual route hypothesis of reading. If there is damage to the deep system, then the ability to pronounce irregular words correctly will be impaired. Words can then only be pronounced by the superficial system, i.e. phonetically based on letter strings. PINT will be therefore pronounced to rhyme with MINT, i.e. a regularization error. Regularization errors are

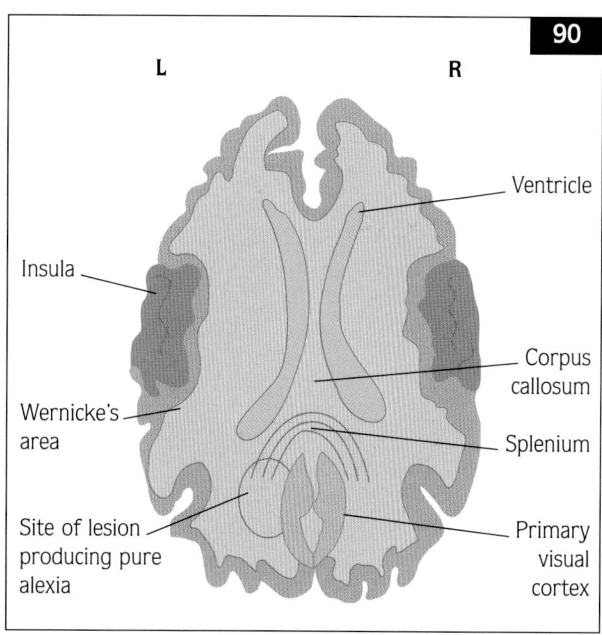

90 Diagram to show alexia without agraphia due to left occipital lesions involving the splenium of corpus callosum.

therefore a sign of damage to the deep semantic system. (Semantics is the referential meaning of words, the database on which one draws to give meaning to conscious experiences.) If the surface system is impaired, words can no longer be processed letter-by-letter. The only way words may be read is therefore through meaning. Patients with such a deficit will be unable to pronounce words for which they do not know the meaning. (They will also be unable to pronounce plausible nonwords, e.g. CHOG, but this only becomes apparent on bedside testing.)

The dysgraphias

Drawing analogies with reading, writing disorders (dysgraphias) may be due to true language impairment, or may be peripheral in origin.

Central dysgraphia

Similar to reading impairment, damage to the deep semantic system results in difficulties with spelling irregular words, e.g. PINT. By contrast, damage to the surface writing system results in patients only being able to spell words they know the meaning of, and they are unable to spell nonwords.

Peripheral dysgraphia

In a patient who has difficulty writing, the preservation of oral spelling informs the clinician that language is not impaired, so the dysgraphia must be due to peripheral mechanisms. In dyspraxic dysgraphia, written letters show errors, often inverted or reversed, with abnormal copying. It usually occurs with dominant parietal lobe damage, e.g. MƎVT instead of MEAT. Should writing exhibit a wide left margin, or a tendency to miss out the first few letters of individual words (e.g. WER instead of FLOWER), this suggests that the dysgraphia is simply one manifestation of a bigger picture of neglect, i.e. neglect dysgraphia.

Dysarthria

Dysarthria refers to impaired articulation of speech in the context of normal language. Pathology at any level below the language centres may be responsible. Damage to cortex or cortico-bulbar fibres (the bulbar upper motor neurones) results in *spastic dysarthria*. Speech is strained, sometimes said to resemble the speech of Donald Duck.

Cerebellar pathology results in *scanning speech*, where syllables are not correctly spaced, and speech is slow. This is called ataxic dysarthria. Basal ganglia disorders result in *monotonous quiet speech*, so-called hypokinetic dysarthria. Damage to X or XII nuclei or nerves results in a *flaccid dysarthria*. Speech is nasal, and ultimately progresses to total anarthria (loss of speech).

CAUSES OF LANGUAGE DISORDER

While the above classification helps to localize where the problems causing language and speech disorder are, the rate of evolution of the symptoms helps to determine the nature of the pathologic process (*Table 14*). For example, sudden onset of speech or language impairment is often due to stroke, which is the commonest cause of speech and language impairment. Twenty to 30% of all strokes have some degree of language or speech impairment, and this can be the only symptom, with no evidence of hemiparesis or other neurological impairment. By contrast, insidious onset and progressive impairment are suspicious of tumour or neurodegenerative disease.

CLINICAL ASSESSMENT

Specific 'focused' history taking

The patient and carer should be asked specifically about problems understanding others' speech and writing, and also whether the patient has a problem

Table 14 Causes of language impairment

Aphasia	❑ Focal lesions – Stroke – Tumour – Abscess ❑ Dementia – Alzheimer's – Fronto-temporal
Dysarthria	❑ Spastic – UMN, e.g. stroke, tumour ❑ Ataxic – Cerebellar lesion ❑ Hypokinetic – Basal ganglia, e.g. Parkinson's disease ❑ Flaccid – LMN, e.g. MND

LMN: lower motor neurone; MND: motor neurone disease; UMN: upper motor neurone.

with speech or written output. Problems in understanding language may first arise during three-way conversations, or when on the phone (due to the lack of nonverbal cues). Enquiries regarding reading and writing should also be made.

Bedside cognitive testing of language

It is essential to cover the following areas: spontaneous speech, naming, comprehension, repetition, reading, and writing.

Spontaneous speech

This is the most important aspect of language examination. In particular, attention should be paid to fluency, grammar, any paraphasias (incorrect words), word finding, and articulation. Fluency refers to phrase length. This should not be confused with pauses due to word-finding difficulty. The nature of any paraphasias may also be illuminating. Phonemic paraphasias (e.g. SPORAGE for ORANGE) occur in damage to anterior language areas, as may neologisms (new words). Semantic paraphasias (e.g. FRUIT or ORANGE for APPLE) are indicative of semantic memory impairment.

Naming

Naming should comprise items of varying degrees of frequency, e.g. nib, hand, as well as watch, as low frequency words may be lost before high frequency words. The type of naming error varies depending on the type of aphasia. Patients with Broca's aphasia produce phonemic paraphasias, while semantic paraphasias may occur in Wernicke's aphasia.

Comprehension

Comprehension needs to be assessed at different levels of complexity, e.g. 'Point to the coin', then 'Put the watch on the floor' then 'Point to the item used for telling the time'.

Repetition

This should be tested for monosyllabic single words, then polysyllabic single words, and finally sentences. Phrases using small grammatical function words, such as 'No ifs, ands or buts', are particularly difficult for patients with conduction aphasia. Impaired repetition indicates perisylvian pathology.

Reading

Impaired reading aloud does not necessarily imply impaired reading comprehension. Asking the patient to read, 'Close your eyes', may test the latter. While reading skills usually parallel spoken language abilities, this is not always the case. If a reading problem is identified, it is important to then establish what type of dyslexia is present. Although this is beyond the scope of the undergraduate, analysis of performance on letter identification, reading exception words and nonwords, and analysis of the type of reading errors allow subclassification of the type of dyslexia.

Writing

Screening for the presence of dysgraphia may be achieved by asking the patient to write a few sentences. If a deficit is detected, then the ability of the patient to write regular and exception words to dictation allows further subdivision of the dysgraphia. If the formation of letters hints at a motor problem in writing, then the subsequent finding of normal oral spelling indicates that this is a peripheral dysgraphia and is not true language impairment.

Investigations

Bedside cognitive testing allows the clinician to determine whether there is language impairment, and what type of dysphasia is present. The choice of instrument that the clinician should use depends on available time.

The Mini-Mental State Examination (MMSE) is a widely used test, originally designed to screen for dementia in the community. On account of its brevity it has several limitations. One major drawback of the MMSE is that the language items are too easy, such that a patient with early language impairment may still perform at ceiling on the language items of the MMSE. The Addenbrooke's Cognitive Examination (ACE) includes and expands on the MMSE. With regard to language, it incorporates timed tests (verbal fluency, producing as many exemplars in 1 minute). Naming, comprehension, repetition, and reading are more fully addressed.

While it is difficult for the clinician to do much beyond this in the busy outpatient clinic, the ideal measure of language performance would encompass a formal neuropsychological assessment. This resource is, however, scarce. Although clinical classification of the aphasia should result in a confident localization of the lesion, imaging is invariably done. Although computed tomography (CT) is more widely available, magnetic resonance imaging (MRI) remains the imaging modality of choice for localizing brain lesions and determining their type. Such structural imaging can be complemented by functional imaging such as single photon emission computed tomography (SPECT), which shows cerebral blood flow. Functional MRI (fMRI) identifies which parts of the brain are active when performing a particular cognitive task, but this is primarily used on a research basis.

Summary

- A logical approach to history taking and clinical examination will allow the student to determine and classify the nature of a language or speech disorder, as well as narrowing the list of diagnostic possibilities.
- It is important to distinguish between true language impairment (aphasia) and disorders of speech articulation (dysarthria).
- All clinicians should be competent at bedside cognitive testing, as back-up neuropsychology is not universally available.
- A competent bedside examination of language should comprise the following areas: spontaneous speech, naming, comprehension, repetition, reading, and writing.

CLINICAL SCENARIOS

Case 1

A 60-year-old right-handed female presented suddenly with inability to speak or to understand language and a right hemiplegia. She was hypertensive, diabetic, and a smoker. As she slowly recovered, she seemed to comprehend language, but still had major difficulties communicating.

Sudden onset hemiplegia and language impairment in a right handed patient are strongly suggestive of a stroke affecting the left hemisphere. The return of comprehension but with significant language output difficulties suggests Broca's aphasia.

On bedside cognitive assessment, she had reduced digit span, and also had markedly reduced verbal fluency. On examining language, spontaneous speech was nonfluent, with impaired articulation and grammatical errors. There were also phonemic paraphasias. Although comprehension was superficially spared, it was poor for command with complicated syntax. Naming was poor, but improved somewhat with phonemic cues. Repetition was poor for sentences. On testing reading, surface dyslexia was seen. Writing involved simplified grammar.

This is all as would be expected in Broca's aphasia. The impairment of repetition shows that this is not transcortical motor aphasia. In summary, the aphasia is characterized by being nonfluent, with impaired repetition and relatively well-preserved comprehension. This is characteristic of Broca's aphasia. CT showed a left fronto-parietal stroke (91). Although she improved gradually over the months, she was left with significant impairment of speech output.

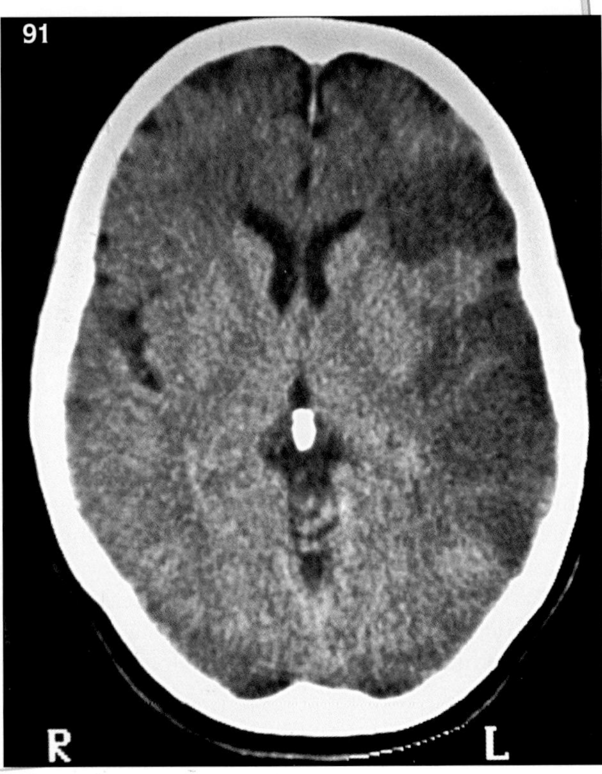

91 Computed tomography scan showing extensive left hemisphere stroke resulting in Broca's aphasia.

CASE 2

A 65-year-old male presented to the Accident and Emergency Department with acute confusion. The patient was unable to give a history, but his family described him as waking up talking gibberish, and unable to understand them. His behaviour otherwise seemed appropriate. He was hypertensive and diabetic, but otherwise well.

Although he initially appeared to be in an acute confusional state, his otherwise normal behaviour suggests that this may be a disorder specifically of language comprehension.

On cognitive assessment, he was talking constantly, and unable to carry out commands. Testing of cognition was difficult on account of lack of patient cooperation. It was, however, noted that spontaneous speech was fluent, but with numerous neologisms. He was unable to obey commands. Naming was markedly impaired, and he could not comply with repetition. Reading and writing could not be assessed.

*It is difficult to assess nonlanguage cognitive function in the presence of language impairment, as conveying what is required relies so heavily on language. However, the neologisms, anomia, and impaired repetition are compatible with a primary language disorder. This constellation indicates Wernicke's aphasia. The combination of fluent aphasia, impaired comprehension, and repetition is characteristic of Wernicke's aphasia. CT confirmed a left hemisphere haemorrhage undercutting Wernicke's area (left superior temporal region) (***92***).*

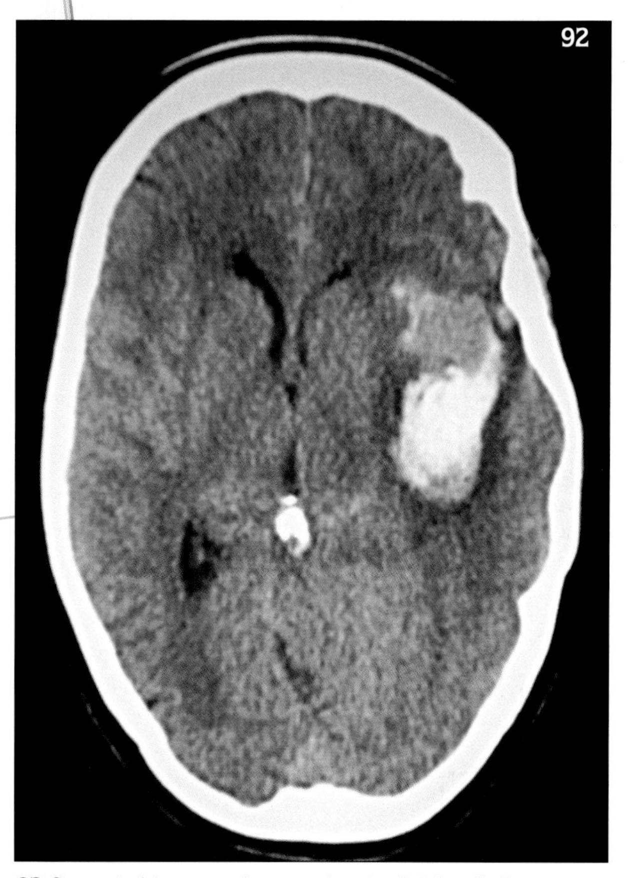

92 Computed tomography scan showing left hemisphere haemorrhage resulting in Wernicke's aphasia.

Case 3

A 55-year-old male and his wife presented to the clinic, complaining that his speech had been gradually deteriorating over the last year. He was still able to understand others' speech, and could read. His own speech was becoming increasingly slurred and unintelligible to others. His writing had also become rather messy, and he felt less steady on his feet.

Slurred speech is in keeping with dysarthria rather than dysphasia. Although dysarthria can be due to lesions at several areas (cerebellum, basal ganglia, cranial nerves), the involvement of writing and gait suggests cerebellar (or possibly basal ganglia) involvement. The tempo of insidious progressive symptoms is compatible with neurodegenerative illness or a slow-growing tumour.

On bedside cognitive testing, his speech was slurred and slow, and syllables were not clearly distinguishable. Naming, comprehension, repetition, and reading were normal. Writing was untidy. There were no other specific cognitive deficits. The neurological examination revealed bilateral papilloedema. There was gaze-evoked nystagmus on left lateral gaze. Finger–nose impairment and truncal ataxia were both evident.

CT scan showed a low-grade tumour in the cerebellum (93). Although this man presented with speech problems, he had a dysarthria rather than aphasia. Other neurological findings were in keeping with his dysarthria being of cerebellar origin.

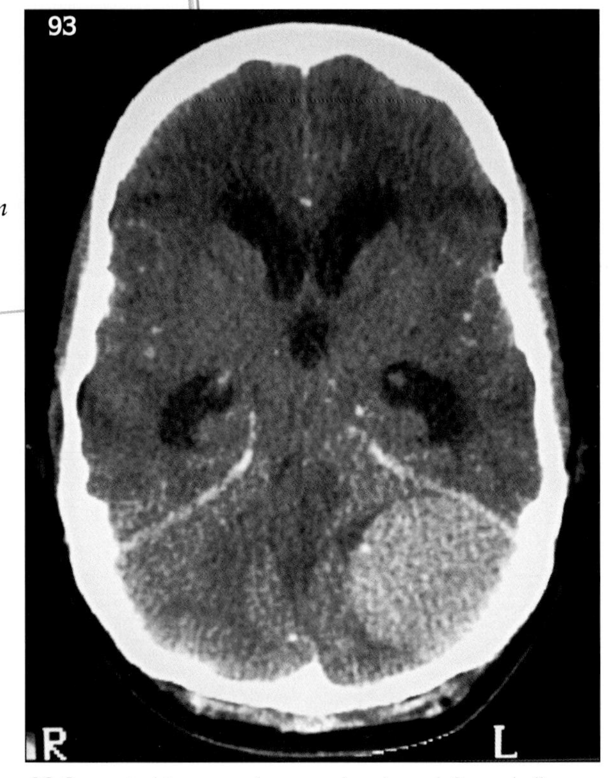

93 Computed tomography scan showing a left cerebellar tumour.

REVISION QUESTIONS

1 The right hemisphere is dominant for language in the majority of left-handers.
2 Phonemic paraphasias (spoonerisms) tend to occur with Broca's aphasia.
3 Repetition ability allows discrimination between conduction aphasia and the transcortical aphasias.
4 Reading ability is often spared in the aphasias.
5 The ability to write, yet be unable to read what has been written, indicates functional rather than organic disease.
6 Slow monotonous speech occurs in extrapyramidal disease.
7 Language impairment cannot be due to stroke unless there is also evidence of hemiparesis.
8 If a patient cannot write, yet has preserved oral spelling, then their symptoms are not organic in origin.
9 The ability to converse by phone is a very sensitive marker of early language dysfunction.
10 Analysis of the type of naming error can identify which part of the language system is impaired.
11 If reading aloud is impaired, then reading comprehension must be impaired.
12 The ability to correctly read irregular words is linked with knowledge of meaning of the word.
13 Normal performance on the Mini-Mental State Examination excludes the possibility of language impairment.
14 Difficulty naming objects occurs in most aphasias.
15 Clinical classification of an aphasia renders subsequent imaging unnecessary.

Answers

1 False.
2 True.
3 True.
4 False.
5 False.
6 True.
7 False.
8 False.
9 True.
10 True.
11 False.
12 True.
13 False.
14 True.
15 False.

Disorders of special senses

VISUAL LOSS AND DOUBLE VISION

James Overell, Richard Metcalfe

INTRODUCTION

Most people take good vision for granted. Such is its importance in everyday life that disturbance or loss of vision, even for seconds, often causes major alarm. It can be very difficult for even the articulate witness to describe visual disturbances, particularly transient episodes. Particular care should be taken when listening to visual complaints. This chapter will consider simple and relatively common disorders of visual sensory and oculomotor function. It assumes that there is no optical or retinal disorder, and does not attempt any discussion of either visual integrative function beyond the primary visual cortex, or more complex disease of the oculomotor system above the brainstem nuclei, concerned with eye movements. The student must remain aware that patients do not respect such artificial constraints.

Once the image of an object is centred on the fovea of the retina, assuming there is no optical defect, the high definition colour-sensitive cones of that region provide neural information to the primary visual cortex. Here, features of the object such as shape, colour, and motion are encoded for use in those parts of the occipito-parietal and occipito-temporal cortices concerned with the integration of vision with other aspects of sensation, both past and present.

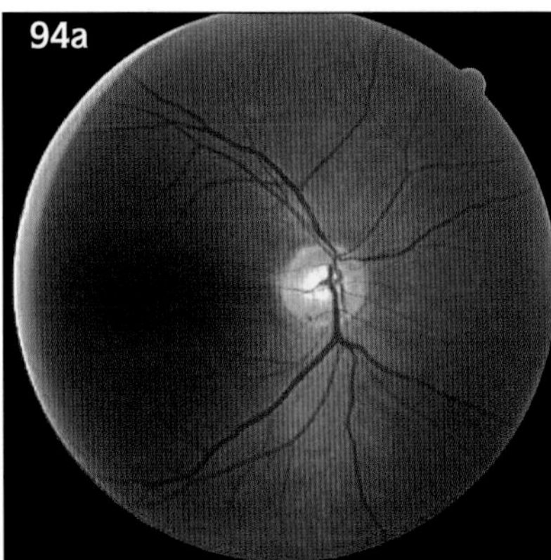

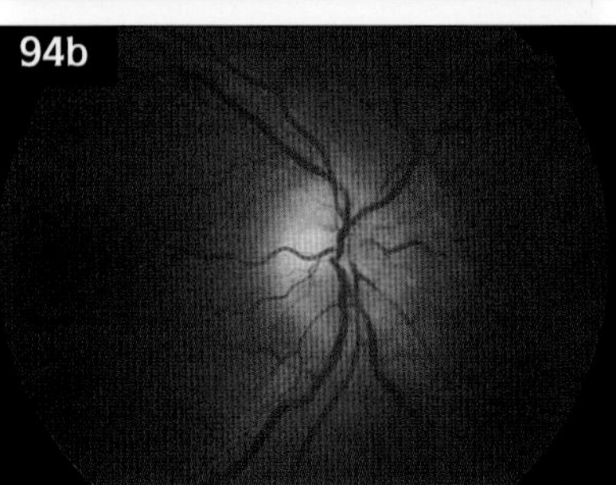

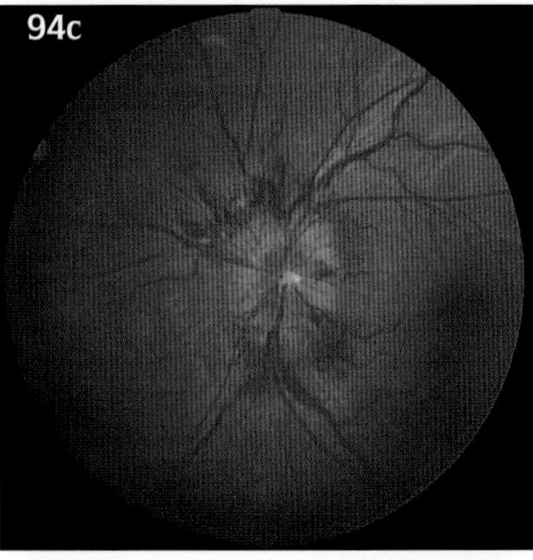

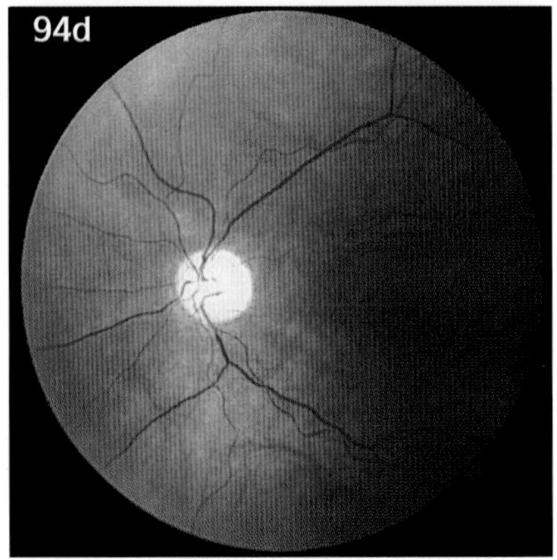

94 Fundoscopy. **a:** normal fundus; **b:** papillitis in a patient with acute optic neuritis; **c:** papilloedema (swelling of the optic disc) in a patient with raised intracranial pressure from a brain tumour; **d:** Optic atrophy in a patient with multiple sclerosis and multiple previous episodes of optic neuritis.

Functional anatomy and physiology

Retina and optic nerve

Light ('information') is detected by the retina, and passed to the optic nerve, the head of which is visible on fundoscopy as the optic disc (**94**). Information from the temporal (outer) visual field is detected by the nasal (inner) portion of the retina, while information from the nasal visual field is detected in the temporal retina (**95**). Similarly, light from the top half of the visual field passes to the bottom half of the retina, and vice versa. Retinal and optic nerve lesions can produce several patterns of visual deficit, the common examples of which are shown in **96**.

Optic chiasm and optic tract

The anatomy of the visual field pathways and resultant visual field defects are shown in **97**. The optic nerve leaves the orbit through the optic foramen and passes posteriorly to unite with the opposite optic

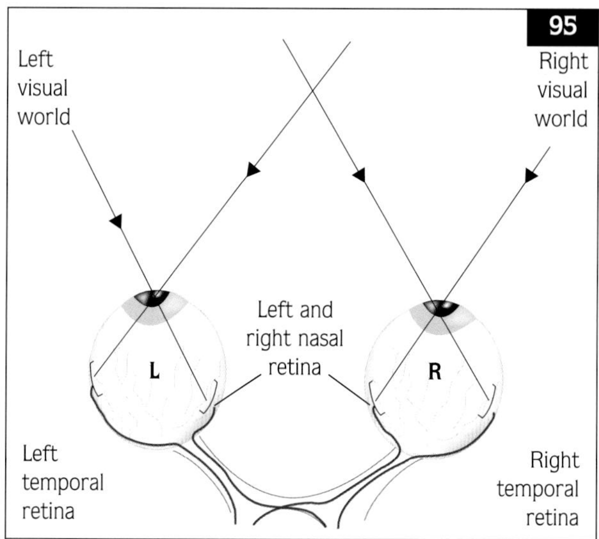

95 Diagram to show the relationship between anatomy and physiology of the visual fields. Light information from the temporal (outer) portion (shown in black) of both left and right visual fields is detected by the left and right nasal retina. Neurones carrying this information go on to decussate in the optic chiasm. Light information from the nasal (inner) portion (shown in red) of both visual fields is detected by the temporal retina on each side.

96 Diagram to show patterns of monocular visual field loss. **a:** central scotoma (a round defect centred at fixation), commonly seen in optic neuritis; **b:** centrocaecal scotoma (a central defect that extends to involve the blind spot), commonly caused by toxins such as alcohol or tobacco; **c:** arcuate scotoma (an arc-shaped defect extending from the blind spot), common in glaucoma.

97 Diagram to show visual field pathways (**a**) and visual field defects (**b**). **A':** monocular visual loss secondary to optic nerve or retinal disease. May be complete or may follow one of the patterns shown in **96**; **B':** bi-temporal hemianopia due to a lesion of the optic chiasm. The upper quadrants are usually affected first; **C':** left homonymous hemianopia from a lesion of the optic tract. The field defect is often incongruous (the shape of the defect is different in the two half fields); **D':** superior left homonymous quadrantanopia from a lesion of the lower fibres of the optic radiation in the temporal lobe; **E':** inferior left homonymous quadrantanopia from a lesion of the upper fibres of the optic radiation in the parietal lobe; **F':** macula-sparing, left homonymous hemianopia from an anterior visual cortex lesion. **1:** retina; **2:** optic nerve; **3:** optic chiasm; **4:** optic tract; **5:** lateral geniculate body; **6:** optic radiation (**7:** lower fibres in temporal lobe; **8:** upper fibres in parietal lobe); **9:** occipital cortex; **L:** left; **R:** right.

nerve at the optic chiasm. Here *partial decussation* occurs, and it is this anatomical arrangement that leads to both *bitemporal hemianopia* from lesions at the chiasm, and to the various types of *homonymous hemianopia*, when the pathology is posterior to the chiasm. Axons that derive from the ganglion cells of the nasal portion of the retina (and which carry information from the temporal field of vision [95]) cross to the contralateral side of the chiasm, and go on to form the optic tract with axons from the temporal side of the ipsilateral retina (**97a**).

> Thus, the left optic tract contains visual information from the right field of vision (nasal field of the left eye and temporal field of the right eye), and the right optic tract contains visual information from the left field of vision (nasal field of right eye and temporal field of left eye).

Visual field defects that derive from lesions at both the chiasm and optic tract are shown in **97b**.

Optic radiation

The optic tract continues posteriorly to the lateral geniculate body, where the axons synapse with cell bodies whose subsequent axons go on to form the optic radiation. These pass backwards, coursing deep through the parietal and temporal lobes. Because the arrangement of axons within the optic radiation continues to follow the distribution that originated in the optic nerve, the superior fibres (in the parietal lobe) contain information from the superior retinal ganglion cells, which comes from the lower half of the visual field. Hence parietal lobe lesions, rather than causing a full hemianopic defect, affect just the inferior quadrant of the homonymous half visual field (a *homonymous inferior quadrantanopia*). Similarly, temporal lobe lesions affect just the superior quadrant (a *homonymous superior quadrantanopia*). These patterns are depicted in **97b**.

Occipital cortex

The two bundles of optic radiation meet again at the temporo-parietal junction, and go on to terminate in the visual cortex of each occipital lobe. Total loss of the visual cortex on one side produces a complete congruous *homonymous hemianopia*. Most commonly, the macular area (central vision), which transmits information to the occipital pole or tip, is spared because so much of the visual cortex subserves this important central vision (**97b**). This is particularly the case in vascular disease because the occipital lobe receives blood from both the middle and posterior cerebral arteries; if the posterior cerebral artery is occluded, the posterior visual cortex continues to receive blood from the middle cerebral artery and so the macula is spared.

Clinical assessment

Focused history taking

Initial localization of the pathological process involves the distinction of monocular from binocular visual loss. Detailed enquiry is worthwhile as very often the history will initially be misleading, and the possibility that the patient may have lost vision *in half of their visual field* rather than *in one eye* will not have occurred to them. Asking about the effect of shutting either eye is helpful. Monocular pathology must lie anterior to the chiasm (**97a**). Unless there is a history suggestive of a process affecting both optic nerves, the pathological process causing binocular vision loss must lie where information from both eyes is in close proximity, either at or posterior to the optic chiasm. The *pattern* of binocular disturbance leads to more precise localization (**97**).

The usual complaint is of loss of all or part of vision (negative symptoms). Transmission of information has been disturbed and the patient sees nothing in all or part of their visual field. There are fewer possibilities when symptoms are positive (for example flashing lights); assuming there is no retinal disorder, such problems are likely to be due to migraine or epilepsy. Common aetiologies of visual loss, divided by anatomical location and speed of symptom onset, are described in *Table 15*. The divisions charted should be applied with some latitude; patients' recollection of their story can be uncertain, and often diagnoses are complicated by coexistent pathology.

Clinical context is the final step in the solution of the clinical problem. Various other aspects of the patient's history lead to modification of the list of possibilities reached on the basis of tempo:

Age of onset: optic neuritis tends to occur between the ages of 20 and 40 years. It may be the first symptom of demyelination. Vascular disease tends to be a disease of older people. Temporal arteritis occurs in patients over 50 years. Tumours can occur at any age, but specific examples present in childhood and young adulthood (for example optic nerve glioma), and in the older age group (for example metastatic carcinoma).

Past history: previous episodes of transient neurological disturbance may have been caused by previous episodes of demyelination (raising the possibility of multiple sclerosis [MS]). Vascular risk factors increase the likelihood that the current complaint has a vascular basis. Atrial fibrillation is a risk factor for embolism both to the middle and posterior cerebral arteries (causing cerebral infarction and hemianopia), and the ophthalmic or retinal artery (causing amaurosis fugax), though this is a problem more commonly seen as a consequence of embolism from a carotid stenosis.

Evolution: sudden and static, or sudden and improving describe acute insults, which are usually vascular, and their aftermath. Level of improvement after a vascular insult varies, but maximal disability is reached at onset, usually over seconds. Anterior ischaemic optic neuropathy (AION), which may be secondary to vasculitis (arteritic), tends to follow this classic vascular pattern.

Sudden and worsening generally describes a situation in which the onset seemed sudden ('I noticed it one day'; 'I woke up with it'), but progression has continued. Generally an active pathological process is continuing to cause clinical worsening, and any progressive problem should raise the suspicion of neoplasia, e.g. chronic progressive monocular visual loss is indicative of ocular nerve compression.

Demyelination will worsen over days before typically showing improvement, which often starts between 1 and 3 weeks after onset.

Associated ophthalmic history: a history of decreased visual acuity and colour vision and pain, especially on moving the eye, suggests optic neuritis. Symptoms following optic neuritis are often worse in the heat or with exercise (Uhthoff's phenomenon).

Altitudinal defects (loss of either the upper or the lower field in one eye) suggest a vascular cause. Often the patient will describe 'a shutter' descending or ascending over their vision. In AION, visual loss tends to be more severe and complete in the arteritic than in the nonarteritic form.

Bitemporal visual field loss caused by chiasmal lesions may be accompanied by more profound visual loss unilateral (suggesting unilateral optic nerve pathology) if the lesion also compresses the optic nerve on one side. Symptoms can develop very insidiously, causing difficulties that are difficult to characterize on history alone. Careful examination of visual fields (see later) is important. Sometimes symptoms caused by instability of the two preserved nasal fields abutting the midline occur, and objects

Table 15 Common aetiologies of visual loss

Onset	Optic disc	Optic nerve	Chiasm/tract	Radiation/occipital lobe
Sudden (seconds to minutes)	❏ Ischaemic optic neuropathy	❏ Ischaemia ❏ Trauma	❏ Pituitary apoplexy ❏ Stroke ❏ Trauma	❏ Stroke
Hours to days	❏ Optic neuritis (papillitis) ❏ Ischaemic optic neuropathy	❏ Optic neuritis ❏ Aneurysm	❏ Pituitary tumour (aggressive) ❏ Toxic ❏ Aneurysm	
Days to months	❏ Glaucoma ❏ Tumour ❏ Sarcoidosis	❏ Tumour (glioma, pituitary tumour, craniopharyngioma) ❏ Sarcoidosis ❏ Thyroid ophthalmopathy ❏ Toxic (alcohol, tobacco)	❏ Tumours (pituitary adenoma, glioma, craniopharyngioma, metastasis)	❏ Tumours (glioma, metastasis)
Months to years	❏ Carcinoma-associated neuropathy	❏ Tumour (meningioma)	❏ Tumour (meningioma)	❏ Tumour (meningioma)

may briefly double or the left side of images may slide in relation to the right. Often close visual work such as threading a needle is impossible.

Papilloedema (optic disc swelling secondary to raised intracranial pressure) may be associated with a history of visual blurring on changing posture (visual obscuration), and loss of peripheral vision. Usually, however, it is asymptomatic. Proptosis indicates an enlarging lesion within the orbit.

Associated neurological history: damage to the optic tract or radiation is often seen in the context of either hemiparesis, aphasia, hemisensory loss, or neglect, and these features both aid the process of localization (see above), and narrow the differential diagnosis. Tumours encroaching on visual pathway structures can cause pain in that area; they may be associated with headache worse in the morning and on lying, stooping, bending, and coughing ('pressure headache').

The presence of 'pressure headache' (and papilloedema) in the absence of structural pathology raises the possibility of cerebral venous thrombosis (causing a blockage to the venous drainage system of the brain) or idiopathic intracranial hypertension, which is often seen in association with obesity.

Temporal arteritis (causing AION) is usually associated with a headache, often temporal and unilateral. Scalp tenderness, jaw claudication, and aching shoulders are specific symptoms that should be sought as supportive evidence.

Migraine can cause various visual disturbances (often positive, see above), which usually precede severe throbbing unilateral headache, photophobia, and nausea.

Hemianopia can be caused by degenerative conditions, such as Alzheimer's disease (AD) and Creutzfeldt–Jakob disease (CJD), but this is uncommon. Agnosia (failure to recognize stimuli in the environment) and syndromes of visual disturbance caused by higher cortical dysfunction (*Table 16*) are more common in these conditions, and occur in the context of cognitive decline and other cortical features such as apraxia and aphasia (in AD) or myoclonus and seizures (in CJD).

Table 16 Visual disturbance resulting from higher cortical dysfunction

Alexia without agraphia (able to write but not read)
- Damage to connections between primary visual cortices and angular gyrus
- Accompanied by right homonymous hemianopia

Balint's syndrome
- Gaze apraxia (inability to direct voluntary gaze)
- Visual disorientation
- Optic ataxia
- Simultanagnosia (loss of panoramic vision)
- Bilateral posterior watershed infarction

Prosopagnosia (inability to recognize faces)
- Bilateral inferior temporal lobe lesions
- May have superior quadrantinopic defects

Central achromatopsia (central colour vision loss)
- Bilateral inferior temporal lobe lesions
- May accompany prosopagnosia

Anton's syndrome (blindness, but denial of blindness)
- Normal pupillary response
- Bilateral damage to occipital and parietal lobes

Table 17 Examination for visual loss

Assessment	Examination
General	Pulse (rhythm, rate)
	Blood pressure
	Lymphadenopathy
	Temporal arteries
Ocular	Proptosis
	Periocular inflammation
	Anisocoria and pupillary response
	Visual fields
	Visual acuity
	Colour vision (Ishihara plates)
Fundoscopy	Anterior chamber
	Venous pulsation and vessels
	Optic disc
	Retina
	Macula
Neurological	
Cranial nerves	Ocular movements
Motor nerves	Lateralized weakness
	Reflexes
	Plantar responses
Sensory system	Vibration and position sense testing
	Lateralized pain and temperature loss
	Sensory inattention and cortical sensory loss

Examinations (*Table 17*)

General examination

Pulse rate and rhythm should be assessed, and blood pressure should be documented. Lymphadenopathy may signify metastatic tumour or sarcoidosis. Temporal arteries should be palpated to determine whether they are patent (temporal arteritis can cause occlusion and pulseless temporal arteries) or thickened, tender or tortuous, which can also be features of arteritis.

Ocular assessment

Proptosis is assessed by standing behind the patient and looking downwards over the patient's brows, comparing the positions of the two corneas relative to each other and to the superior orbital rims. Pupils should be assessed in a step-by-step process. Minor degrees of anisocoria (pupillary inequality) are common in the general population; acquired (new) anisocoria indicates a disruption of efferent supply (sympathetic or parasympathetic) to that pupil. The direct light response is first assessed by shining a bright light into one pupil (**98a**). The light source is then removed and the procedure repeated with the examiner concentrating on the other pupil to assess the consensual response (**98b**). A brisk constriction of the pupil should be seen in both eyes when light is shone in either. Finally, the swinging light test should be performed to determine the presence of a relative afferent pupillary defect (RAPD), or Marcus Gunn pupil (**98c**). An optic nerve lesion will disturb the pupillary light reaction (causing an RAPD) often permanently, and will usually reduce visual acuity. Asking the patient to fix on a far and then a near target assesses pupillary responses to accommodation: the pupils should constrict and the eyes should converge.

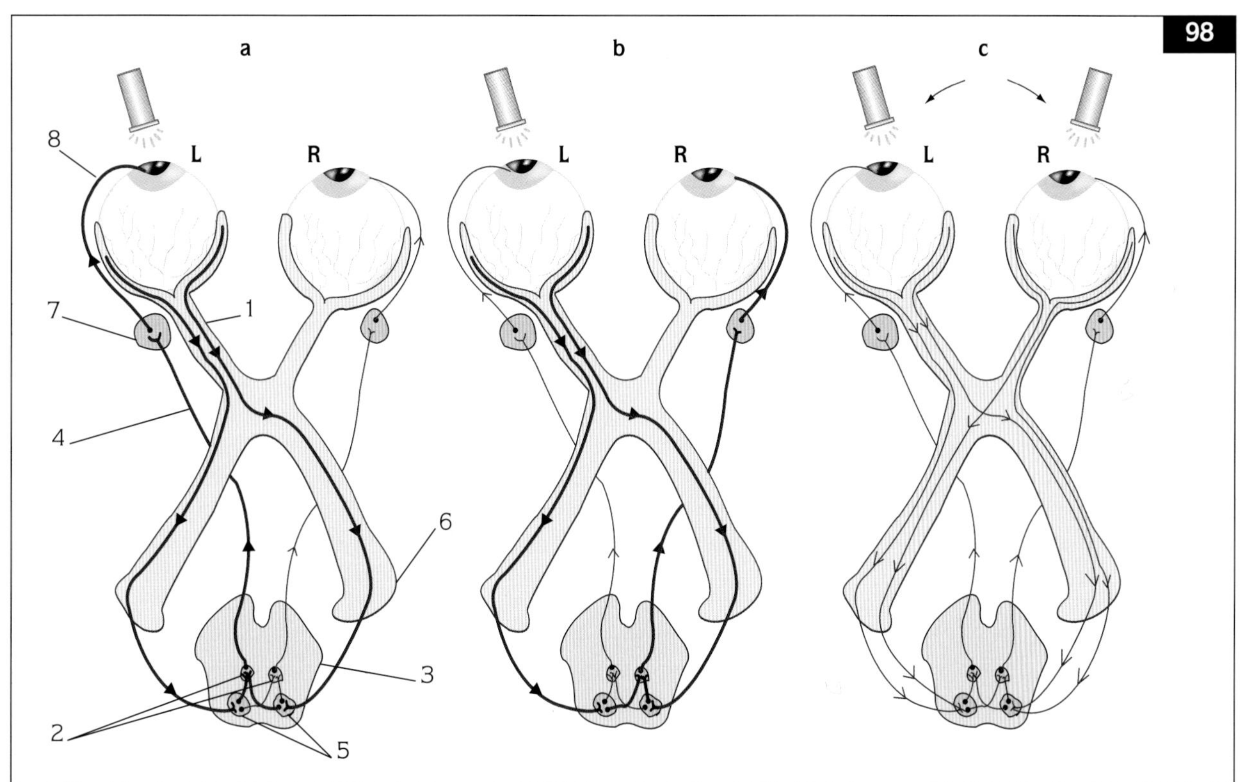

98 Diagram to show pupillary response testing. The direct light response (**a**) impulses are conveyed in the left optic nerve (**1**) to both Edinger–Westphal nuclei (**2**) in the midbrain (**3**). From here efferent fibres pass in the oculomotor nerve (**4**) to constrict the left pupil. Since impulses from the left eye are relayed to both nuclei, efferent impulses also pass in the right oculomotor nerve to constrict the right pupil, the 'consensual light response' (**b**). The swinging light test (**c**) assesses the relative power of the right and left afferent response. Light is rapidly alternated between right and left eyes, and the response from an eye affected by an optic nerve lesion will be shorter, slower, and less complete. **5:** superior colliculi; **6:** lateral geniculate body; **7:** ciliary ganglion; **8:** ciliary nerve.

Visual fields are assessed by the technique of confrontation (**99**). The examiner should be directly in front of the patient, sitting about 1 metre away. An initial screening examination to detect homonymous hemianopic defects is useful, particularly if such a problem is suggested by the clinical history. Static and moving targets are presented in the four quadrants of binocular vision (**99a**). If fields have been found to be intact by this technique, simultaneous binocular targets are presented and the patient is asked which they see: only seeing one indicates a deficit of visual attention, seen in lesions of the nondominant parietal lobe (**99b**). More detailed testing should follow, particularly if the history suggests a chiasm or optic nerve disorder; the patient's left eye visual field will correspond with the examiner's right eye visual field. The examiner and the patient each close or cover one eye, and concentrate on the opposite pupil. The patient is then asked to indicate when they can see a visual target, and a red pin is advanced diagonally across each visual quadrant, half way between examiner and patient. The examiner's field is thus compared to that of the patient (**99c, d**). In the temporal field of either eye the normal visual field of both examiner and patient will extend beyond the reach of even the longest arm, and so the target is usually advanced from a position slightly behind the patient. This is well within the examiner's visual field, and so an absolute comparison of examiner and patient is impossible (in this part of the visual field), but asymmetry and abnormalities become evident with experience.

For central defects (central scotoma) a small pin is used to map out any area of visual loss. In AION, visual field loss tends to be altitudinal and has a sharp demarcation at the horizontal meridian, whereas optic neuritis is commonly associated with a central area of field loss (scotoma) (**96**). In the temporal portion of the visual field lies the physiological blind spot: again a pin is used to compare the size of this area between examiner and patient. This technique requires cooperation on the part of the patient, practice by the examiner, and the patience of both. The patient's gaze must not deviate from the examiner's pupil (**99e**). Papilloedema causes an enlarged blind spot and constriction of the visual field. Visual fields are more accurately tested with a Goldmann perimeter machine or other types of visual analyser. This is useful to confirm findings from confrontation, especially the presence of central field defects or an enlarged blind spot, and also to assess change in visual fields over time.

Visual acuity should be tested in each eye with a Snellen chart (for far vision) and a near reading card for near vision. Each assessment is recorded in a standard way. For neurological purposes it is important that the patient wears glasses that they have been prescribed, to correct any refractive error. If these are unavailable, then looking through a small pinhole in a piece of paper or card will eliminate major refractive errors. If patients are severely visually impaired, an assessment of whether they can see how many fingers the examiner is holding up, or can appreciate movements of the hand or a light shone in the eye, is performed. Colour vision is assessed using specialist colour charts known as Ishihara plates. These were designed to detect congenital colour vision disorders, but are also useful for acquired defects.

Fundoscopy is a key skill in visual assessment. It is easier when the pupil has been dilated pharmacologically. The ophthalmoscope is held in the examiner's right hand, and the examiner's right eye is used to examine the patient's right eye. The left hand and eye are used for the patient's left eye. The patient is asked to fixate on a distant target and keep both eyes open, and a strong positive lens is initially used to examine the anterior chamber. The retina is then brought into focus by reducing the lens strength. The setting required to examine the retina will depend on any refractive errors that the patient and/or examiner may have. The retinal vessels are traced back to the optic disc, and examined for nipping (which indicates hypertensive eye disease) and venous pulsation (which is lost early in disc swelling). The clarity of the disc edge is then assessed, along with the disc colour and pallor. The retina is examined for haemorrhages and exudates (seen in hypertension and diabetes) by systematically panning from disc to periphery in a clockwise manner around the fundus. Finally, the light beam of the ophthalmoscope is set to narrow and the patient is asked to look directly into the light, which brings the macula into view. Lesions in this area tend to cause serious loss of vision.

A normal optic disc is shown in **94a**. Myopia makes the disc look enlarged and pale, and hypermetropia makes it look pink and small. Fundal examination in the acute phase of optic neuritis is usually normal but sometimes shows swelling of the optic nerve head (papillitis) (**94b**). Swelling may also be seen in AION, often associated with pallor and haemorrhages in the arteritic form. Optic disc

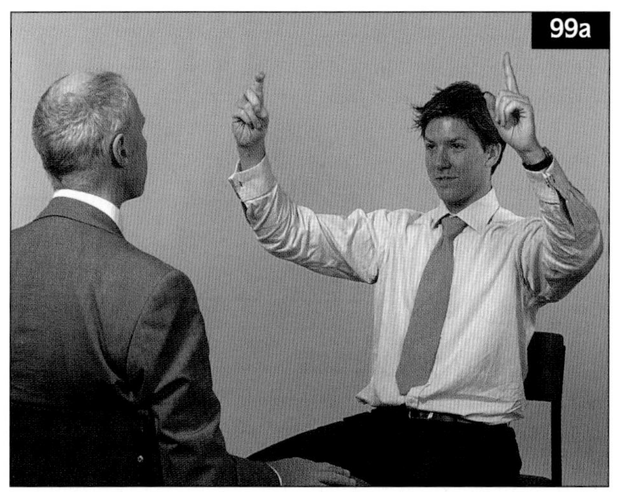

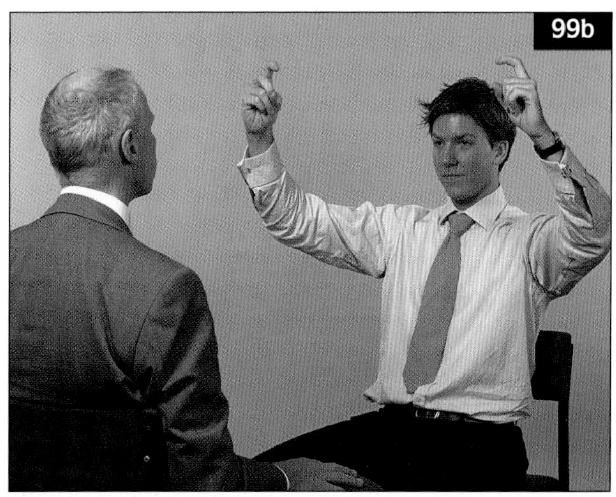

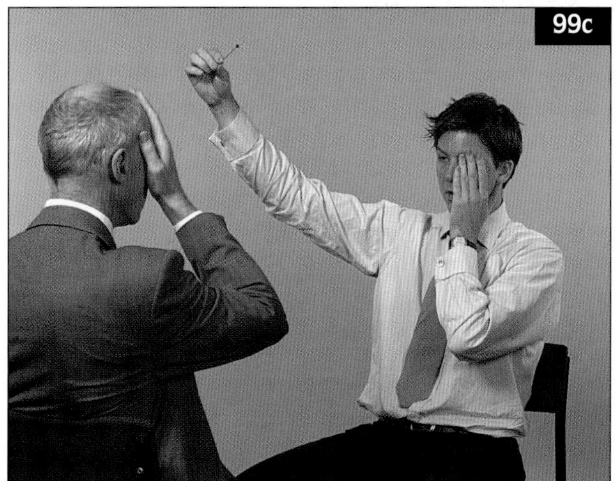

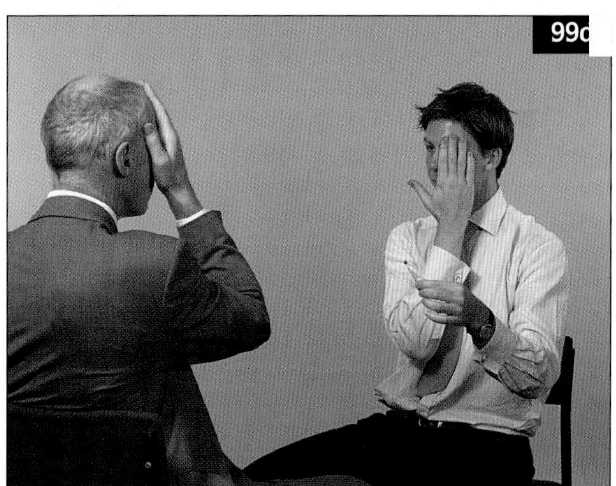

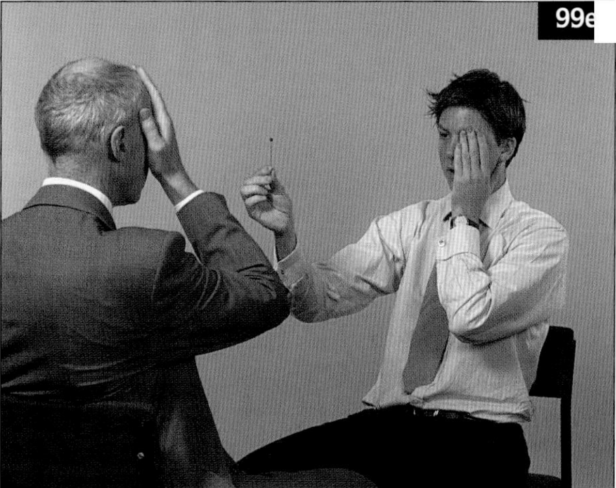

99 Visual field testing. The initial screening assessment to detect (gross) hemianopic defects involves presenting targets separately in the fields of binocular vision (**a**). Simultaneous bilateral targets are presented to test for visual inattention (**b**). During uniocular testing, a target is advanced diagonally from periphery to centre across each visual field (**c, d**). Small central defects (scotoma) and the size of the physiological blind spot are assessed as shown in (**e**).
a: binocular (screening) testing: a moving target in the patient's upper left field; **b:** testing for visual inattention; **c:** uniocular testing: the upper temporal field of the left eye; **d:** uniocular testing: assessing the lower nasal field of the left eye; **e:** mapping out the blind spot of the left eye.

swelling in the presence of normal visual acuity is typically papilloedema (**94c**), which should be presumed to be due to raised intracranial pressure unless proved otherwise. Optic atrophy (**94d**) is the end stage of a range of different optic nerve pathologies.

> Fundal and pupillary examination in patients with visual defects caused by pathology posterior to the chiasm that has not caused any brain swelling will be normal.

Neurological examination

Cranial nerves III, IV, and VI should be examined carefully in all cases of visual loss (see later for details). Diplopia is sometimes mistaken for visual loss or blurring and *vice versa*. Lesions posterior to the chiasm will often be associated with lateralized weakness, and so testing for tone and power may help in localization (see page 148). Reflex asymmetry or an extensor plantar may be present in the absence of motor weakness. Long tract motor signs may indicate previous lesions in other parts of the nervous system in a patient with optic neuritis (indicating MS) or AION (indicating possible previous vascular events). Similar principles apply to the sensory examination (see page 214). Testing for sensory inattention is important in patients with a visual deficit that is hemianopic, and other features of cortical sensory loss such as astereognosis (inability to recognize objects by touch) and agraphaesthesia (inability to recognize numbers traced on the palm) may be present. Various syndromes of higher cortical dysfunction are associated with visual disturbance (*Table 16*).

Investigations

These are guided by history and examination findings. Specific tests that are useful in certain situations are illustrated in *Table 18*.

Table 18 Clinical syndromes and their investigation

Acute monocular visual loss	FBC, ESR, CRP, glucose, cholesterol ECG Carotid Doppler Echocardiography
Subacute monocular visual loss	FBC, ESR, CRP, glucose, cholesterol, vitamin B_{12} VER MRI Lumbar puncture for OCB Mitochondrial DNA analysis (Leber's hereditary optic neuropathy)
Progressive monocular visual loss	VER MRI of orbits, orbital apex, and chiasm
Binocular visual loss	
Chiasm	MRI suprasellar space, pituitary fossa, and sphenoid sinus
Homonymous	CT or MRI of parietal, occipital, and temporal lobes ECG FBC, ESR, CRP, glucose, cholesterol Carotid Doppler Echocardiography EEG (if suggestive of visual seizure)
With associated higher cortical dysfunction	CT or MRI Neuropsychological evaluation
Functional visual loss	VER Goldmann perimetry

CRP: C reactive protein; CT: computed tomography; ECG: electrocardiogram; EEG: electroencephalogram; ESR: erythrocyte sedimentation rate; FBC: full blood count; MRI: magnetic resonance imaging; OCB: oligoclonal bands; VER: visual evoked response. This table excludes the investigation of ophthalmological disorders. In case of doubt, always consult an ophthalmologist.

CLINICAL SCENARIOS

CASE 1

A previously healthy, 28-year-old female computer programmer noticed that she was having difficulty seeing fine lines and small computer text with her left eye. The symptoms progressed slowly over the next day, so that she had difficulty discriminating between letters in newspaper headlines.

These symptoms denote a clear history of a monocular alteration of vision in a young patient with no previous visual or neurological problems. The manner in which the problem has been noted (reading or looking at a screen) and has progressed suggests a subacute onset (hours to days).

Two days after the onset of her symptoms she noted altered perception of colours and developed pain in her left eye, but no swelling or redness. The pain was worse with eye movement or pressure on the globe.

These complaints are more specific, and suggest optic neuritis.

On examination, her Snellen visual acuity was 6/36 in the left eye and 6/5 in the right eye. Confrontation visual fields were normal on the right, but demonstrated a central scotoma on the left. Colours were less intense in the left eye, and she could only read 7/13 Ishihara plates in that eye. There was an afferent pupillary defect on the left. Fundoscopy was normal bilaterally. The rest of her neurological examination was normal.

Afferent pupillary defects occur with any optic nerve injury. Similarly, marked reduction in visual acuity, central scotoma, and altered colour vision merely denote optic nerve injury, rather than its cause, but the combination of features is characteristic of optic neuritis. Examination will usually be normal in optic neuritis, but in about one-fifth of cases papillitis (swelling of the optic nerve head) will be seen. Eventually the disc will appear pale (optic atrophy), especially the temporal aspect. The fact that the rest of the neurological examination was normal is extremely important, because optic neuritis is a common presentation of MS, and a previous neurological event at a different site may have been subclinical (i.e. may not have caused symptoms).

Lumbar puncture was normal. Visual evoked potentials were delayed in the left eye but normal on the right. Magnetic resonance imaging (MRI) was normal.

MRI shows no evidence of previous episodes of demyelination, and oligoclonal bands (which are commonly detected in MS and reflect immunoglobulin response to central nervous system [CNS] antigens) are not present. This diminishes the likelihood that the optic neuritis was secondary to underlying MS, and makes it less likely that the patient will go on and have further episodes of optic neuritis or CNS inflammation / demyelination elsewhere. It does not, however, guarantee freedom from further episodes.

She was not treated, and after 2 weeks her visual symptoms gradually improved. After 3 months, her vision was 6/6 in both eyes, and the central scotoma was gone. Colour perception remained slightly reduced on the left.

CASE 2

A 62-year-old male retired postman awoke with 'darkened', impaired vision in the upper half of the visual field of his left eye 3 days prior to evaluation. He described the onset of symptoms as 'like a shade being pulled down' over the visual picture. He did not complain of eye pain.

While the problem is again monocular, there are other specific features here, and the patient is much older than in Case 1. Patients that wake with symptoms may have developed them suddenly or over hours (they don't know, they were asleep). Vascular problems are, however, common on waking. Altitudinal defects (from the bottom up, or the top down) are common in vascular disorders of the optic nerve head.

He had noted a headache for 6 weeks beforehand, and had consulted his general practitioner (GP) on three occasions about this. He was told that he was suffering from tension headache, and was prescribed simple analgesics. When questioned specifically he reported pain at each side of his jaw when he ate, especially towards the end of the meal. He was hypertensive, and on treatment with a beta-blocker. He had never smoked.

This shows the importance of background history, and the patient being given the opportunity to relate it. Symptoms that his GP has diagnosed as tension headache take on a new importance when considered in the context of his visual loss. Jaw claudication as described above is pathognomonic of temporal arteritis, which usually causes troublesome headache. The concern in temporal arteritis is the development of arteritic AION, and this must be the suspicion even before the patient is examined.

Examination revealed corrected visual acuity of 6/9 in the right eye and 6/36 in the left eye. The temporal arteries were nonpulsatile, thickened, and tender; there were no carotid bruits. A left afferent pupillary defect was present. The left optic nerve head demonstrated diffuse, pale swelling (**100**); small haemorrhages were visible at the superior disc margin and retinal arteriolar narrowing was noted. Confrontation testing revealed a superior altitudinal visual field defect in the left eye. The remainder of the neurological examination was normal.

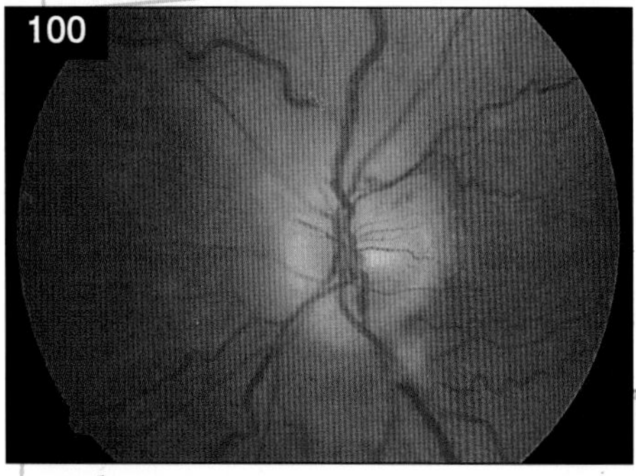

100 Pallid oedema of the optic disc.

The reduced visual acuity in the left eye is consistent with optic nerve injury, and not secondary to a refractive error (because refractive deficits were corrected). The afferent pupillary defect confirms an optic nerve problem.

Temporal arterial pulsation is sometimes difficult to feel in normal patients, but in this case thickening and tenderness imply an inflammatory process occurring in the vessel that may also have led to occlusion and pulselessness. Disc swelling is classically pale in AION, but may be hyperaemic (red and swollen), particularly in the nonarteritic form. The disc swelling is most often diffuse, with a segment of more prominent involvement frequently present. The field defect suggests an anterior problem (since it is monocular and altitudinal). The normal neurological examination provides further reassurance that the problem is anterior.

Full blood count revealed mild normochromic, normocytic anaemia, and a raised erythrocyte sedimentation rate (ESR) of 89 mm/hr in the first hour. Methylprednisolone (1 g) was infused intravenously immediately after the receipt of the ESR result, and the following day his headache had resolved. Further doses of methylprednisolone over the subsequent 2 days were followed by high-dose oral prednisolone. Left temporal artery biopsy conducted on the second day of admission revealed areas of intimal proliferation with a tunica media infiltrated with lymphocytes, plasma cells, epithelioid cells, and multinucleated giant cells, consistent with a diagnosis of temporal arteritis.

It is important to recognize temporal arteritis quickly, and to treat it on suspicion, because continued ischaemia (of the same or of the other eye) could further jeopardize sight.

Over the next week visual acuity stabilized at 6/24 on the left. At 2 months following onset of visual loss, the optic disc became atrophic, worse in the inferior half, with complete resolution of disc oedema. Oral prednisolone was subsequently reduced over the ensuing weeks and months with no return of visual disturbance.

Case 3

A 56-year-old male with lifelong myopia had a number of 'near misses' while driving his car and his wife noticed that he was apparently not seeing vehicles approaching from the left which were very obvious to her. He had no difficulty seeing road signs or with reading but was persuaded to go to see his optician to check his glasses prescription.

The symptoms suggest a loss of the peripheral visual field that could be due to a large number of different causes. For example, glaucoma results in loss of peripheral vision, secondary to raised intraocular pressure at the optic nerve head, and retinitis pigmentosa causes similar loss due to a retinal degeneration. The difficulty seeing to the left would be consistent with a left homonymous hemianopia due to a lesion affecting the right optic tract, radiation, or visual cortex. The fact that the patient did not notice a specific time of onset argues against a sudden lesion such as a right occipital lobe infarct.

His optician found normal corrected visual acuity, a normal fundal appearance, and normal intraocular pressures. He did find some peripheral visual field defects in both eyes and recommended a referral to an ophthalmologist.

The findings of the optician suggest that the problem is not ocular, and suggest that the problem is not confined to one optic nerve or pathway. They do not localize the lesion, but they exclude anterior causes: the problem is binocular, and is therefore either at the chiasm or posterior to it.

The ophthalmologist confirmed the visual acuity findings and arranged visual field testing (**101**). The patient had no other complaints or problems and the past medical, family, and social histories were unremarkable.

(Continued overleaf)

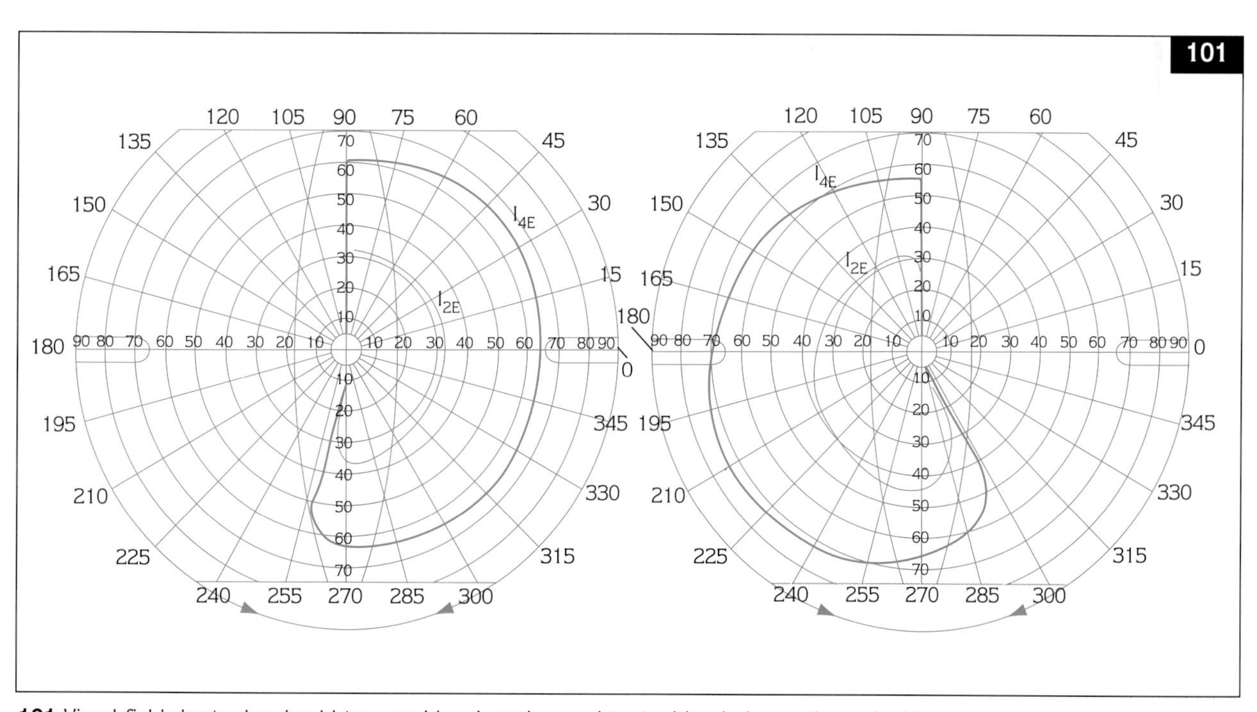

101 Visual field charts showing bi-temporal hemianopia, consistent with a lesion at the optic chiasm.

Case 3 *(continued)*

*The visual fields show a bitemporal field defect that is consistent with a lesion at the optic chiasm. Subsequent MRI showed a meningioma pressing on the optic chiasm (**102**). Lesions of the optic chiasm, most commonly arising from the pituitary gland, classically produce a bi-temporal hemianopia due to interruption of the crossing fibres in the chiasm. This can involve peripheral and/or central retinal fibres. If the lesion affects the anterior chiasm then one optic nerve and the crossing fibres from the nasal retina of the other eye may be affected, whereas a posterior placed lesion may produce an incongruous hemianopia due to optic tract involvement.*

The lesion was successfully removed with considerable resolution of visual field loss.

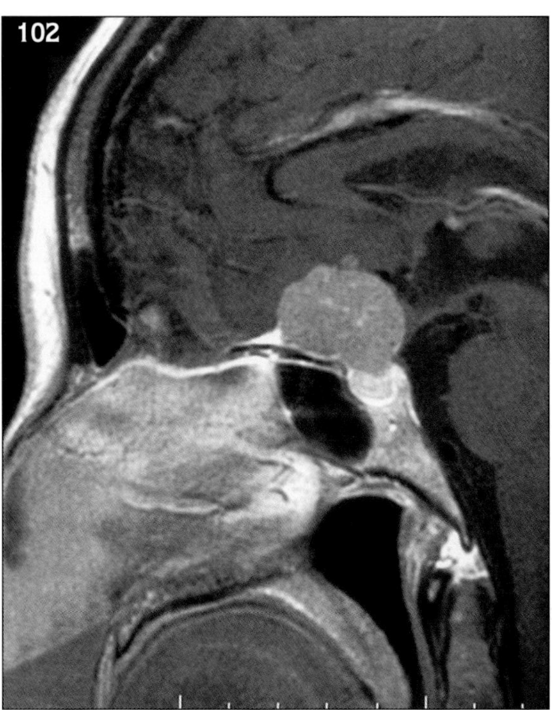

102 Magnetic resonance image showing a meningioma, pressing on the optic chiasm from below.

Case 4

A 74-year-old male retired lawyer with a history of hypertension and hypercholesterolaemia presented to the Accident and Emergency Department complaining of visual loss to the left, which had developed suddenly while he was gardening 6 hours previously. The visual loss was present when he shut either eye.

The background of vascular risk and sudden onset immediately raises suspicion of a vascular cause. The history also suggests that the problem is binocular (because it was present when he shut either eye), and hemianopic ('to the left'). Often the history will be much more vague ('there's something wrong with my vision'), and this useful information will only be available after careful probing.

He had no other symptoms at the time of visual loss, but had recently been discharged from a neighbouring hospital. He had presented there with vomiting and imbalance 4 weeks previously, and had been diagnosed with an ischaemic cerebellar stroke after having a brain scan. He had slowly recovered, had been started on aspirin and increased antihypertensives, and had received a course of physiotherapy.

His symptoms at the time of this first event are certainly suggestive of posterior circulation stroke, and the slow recovery after sudden initial presentation is consistent with this diagnosis. The fact that both events occurred in quick succession suggests they may be connected. Moreover, if the visual defect is consistent with the suggested deficit of hemianopia, both could result from posterior circulation ischaemia, since infarction of the posterior cerebral artery causes occipital lobe infarction and hemianopia.

Examination revealed xanthelasma and hypertension (176/92 mmHg [23.5/12.3 kPa]). Corrected visual acuity was 6/9 in each eye, and pupillary and fundal examination was normal. Confrontation visual field testing revealed a left homonymous hemianopia. Goldmann perimetry subsequently showed this to spare the macula. The remainder of the neurologic examination revealed past pointing and intention tremor, most marked in the left upper limb. He was mildly ataxic on heel-to-toe walking.

(*Continued on page 117*)

Case 4 *(continued)*

He has physical markers of vascular risk (xanthelasma and hypertension). The visual deficit is homonymous and hemianopic, which places the lesion in the optic tract, radiation, or cortex. In keeping with this, examination of optic nerve function (acuity, pupils, and fundi) is normal. The congruous nature and fact that the macula is spared suggest an anterior visual cortex lesion. His cerebellar signs are likely to be sequelae of the first event 4 weeks previously.

Computed tomography (CT) scanning revealed two discrete infarctions (**103a, b**). The first, older and more circumscribed, was located in the left cerebellar hemisphere. The second, poorly defined and associated with some swelling, affected the right occipital lobe in the territory of the posterior cerebral artery. Angiography revealed atherosclerosis of the basilar artery, a proximal embolic source for both of these arterial lesions. Echocardiography was normal. The patient was treated with antithrombotics to protect against further events.

Proceeding to vascular imaging is important because two events occurred in the same vascular system. It was important to investigate for a common proximal embolic source (in this case atherosclerosis in the basilar artery).

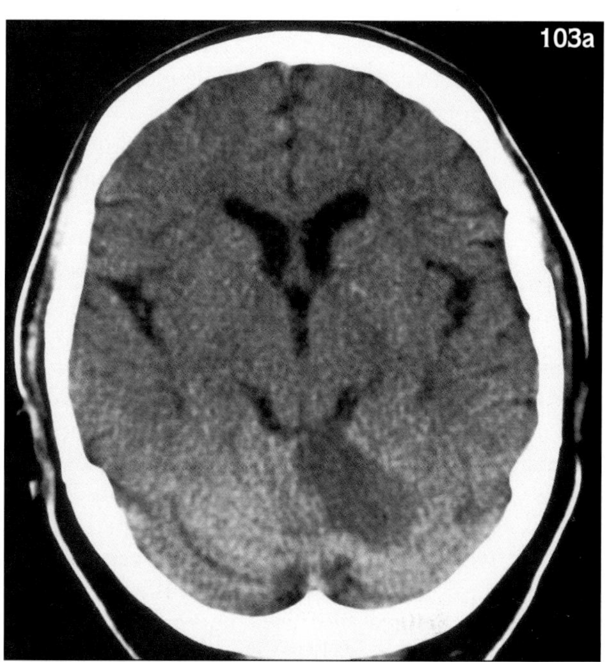

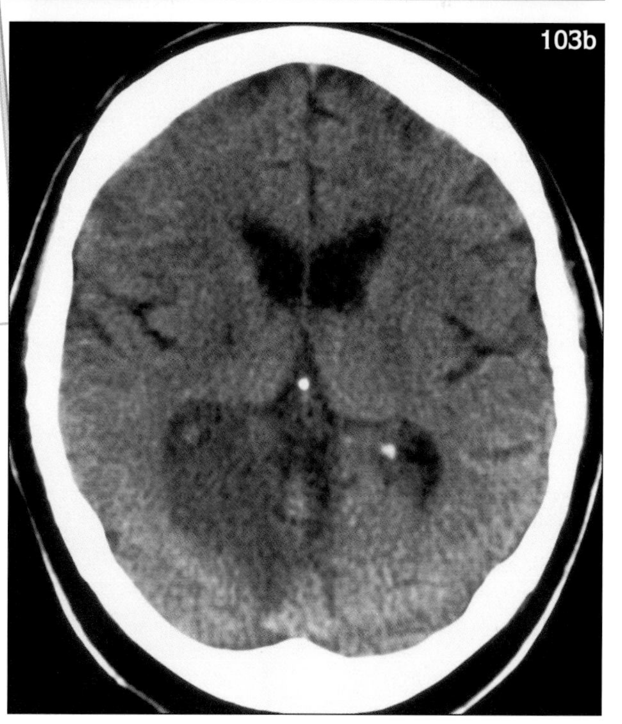

103 Computed tomography scan of vascular disease. **a:** older infarction in the territory of the left superior cerebellar artery; **b:** newer infarction in the territory of the right posterior cerebral artery.

Double vision

Diplopia means double vision. Diplopia can be horizontal (one image beside the other) or vertical (one image on top of the other). Abnormalities of the ocular media (e.g. cornea and lens) create monocular diplopia, in which when the patient covers the normal eye the double vision persists. Misalignment of eyes causes binocular diplopia; covering either eye abolishes the double vision. Neurological causes of double vision are almost exclusively binocular. The physical examination usually reveals the location of the abnormality, and the history indicates its aetiology. Disorders of the extraocular muscles, III, IV, and VI cranial nerves and brainstem oculomotor pathways cause binocular diplopia. Rarely, cerebral cortical lesions can cause multiple images (polyopia). Many patients with misalignment of the eyes beginning in childhood (secondary to strabismus or 'squint') do not experience diplopia because the image from the deviated eye is suppressed (amblyopia or 'lazy eye').

Functional anatomy and physiology

Extraocular muscles

Six muscles control eye movement. Each moves the eyeball or globe in a specific direction. These directions of action are illustrated in **104**, along with the specific nerve supply of each muscle (see later). Vertical is more complex than horizontal gaze with the oblique muscles moving the eye up and down when it is turned in (ADduction) and the recti moving the eye up and down when it is turned out (ABduction). If an extraocular muscle is weak, movement of the eye in the direction of the muscle's action will be impaired, and the patient will see double when looking in that direction, because conjugate eye movement has been disrupted. The false image lies outermost and comes from the underacting eye (**105**). Extraocular muscles may be affected directly by muscle (e.g. myositis) or neuromuscular junction (NMJ) disorders (e.g. myasthenia gravis) that make the muscles weak or restricted.

Orbit

The optic nerve enters the orbit through the optic foramen, alongside the ophthalmic artery. The nerves that supply ocular movement (see below) enter the orbit through the superior orbital fissure. Orbital apex anatomy is illustrated in **106**. Masses (which may be inflammatory, infective, or neoplastic) in the orbit may displace the globe (causing proptosis or forward displacement of the globe), may mechanically interfere with the extraocular muscles, or may compress the nerves supplying ocular movement, so causing cranial nerve palsy. They may also cause visual loss, due to interference with the optic nerve at the orbital apex.

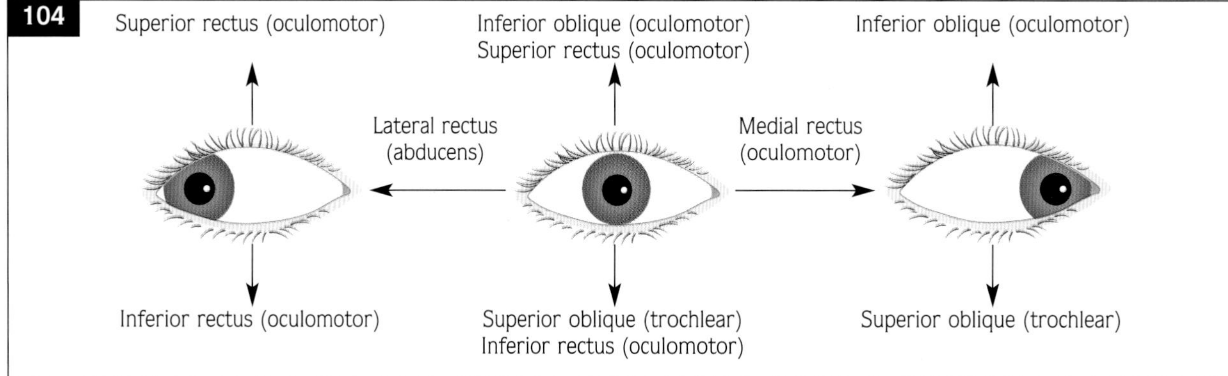

104 Diagram to show the line of action of individual ocular muscles and their nerve supply. Medial and lateral rectus move the eye medially and laterally, respectively. With the eyes in midposition, superior rectus and inferior oblique move the eye up, and inferior rectus and superior oblique move the eye down. The oblique muscles move the eye up and down when it is turned in (medially). The recti move the eye up and down when it is turned out (laterally).

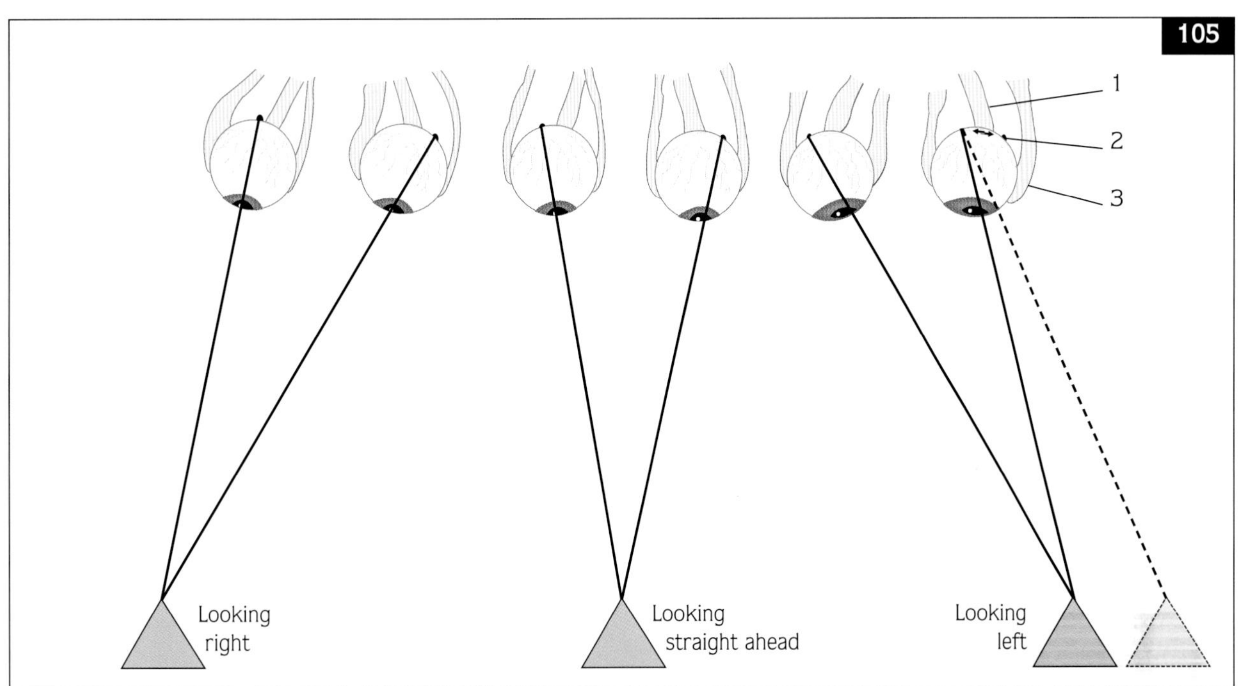

105 Diagram showing left abducens palsy, illustrating the mechanism of diplopia. When looking right and straight ahead, the extraocular muscles adjust the alignment of the eyes to maintain centring of the visual object on the macula. Since the left eye cannot look out (abduct), the image cannot be maintained on the macula of the left eye when the patient looks left. Thus the image falls on the nasal retina and is projected into the temporal half field. **1:** optic nerve; **2:** macula; **3:** extraocular muscles.

106 Diagram to show the neuromuscular anatomy of the orbit and orbital apex. The orbital apex is shown in cross-section in the box. **1:** superior oblique, supplied by the trochlear nerve (**2**); **3:** optic nerve; **4:** superior orbital fissure; **5:** superior rectus and **6:** medial rectus (supplied by the oculomotor nerve); **7:** superior and inferior divisions of the oculomotor nerve; **8:** lateral rectus, supplied by the abducens nerve (**9**); **10:** optic foramen; **11:** ophthalmic artery.

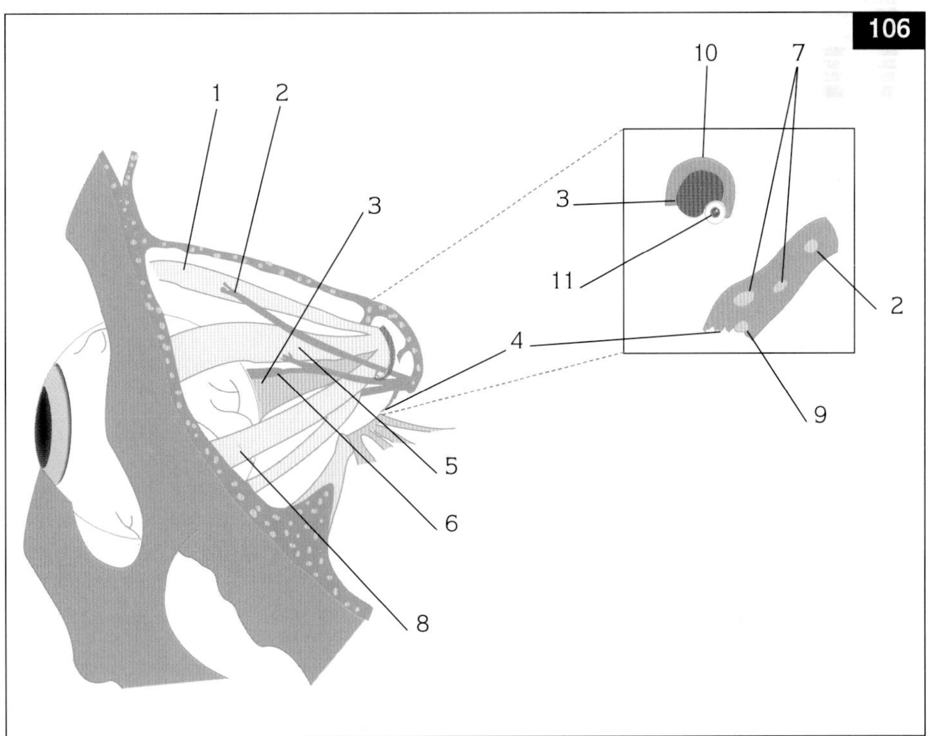

Cranial nerves

Three nerves supply the muscles that serve eye movement. Their anatomical path towards the orbital apex (**106**) is shown in **107**.

The oculomotor (III) nerve is the major nerve supplying eye movement, controlling the superior, inferior and medial recti, and the inferior oblique (**106, 107**). It also innervates levator palpebrae superioris (which elevates the eyelid) and carries the parasympathetic nerve supply to the pupil. On leaving the midbrain anteriorly, the nerve passes through the interpeduncular cistern in close relation to the posterior communicating artery and runs through the cavernous sinus. From here it enters the orbit through the superior orbital fissure.

The trochlear (IV) nerve supplies the superior oblique muscle, which depresses the eye when it is turned in (or ADducted, (**106, 107**). It emerges dorsally from the midbrain and passes laterally around the cerebral peduncle to enter the cavernous sinus. From here it enters the orbit through the superior orbital fissure.

The abducens (VI) nerve supplies the lateral rectus muscle, which ABducts the eye (**106, 107**). After emerging from the pons, the nerve runs anterior to the pons before piercing the dura at the basilar portion of the occipital bone. Under the dura the nerve runs up the petrous portion of the temporal bone and, at its apex, passes through to the lateral wall of the cavernous sinus. From here it enters the orbit through the superior orbital fissure.

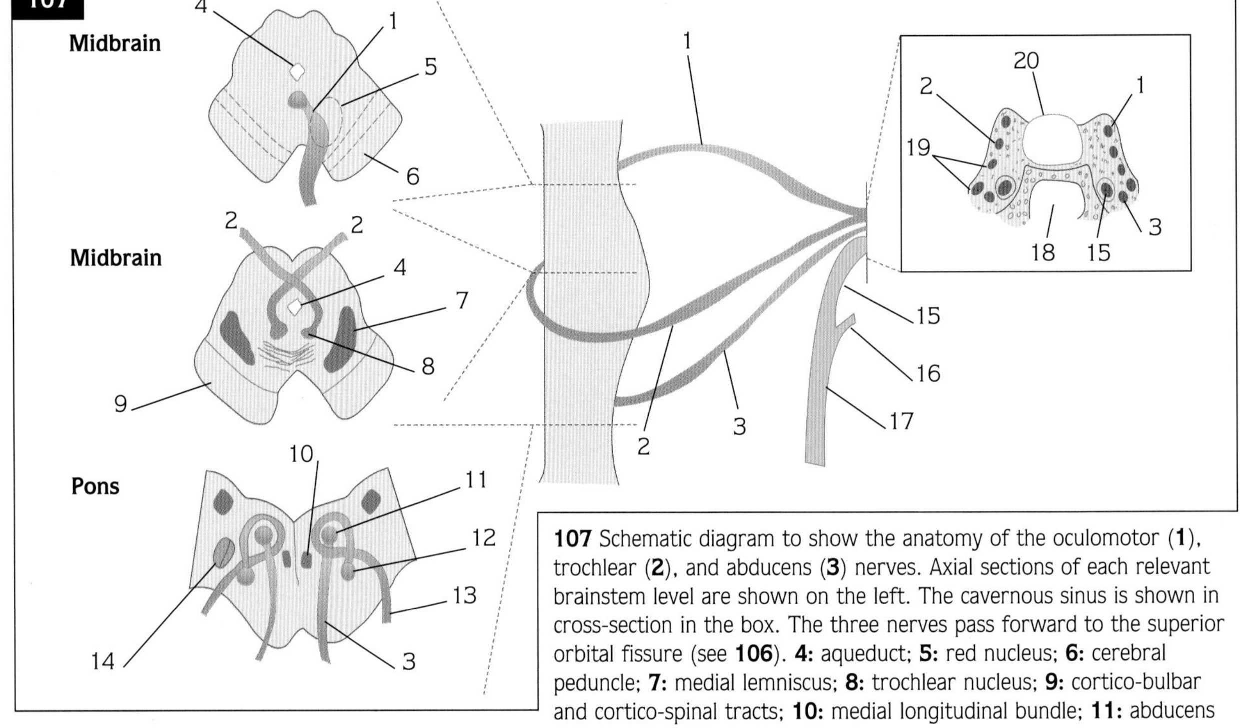

107 Schematic diagram to show the anatomy of the oculomotor (**1**), trochlear (**2**), and abducens (**3**) nerves. Axial sections of each relevant brainstem level are shown on the left. The cavernous sinus is shown in cross-section in the box. The three nerves pass forward to the superior orbital fissure (see **106**). **4:** aqueduct; **5:** red nucleus; **6:** cerebral peduncle; **7:** medial lemniscus; **8:** trochlear nucleus; **9:** cortico-bulbar and cortico-spinal tracts; **10:** medial longitudinal bundle; **11:** abducens nerve nucleus; **12:** facial nerve nucleus; **13:** facial nerve; **14:** trigeminal nucleus and tract; **15:** internal carotid artery; **16:** external carotid artery; **17:** common carotid artery; **18:** sphenoidal sinus; **19:** trigeminal nerve; **20:** pituitary.

Many diseases or disorders can disrupt cranial nerve functions, so causing diplopia. The nerves may be compressed by neoplasms occurring at any point along their anatomical path, by aneurysms of adjacent vascular structures (for example a posterior communicating artery aneurysm causing a third nerve palsy), or by raised intracranial pressure causing transtentorial herniation. Their blood supply may become disrupted (microvascular occlusion), and they may be affected by inflammatory and infective disorders. As they pass into the cavernous sinus and superior orbital fissure, function may be disrupted by inflammatory masses, neoplasm, aneurysms, fistulae (between carotid artery and cavernous sinus), or by thrombosis of the cavernous sinus itself.

Brainstem

Each of the three cranial nerves supplying eye movement (III, IV, VI) originates in the brainstem.

The oculomotor nucleus lies immediately anterior to the cerebral aqueduct in the midbrain at the *level of the superior colliculus* (**107**). Nerve fibres pass anteriorly through the red nucleus and substantia nigra to emerge medial to the cerebral peduncle.

The trochlear nucleus lies immediately anterior to the cerebral aqueduct in the midbrain at the *level of the inferior colliculus* (**107**). The nerve passes posteriorly to decussate in the dorsal midbrain. It emerges on the posterior aspect of the midbrain.

The abducens nucleus lies in the floor of the fourth ventricle within the inferior portion of the pons (**107**). It lies in close relation to the facial nerve nucleus and facial nerve axons loop around it. The nerve passes anteriorly to emerge from the brainstem on the anterior surface of the pons without decussating.

Vertical and horizontal movements are initiated via gaze centres in the brainstem, and the actions of the three nerves supplying ocular movement are united to produce a coordinated response. So when, for example, the left eye adducts (to look right), an action of the left medial rectus, the right eye abducts (to look right), an action of the right lateral rectus.

Brainstem lesions can cause diplopia by affecting the cranial nerve nucleus, or the cranial nerve fascicle (nerve trunk). Common aetiologies include demyelination and ischaemia or infarction. Infections (encephalitis or abscess), haemorrhage, and neoplasm may also affect the brainstem. Often nonocular symptoms or signs, as a result of disturbance of closely related structures, will accompany the eye movement problem. Lesions affecting the structures which control coordinated gaze (for example the medial longitudinal fasciculus) can also produce the symptom of diplopia, though they frequently do not.

Clinical assessment

Focused history taking

Initial confirmation that the problem is indeed diplopia must be obtained. Often patients use the term 'visual blurring' or shadowing to mean a variety of complaints. Diplopia means seeing two objects; these may not be equally distinct, but there are two.

The clinician should then ascertain the effect of eye closure. Binocular diplopia is caused by misalignment of the images obtained from each eye; it will be abolished by closure of either eye. The presence of this feature (or confirmation of its presence on examination) establishes the cause of the diplopia as neurological. Monocular diplopia will continue when the normal eye is covered and disappear when the abnormal eye is covered.

The direction of the diplopia must be investigated. Disorders of muscles or nerves supplying muscles, that act in a vertical (up and down) plane will cause vertical diplopia, while problems with those that act in a horizontal (side-to-side) plane will cause horizontal diplopia. Diplopia is maximal in the direction of action of a paretic muscle. Thus trochlear nerve palsy causes vertical diplopia maximal on down gaze, for example when going down stairs, because it affects the superior oblique muscle, which makes the eye look down when ADducted.

Sudden onset implies a vascular or traumatic cause. An expanding aneurysm causing compression of a cranial nerve tends to occur suddenly or worsen over hours. Gradual onset over days may occur in infective, inflammatory, or demyelinating disorders. Gradual onset over weeks commonly occurs in neoplastic processes.

Progressive, relentless worsening implies a progressive pathology: an expanding aneurysm, a growing tumour, or worsening cavernous sinus thrombosis. Vascular (arterial) occlusion causing microvascular cranial nerve palsy or brainstem stroke, tends to occur suddenly, and either remains static or improves. Myasthenia, causing extraocular muscle weakness, tends to worsen as the day goes on or as a specific task (for example reading) continues. Inflammatory diseases may have a progressive or varying course.

Myasthenia and demyelination are usually painless. Microvascular occlusion of a cranial nerve *may* be accompanied by retro-bulbar pain. Local infective or inflammatory diseases tend to be accompanied by pain; thus granulomatous inflammation at the superior orbital fissure or cavernous sinus in the Tolosa–Hunt syndrome causes multiple cranial nerve palsies with severe pain. Encephalitis and meningitis are usually accompanied by more diffuse headache. Expanding aneurysmal or neoplastic pathologies produce pain: painful third nerve palsy should be assumed to be due to compression by an aneurysm of the posterior communicating or basilar artery until proved otherwise.

Other ocular symptoms should be investigated. Proptosis and periocular oedema imply the presence of an orbital or retro-orbital mass that may be infective or inflammatory. It may also be caused by carotico-cavernous fistula (in which case it may be pulsatile), cavernous sinus thrombosis, and thyrotoxic eye disease, which causes enlargement of extraocular muscles. Loss of vision (see earlier) accompanying diplopia occurs in the context of diseases of the orbit that affect ocular movement, such as inflammatory or granulomatous conditions, primary and metastatic tumours, orbital cellulitis, and orbital wall fractures. Weakness of eye closure is a clue that a NMJ or muscle disease causing extraocular muscle weakness may be the cause of the diplopia.

Ptosis can accompany disorders of the extraocular muscles, for example myasthenia gravis (often fatiguable) or chronic progressive external ophthalmoplegia (progressive). Rarely, it accompanies diseases that affect the cavernous sinus, because sympathetic fibres to the eyelid and pupil are intimately associated with the internal carotid artery, which passes through the cavernous sinus. In this instance, pupillary constriction may also be present (Horner's syndrome). Ptosis is also a feature of third nerve palsy, because the third nerve supplies fibres to the levator palpebrae superioris, which elevates the eyelid.

Pupillary dilatation occurs as a feature of third nerve palsy, due to disruption of parasympathetic supply to the pupil: it tends to be an early feature of third nerve palsy if this is secondary to compression by aneurysm or infiltration. Microvascular third nerve palsy usually spares pupillary reactions. This difference in presentation is explained by the superficial arrangement of pupillary fibres within the nerve trunk: they are affected first by extrinsic compression and tend to be spared by central nerve trunk infarction.

Other neurological symptoms can occur. Facial sensory disturbance (V nerve dysfunction) in combination with diplopia suggests either brainstem or cavernous sinus disease. Facial weakness occurs with diplopia in two contexts. Unilateral dysfunction of facial power may accompany abducens nerve palsy or internuclear ophthalmoplegia in brainstem lesions because of the close proximity of the two structures in the pons. Neuropathies, NMJ disorders (myasthenia) and myopathies may result in facial and extraocular muscle weakness. In these instances, the facial weakness will usually, but not always, be bilateral. Hemiparesis or hemisensory loss again usually implies damage to the motor or sensory tracts that pass through the brainstem in close proximity to nerves III, IV, and VI. Ataxia in combination with diplopia can occur due to damage to the cerebellar peduncles or lobes from an ischaemic or demyelinating event that has also affected the structures involved in eye movement. It may also occur due to Wernicke's encephalopathy (caused by acute thiamine deficiency, and often seen in alcoholics), when it will usually be accompanied by confusion and amnesia.

It is important to establish the patient's medical history and background. Vascular disorders, such as microvascular cranial nerve palsy, tend to occur in the context of vascular risk factors (age >60 years, diabetes, hypertension, hyperlipidaemia). Inflammatory disorders of the orbital apex or cavernous sinus tend to occur in middle age. Expanding aneurysms causing cranial nerve palsy, myasthenia, metastatic and most primary neoplasms tend to occur in middle and old age. Demyelination is usually a disease of young adults, and previous episodes suggestive of transient neurological disturbance may have occurred in the past.

Examinations

Focused examination

Directed clinical examination of the patient presenting with diplopia is summarized in *Table 19*. Other aspects of the history may have raised questions that need to be answered by a more comprehensive general or neurological examination.

General examination

Arrhythmias may suggest cardiac disease or embolic source, and tachycardia occurs in the context of systemic infection in association with fever. Hypertension is the major risk factor for stroke, aneurysm formation, and microvascular cranial nerve palsy. Raised intracranial pressure impairs consciousness, increases blood pressure, and slows the pulse (Cushing's response). A goitre should raise suspicion of thyroid eye disease or myasthenia, which can occur in association with thyroid disorders. Lymphadenopathy occurs in metastatic neoplasm and lymphomas, sarcoidosis, and lupus. Patients with paretic eye muscles often compensate for their problem by tilting or turning their head away from the direction of action of the paretic muscle, since this minimizes the diplopia they experience. This is discussed further below.

Table 19 Examination for diplopia

Assessment	Examination
General	Pulse (rhythm, rate)
	Blood pressure
	Goitre/lymphadenopathy
	Compensatory head position
Ocular	Visual acuity
	Fundoscopy
	Visual fields
	Anisocoria and pupillary responses
	Ptosis/eyelid retraction
	Periocular inflammation
	Proptosis
Diplopia	Monocular occlusion
	Range of motion
	Cover test (tropia)
	Saccades
	Doll's eye test
Neurological	
Cranial nerves	Facial weakness/palsy
	Facial sensory loss and corneal reflex
	Hearing
Motor system	Lateralized weakness
	Reflexes
	Plantar responses
Cerebellar system	Finger-to-nose testing
	Rapid alternating movement testing
	Heel-shin testing
Sensory system	Vibration and position sense testing
	Lateralized pain and temperature loss

Ocular assessment

Visual fields, fundi and acuity should be assessed as discussed in the first section of this chapter. Pupillary size, anisocoria (unequal pupils), and response to light and accommodation are assessed. Pupillary dilatation can be subtle, and may not be fixed (in other words the response is sluggish and abnormal, but present). It occurs in (complete) third nerve palsies (because the third nerve carries parasympathetic nerves which constrict the pupil), and should raise suspicion of a compressive aetiology because pupillary fibres lie superficially in the nerve trunk and are often affected first. Horner's syndrome (a small pupil [miosis] more evident in the dark and ptosis) indicates disruption of sympathetic nerve supply to the eye and, in the context of diplopia, raises suspicion of pathology at the cavernous sinus/superior orbital fissure or brainstem. Ptosis (drooping of the eyelid) should be looked for and the palpebral aperture (distance between the eyelids) measured with a ruler to compare the two sides. Asking the patient to look upwards for 30 seconds before returning to the primary position and remeasuring assesses fatiguable ptosis. Cogan's lid twitch sign is a useful addition: the patient is asked to look down for 10 seconds, and then quickly up to a central target; the upper eyelid overshoots its normal position and then comes down like a shutter to its resting state. Fatiguable ptosis indicates a NMJ disorder, most commonly myasthenia. It is often, but not exclusively, bilateral. It also occurs congenitally and in chronic progressive external ophthalmoplegia. Unvarying ptosis may be due to mechanical disorders, a Horner's syndrome (incomplete and with miosis) or oculomotor nerve palsy (typically more severe, and with a normal or dilated pupil). Lid retraction occurs in thyroid eye disease, in association with lid lag (lagging behind of the eyelid as it is shut). Proptosis is best assessed by standing behind the patient and looking downwards over the patient's brows, comparing the positions of the two corneas relative to each other and the superior orbital rims.

Diplopia examination

A specific diplopia examination should also be performed. Monocular occlusion is performed initially, either looking straight ahead or in whichever direction the diplopia occurs, to determine whether this does abolish the double vision. For range of motion (duction testing) the patient is asked to a) look at the target, b) follow the target with their eyes and not by moving their head, c) and to report if they see double at any point. These instructions should be clear and often need to be reiterated. The target (preferably a light to allow observation of the corneal light reflex) is held at arm's length from the patient's eyes. It is moved upwards, downwards, to the left, to the right, and then upwards and downwards when the patient is looking to the left and to the right. After testing with both eyes open (versions), it is useful to test each eye separately, the other being covered by the examiner's hand (ductions). Often, duction failure (loss of movement) of the eye in a certain direction or series of directions is obvious. The common patterns of ophthalmoplegia (failure of eye movement) associated with III, IV, and VI cranial nerve palsies are demonstrated in **108**. Also illustrated is the pattern seen in internuclear ophthalmoplegia; although this often does not cause diplopia, it is an important pattern to recognize, and denotes a lesion of the medial longitudinal fasciculus in the brainstem.

If double vision is present, the examiner should establish in which direction the images are maximally separated. In this position the most peripheral (outermost) of the two images is the false image (**105**). By covering the eyes alternately and asking the patient to say when the outermost (normally also the faintest) image disappears, it is possible to establish which eye is at fault ('the bad eye'). The weakened muscle is that which normally moves the bad eye in the direction in which maximal diplopia occurs.

A tropia is a misalignment of the eyes during binocular vision. The cover test is a useful addition, as it will detect subtle misalignment that may be associated with diplopia, but which is not evident when testing for range of motion as described above. The patient is asked to fixate on a target straight ahead, one eye is covered and the examiner watches the other eye. If that eye makes a refixation movement, it was not aligned on the target. If the eye moves nasally (in), it was misaligned temporally (out) and so on.

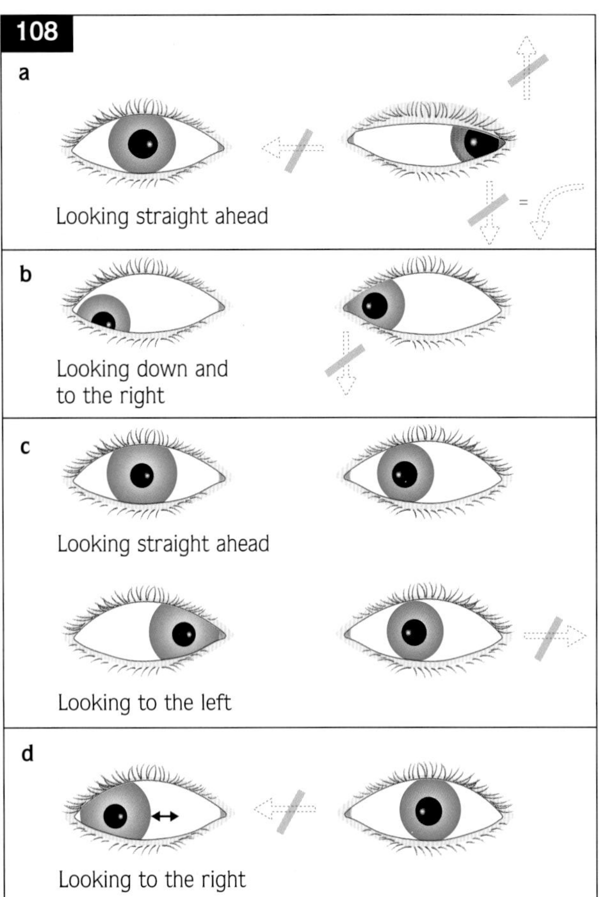

108 Diagram to show the common patterns of ophthalmoplegia. ←/: indicate the movements that are lost in each presentation. **a:** left oculomotor palsy: there is ptosis, pupillary dilatation, and diplopia in all directions except on lateral gaze (since lateral rectus function is intact). When the patient attempts to look down, the eye intorts (inwardly rotates, ↘). Superior oblique (intact since it is supplied by the trochlear nerve) has a rotatory action when the eye cannot be adducted; **b:** left trochlear palsy: frank diplopia occurs when the patient looks down and away from the side of the affected eye; **c:** left abducens palsy: diplopia is maximal when looking to the paralysed side; **d:** left internuclear ophthalmoplegia is a disorder of conjugate gaze, causing the eyes to move independently on lateral gaze. On lateral gaze away from the side of the lesion (which lies in the medial longitudinal fasciculus) the adducting eye fails to adduct, and the abducting eye demonstrates coarse jerky nystagmus (←→). **a:** Looking straight ahead; **b:** Looking down and to the right; **c:** Looking straight ahead; Looking to the left; **d:** Looking to the right.

Different patterns are illustrated in *Table 20*. If the eye does not refixate, the same procedure is carried out for the other eye, after a momentary pause to allow binocular vision to be re-established. Nonparalytic strabismus beginning in childhood commonly causes tropia; in this situation there is no diplopia, because the image from the deviated eye is suppressed or vision in one eye is poor (amblyopic). If the patient has a nerve or muscle weakness causing diplopia, the tropia increases when the patient is asked to look in the direction of action of the paretic muscle. Testing for phorias (misalignment of the eyes during monocular vision), which do not cause diplopia under normal conditions, is beyond the scope of this text.

Saccades are rapid conjugate voluntary eye movements between objects. The examiner holds their right fist 30° to the patient's left, and their left palm 30° to the patient's right. The patient is then asked to look quickly back and forth between the fist and the palm. The test is repeated with the fist held 30° above the patient's line of vision and 30° below it. Normal saccades have high velocities and are accurate. Any ophthalmoplegia will cause slowing of saccades: the examiner detects that the paralysed eye reaches the target after the normal eye when the patient is asked to look in the direction of action of a weak muscle. This again is a more sensitive sign than range of motion testing. It is particularly useful in the detection of internuclear ophthalmoplegia.

The Doll's eye test (vestibulo-ocular reflex) is useful for evaluating eye movements when the patient is unconscious, but is also helpful in the distinction of supranuclear gaze palsy from nuclear gaze palsy. The examiner rapidly oscillates the head horizontally and vertically. The normal response is for the eyes to rotate in the opposite direction, maintaining fixation. If a gaze palsy has been identified on range of motion testing, but on Doll's eye testing the eyes move normally in the 'paralysed' direction, then the problem must lie in structures that control voluntary gaze, superior to the cranial nerve nucleus that actually subserves movement, with vestibular input being preserved.

Neurological examination

Cranial nerves V and VII should be examined carefully. Cranial nerve V lies near the floor of the fourth ventricle in the lateral part of the pons and so may be affected by pontine lesions that also affect the medial longitudinal fasciculus (causing internuclear ophthalmoplegia), and cranial nerve VI. Only the first (ophthalmic) division of the trigeminal nerve will be affected in cavernous sinus lesions, and the corneal reflex will often be depressed. Cranial nerve VII loops around the VI nerve nucleus, and so is commonly affected by processes disturbing the VI nerve and nucleus in the pons. A contralateral hemiplegia may accompany this pattern. It is also important to examine facial power in patients suspected of having myasthenia or generalized neuropathy or myopathy: often facial weakness will be bilateral, and this can make it more difficult to detect since there is no asymmetry. Asking the patient to screw their eyes up tight and to whistle can uncover mild bilateral weakness in this situation.

Table 20 Classification of tropia

Type	Misalignment	Cover test
Exotropia	Temporal (outward)	Nasal movement
Esotropia	Nasal (inward)	Temporal movement
Hypertropia	Superior (upward)	Downward movement
Hypotropia	Inferior (downward)	Upward movement

A motor system examination should be performed (see page 148). Long tract signs may occur in pontine or midbrain lesions because the cortico-spinal tracts run through these structures in close proximity to cranial nerve nuclei and fascicles. Lower motor neurone weakness may occur in the context of generalized neuropathies that affect eye movement and skeletal muscle power (for example Guillain–Barré syndrome), and both NMJ disorders (e.g. myasthenia) and myopathies may affect limb power as well as eye movements.

The integrity of the cerebellar system is also assessed (see page 176). The patient should be tested for upper limb cerebellar signs (finger-nose-finger test and rapid alternating movements [dysdiadocho-kinesis]), lower limb cerebellar signs (heel-shin test) and asked to tandem walk. Abnormalities indicate disease of the cerebellum or its connections, and tend to occur ipsilateral to any cerebellar lesion. It is commonly seen in association with diplopia or eye movement disorders in alcoholics who have developed Wernicke's syndrome and in multiple sclerosis (MS).

In the sensory system (see page 214), lateralized sensory disturbance may occur in brainstem disease. Peripheral loss of pain and temperature sensation is commonly seen in neuropathies. Posterior column sensation (vibration) is often particularly affected by spinal MS, that may be subclinical.

Investigations

These are guided by history and examination findings. Specific tests that are useful in certain situations are illustrated in *Table 21*.

SUMMARY

- ❏ The speed of onset of visual symptoms is the best indicator of the underlying pathology.
- ❏ Monocular visual loss is caused by pathology anterior to the optic chiasm.
- ❏ Lesions at or posterior to the optic chiasm affect the visual fields in both eyes.
- ❏ Neurological diplopia is binocular.
- ❏ A painful third (oculomotor) nerve palsy is a neurological emergency due to an aneurysm until proven otherwise.
- ❏ Neurological diplopia can be caused by nerve, muscle, or neuromuscular junction disorders. Think about the latter two if the first doesn't fit.

Table 21 Investigation of clinical syndromes

Isolated diplopia		
Acute diplopia		Glucose, FBC, ESR, CRP, ANA, RF, ENA, cholesterol
		CT +/- MRI
		Angiography
Subacute diplopia		AChRAb
		Tensilon test, EMG
		Infection screen (Lyme, tuberculosis)
		TFT, thyroid autoantibodies
		ESR, CRP, ANA, RF, ENA, ACE
		CSF including OCB and pressure
		MRI +/- gadolinium
		Angiography
Chronic progressive diplopia		AChRAb
		Tensilon test, EMG
		TFT, thyroid autoantibodies
		CSF including OCB
		MRI +/- gadolinium
Nonisolated diplopia		
Diplopia	+ signs of raised intracranial pressure	MRI or CT +/- contrast
	+ proptosis and/or papilloedema	MRI (with gadolinium) of orbits, orbital apex and cavernous sinus
	+ combination (2 or more) of Horner's, III, IV, V, or VI palsy	MRI (with gadolinium) of orbits, orbital apex and cavernous sinus
	+ multiple other cranial nerve palsies	MRI (with gadolinium) of posterior fossa and meninges CSF
	+ brainstem or long tract signs	MRI (with gadolinium) of posterior fossa
	+ generalized weakness or bulbar weakness	AChRAb, Tensilon test, NCS, EMG

ACE: angiotensin-converting enzyme; AChRAb: anti-acetylcholine receptor antibody; ANA: antinuclear antibody; CRP: C-reactive protein; CSF: cerebrospinal fluid; CT: computed tomography; EMG: electromyography; ENA: extractable nuclear antigen; ESR: erythrocyte sedimentation rate; FBC: full blood count; MRI: magnetic resonance imaging; NCS: nerve conduction study; OCB: oligoclonal bands; RF: rheumatoid factor; TFT: thyroid function test.

CLINICAL SCENARIOS

CASE 1

A 30-year-old female with no relevant past medical history presented with acute, binocular, horizontal diplopia and severe headache.

Almost every word here is important in narrowing a differential that initially seems unmanageably broad. This is an acute (therefore, in the absence of trauma, probably vascular and unlikely to be tumour related) event in a young woman with no previous history (therefore unlikely to have generalized vascular disease or vascular risk factors). Thus the vascular event is less likely to be an infarction (though it could be), and more likely to be related to an aneurysm or vascular malformation. The diplopia was binocular (therefore neurological), horizontal (therefore, if neural rather than muscle, the problem affects nerves that move the eye in a horizontal plane [oculomotor or abducens]), and was associated with severe headache (which makes demyelination and myasthenia unlikely).

On examination, there was a partial ptosis on the left and a dilated and unreactive left pupil. The left eye was abducted when looking straight ahead. Eye movement testing revealed moderate underaction of adduction, elevation, and depression of the left eye. The right eye moved normally. There was intorsion of the left eye in down gaze, suggesting an intact fourth cranial nerve. The rest of the neurological examination, including fundal examination, was normal. Blood pressure and blood glucose testing were normal.

These are the physical signs of complete oculomotor palsy. Microvascular oculomotor palsy (often secondary to hypertension or diabetes) normally spares the pupil. The fact that these very distinct signs are present in isolation is important: posterior circulation stroke would affect other structures and so cause other signs, as would lesions in the cavernous sinus or orbital apex.

A diagnosis of an isolated, pupil-involved, left third nerve palsy was made. A CT scan of the head was normal, but a CT cerebral angiogram revealed an aneurysm of the left posterior communicating artery (**109**). This was successfully obliterated by insertion of a coil the following day.

Painful acute oculomotor palsy should always prompt urgent investigation and vascular imaging: the presence of pain in this situation implies that the aneurysm is expanding and may rupture.

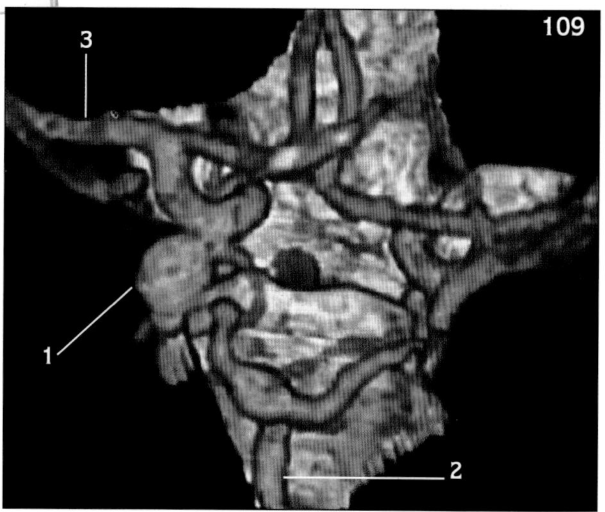

109 A computed tomography angiogram showing an aneurysm of the left posterior communicating artery (**1**). **2:** basilar artery; **3:** left middle cerebral artery.

Case 2

A 72-year-old male with a history of hypertension and diabetes presented with acute, painless, binocular, horizontal diplopia worse on looking to the left.

This is a completely different context to Case 1. One of the key skills of a good physician is to appreciate that 'common things are common', while always looking for warning signs that might push him or her away from the common and straightforward answer and towards a less obvious diagnosis. This could have the same cause as Case 1, and that would always be something that the astute doctor would have in mind. However, a number of features make a more benign aetiology more likely. This is a patient with a considerable vascular risk profile and his problem is painless. The problem again sounds vascular, but an ischaemic basis is more likely in this type of patient.

On examination, his blood pressure was 190/96 mmHg (25.3/12.8 kPa) and his random blood glucose was 13.4 mmol/l (241 mg/dl). The left eye was slightly adducted when looking straight ahead. On testing eye movements, he was unable to abduct the left eye, and saw two images side by side when asked to look to the left. The outer, more faint image disappeared when the left eye was occluded. The remainder of the cranial nerve tests and ophthalmologic and general examinations were normal.

It is important to appreciate the general medical context in which neurological events occur; this patient's hypertension and diabetes are both poorly controlled. Eye abduction is an abducens nerve function, and diplopia occurs on looking in the direction of action of the left abducens nerve. The fact that the false image disappears on occluding the left eye confirms that this is a problem with left lateral rectus (supplied by the left abducens nerve), not right medial rectus (supplied by the right oculomotor nerve), which also acts in this direction. No oculomotor functions are affected and the pupils are normal, further reassurance that the diagnosis as in Case 1 is unlikely. Again the problem is isolated, making structural pathology in the brainstem or cavernous sinus unlikely.

A diagnosis of an isolated, presumed microvascular left sixth nerve palsy was made. A CT scan of the head was normal. He was started on low-dose aspirin, and his hypertension and diabetes were controlled by additional antihypertensives and gliclazide. For 2 weeks the patient wore a patch over the left eye to alleviate his symptoms, but by 4 weeks both his symptoms and signs had completely resolved.

Microvascular nerve palsy generally has a benign prognosis, and patients normally recover fully. Patches are a simple and useful short-term measure to obliterate the false image.

Case 3

A 54-year-old male was referred to his local Ophthalmology Department complaining of double vision. This had come on quite suddenly, but image separation (which was horizontal) increased over 48 hours. He had no other complaints. He had hypertension (which was well controlled), but had been otherwise well in the past.

If this is binocular diplopia (as seems likely), the patient will need to be examined to identify the affected muscles. Horizontal image separation suggests involvement of the medial and/or lateral rectus. Diplopia noted to be worse on lateral gaze to the right or left can give clues as to the affected muscles, but this information is not available here.

On examination, the abnormalities were confined to the left eye. The left eye was turned out in the primary position (exotropia) and there was weakness of ADduction, elevation and depression. There was a partial ptosis but the pupil was normal.

This looks like an isolated third nerve palsy, sparing the pupil and therefore likely to be due to ischaemia of the nerve and is perhaps related to his hypertension.

(Continued on page 129)

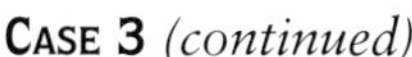

CASE 3 *(continued)*

Blood glucose (to investigate for diabetes), inflammatory markers (to investigate for arteritis), and angiography (to investigate for a compressive vascular lesion) were all normal. On review 3 weeks later, the symptoms had improved and, presuming that this was indeed due to microvascular disease of the nerve, he was told that there was a good chance of complete recovery.

Most ischaemic mononeuropathies do recover well and at the present time there is nothing to suggest any other disorder.

One month later, his diplopia had returned with both horizontal and vertical image separation and drooping of both eyelids. On examination, he had weakness of varying degrees affecting all eye movements, bilateral ptosis, and also weakness of eye closure. His symptoms were worse at the end of the day.

It appears that the initial diagnosis was incorrect. He now has widespread weakness, which cannot be explained by a disorder of one or even two or three nerves. This, together with the weakness of eye closure, suggests a disorder of muscles and the diurnal variation is highly suggestive of ocular myasthenia. The initial presentation had been deceptive.

This diagnosis was confirmed by a dramatic response to intravenous edrophonium (Tensilon test) and single fibre electromyography. He was subsequently treated with steroids and azathioprine, resulting in a good clinical response.

REVISION QUESTIONS

1 Five lesion sites (a–e) and five visual loss patterns (1–5) are stated below. Match the site with the visual deficit that a lesion at that site commonly produces:

a Right optic nerve.	1 Left incongruous homonymous hemianopia.
b Optic chiasm.	2 Left macular sparing homonymous hemianopia.
c Right optic tract.	3 Right central scotoma.
d Right temporal optic radiation.	4 Bitemporal hemianopia.
e Right visual cortex.	5 Left superior homonymous quadrantinopia.

2 Which of the following statements about the medical history of a patient with visual loss are true:

a Binocular visual loss will be abolished by shutting one eye.
b Optic neuritis characteristically occurs in patients over 60 years.
c Tumours tend to cause progressive visual disturbance over days or months.
d Migraine causes monocular or binocular visual disturbance normally followed by severe headache.
e Temporal arteritis usually causes a hemianopic visual disturbance.

3 During a focused assessment for visual disturbance:
   a A left relative afferent pupillary defect suggests disease of the left optic nerve.
   b Visual field testing may be omitted if visual acuity is normal.
   c An enlarged blind spot and constriction of the visual field are features of papilloedema.
   d Finding associated lateralized motor weakness and upper motor neurone signs suggests that the lesion lies in the optic chiasm.
   e ESR and carotid Doppler should be ordered to investigate acute monocular visual loss in a 70-year-old male.

4 Neurological diplopia:
   a Is abolished by shutting either eye.
   b Always results in images appearing side by side.
   c Can be caused by a lesion affecting the oculomotor, trochlear, or abducens nerves, or the muscles that they supply.
   d Occurs only as a symptom of brainstem disease.
   e Remains a lifelong problem for patients with congenital strabismus ('squint').

5 Which of the following statements about the history of a patient with diplopia are true?
   a Isolated trochlear palsy causes vertical diplopia maximal when looking down.
   b Myasthenic symptoms will be most marked when the patient wakes up.
   c Proptosis suggests aneurysmal expansion causing diplopia.
   d Unilateral ptosis indicates that the patient must be suffering from an oculomotor nerve palsy.
   e Diplopia is maximal in the direction of action of a paralysed muscle.

6 Which of the following investigation and management plans, formulated by a Casualty officer, would you agree with?
   a A patient with a painful complete oculomotor nerve palsy (pupil involved) was reassured and sent home for review in the neurology clinic the following week.
   b A patient with diplopia and ophthalmoplegia which worsened as the day progressed was referred for a Tensilon Test.
   c A patient with a sudden abducens nerve palsy and a history of hypertension, whose CT scan was normal, was started on aspirin, given a patch to wear over his right eye, and reassured. Plans were made for clinic review.
   d A 20-year-old patient was found on examination to have a left internuclear ophthalmoplegia and a relative afferent pupillary defect in the right eye. The patient was told that he had probably suffered a stroke and was referred for a CT scan.
   e A patient with symptoms of unilateral pain behind the eye, and a combined oculomotor and abducens palsy and tingling on their forehead, was referred for an MRI scan of their orbital apex and cavernous sinus.

Answers

1 a with 3
   b with 4
   c with 1
   d with 5
   e with 2

2 c,d

3 a True.
   b False.
   c True.
   d False.
   e True.

4 a True.
   b False.
   c True.
   d False.
   e False.

5 a, e

6 b, c, e

DIZZINESS AND VERTIGO

James Overell, Richard Metcalfe

INTRODUCTION

Dizziness and vertigo are common problems both in primary and secondary care. Both are terms that mean different things to different people, and the initial objective of the physician must be to identify the exact nature of the patient's complaint. This requires patience, careful listening and questioning, and a willingness not to jump to a (often incorrect) conclusion. Even after a measured assessment of the problem, both dizziness and vertigo have a number of diverse aetiologies: serious and life-threatening problems such as cardiac dysrhythmia need to be distinguished from the more common vestibular disorders. Anxiety may be both a cause and an effect of dizziness, and patients with chronic problems often develop a vicious cycle of anxiety and dizziness that can be difficult to disentangle, and may prevent resolution of symptoms long after any pathological problem has resolved (**110**).

Sensory inputs (visual, vestibular, and joint position – see below) are normally combined to provide an accurate model of the physical world. Symptoms can normally occur in the healthy individual when exposed to an unusual *combination* of sensory inputs triggered by exposure to odd visual stimuli, such as flickering images on screen or fast-moving traffic. This leads to a mismatch between visual, vestibular, and proprioceptive inputs, and to symptoms that are termed visual vertigo. These occur in the absence of demonstrable vestibular disease. This phenomenon is the basis for the lay perception of vertigo as meaning 'being scared of heights': a mismatch between sensory inputs causes troublesome symptoms at the top of tall buildings. Medical meanings are discussed below.

Dizziness is a broad and nonspecific term describing an unpleasant sensation of imbalance or altered orientation in space. When using the term 'dizziness', patients may mean that they are suffering from vertigo, disequilibrium, presyncope, or symptoms that stem from psychological disturbance. Vertigo describes an illusion of movement in relation to the environment. It is usually rotatory (a sensation of 'spinning round the room' or 'the room spinning around me'), but also sensations of body tilting, swaying, or forceful movement (impulsion) may occur. Disequilibrium is a sensation of altered static (standing) or dynamic (walking) balance; common terms used by patients are unsteadiness and loss of balance, and they may fall as a consequence. Ataxia means an unsteady gait, often described as 'walking as

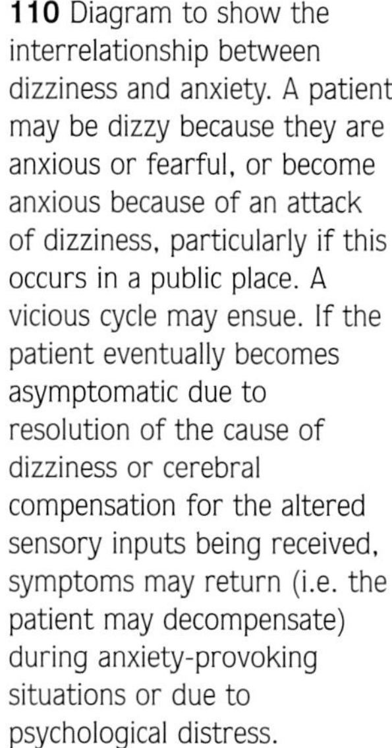

110 Diagram to show the interrelationship between dizziness and anxiety. A patient may be dizzy because they are anxious or fearful, or become anxious because of an attack of dizziness, particularly if this occurs in a public place. A vicious cycle may ensue. If the patient eventually becomes asymptomatic due to resolution of the cause of dizziness or cerebral compensation for the altered sensory inputs being received, symptoms may return (i.e. the patient may decompensate) during anxiety-provoking situations or due to psychological distress.

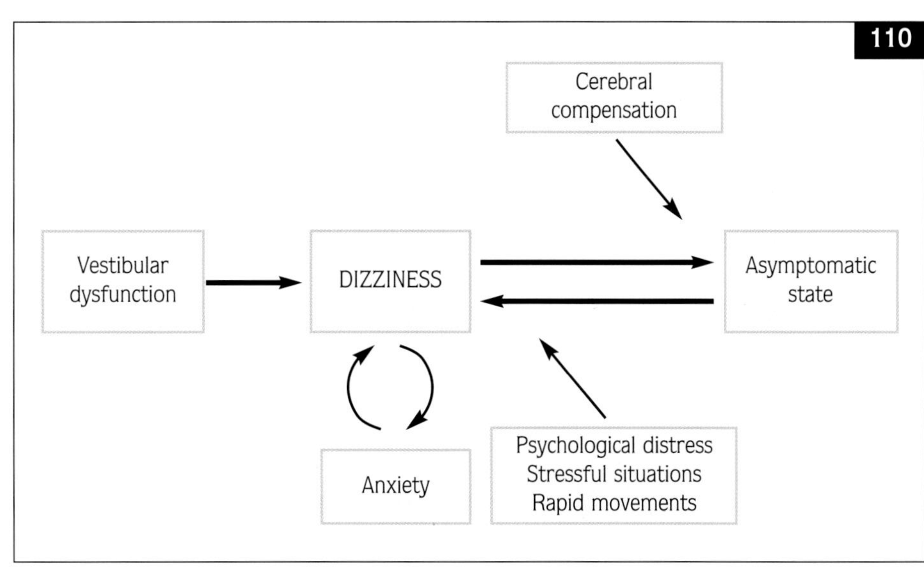

though I am drunk'. Presyncope is a sensation of impending loss of consciousness (or syncope). The terms 'light-headedness', 'feeling faint', or 'feeling woozy' are often used to describe this sensation. It is commonly associated with sweating, nausea, pallor, visual dimming or blurring, and generalized weakness. Anxiety may cause aspects of all the sensations described above, but generally causes a vague 'giddy', 'woozy', or light-headed sensation that is typically protracted with periodic exacerbations. It may cause patients to hyperventilate, and this can result in presyncopal and other frightening sensations. Anxiety may exacerbate symptoms from other causes or lead to decompensation and recurrence of symptoms in patients who have recovered (**110**).

Functional anatomy and physiology

The vestibular system is a special sensory system that detects rotational and linear acceleration. Along with inputs from the visual system and joint and body position sense from the proprioceptive system, body orientation in space (equilibrium) is maintained. Loss of any one of these three systems will produce clinical symptoms referable to that system (for example functional loss of the vestibular system will produce vertigo), but loss of two of the systems will produce profound imbalance and falling. Thus a patient with severe proprioceptive disturbance will fall if vision is eliminated (the basis for the Romberg sign, see below). Mild impairment of all three systems is a common cause of dizziness in older patients ('multisensory disequilibrium of the elderly').

The vestibular apparatus is a series of intercommunicating sacs and ducts filled with endolymphatic fluid, otoliths (granules), and hair cells, the movement of which generates sensory action potentials. The functional units of the system are divided into the utricle, the saccule, and the semicircular canals. The semicircular canals are arranged in three different planes; this arrangement ensures that angular movement in any direction results in displacement of the hair cells imbedded in the endolymph (**111a, b**). Linear acceleration results in displacement of otoliths within the utricle and/or saccule, which again is detected by the hair cells. Action potentials from the hair cells are transmitted to the vestibular division of the VIIIth cranial nerve. This travels (along with acoustic information transmitted from the cochlea) through the

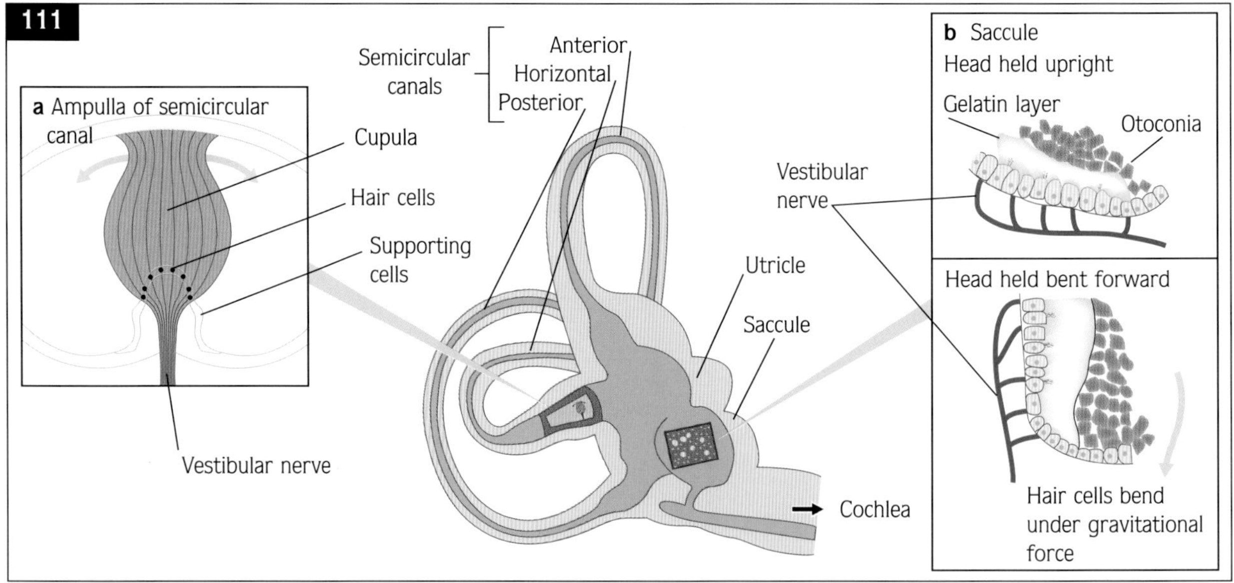

111 Diagram of the vestibular apparatus, comprising the semicircular canals, the utricle, and the saccule. The six semicircular canals (three on each side) work as three matched pairs in three planes. **a:** The ampulla, a swelling at the end of each canal, contains the sensory apparatus, comprising the cupula and hair cells. As the head moves, movement of endolymph causes the cupulae on both sides of the head to bend in opposite directions. The difference in activity between the paired ampullae results in the sensation of movement. **b:** The utricle and saccule contain the otolith organs. The organ in the saccule senses angular acceleration of the head. Forward movement forces the crystals to attempt to slide down the slope, proportional to the speed and angle of the movement. This displaces the hair cells, which is transmitted in turn to the vestibular nerve.

petrous temporal bone to the internal auditory meatus. From here the VIIIth cranial nerve passes through the subarachnoid space in the cerebellopontine angle to synapse in the vestibular nuclei (located on the floor of the fourth ventricle at the pontomedullary junction) and cerebellum. This arrangement is illustrated in **112**.

The vestibular nuclei project the sensory information to the following functional systems:

- Cerebellum. Spatial and motion sensation from the vestibular system is transmitted to the cerebellum, which is the functional centre for balance and coordination. Ataxia (see below) occurs as a result of disturbed sensory input to this system.
- Parieto-temporal cortex. These projections are responsible for the conscious perception of motion and spatial orientation. A disturbance in the inputs to this system will produce the sensation of vertigo. Such a disturbance may be due to disordered vestibular afferent information (for example discordant information from the two vestibular apparatuses), or a conflict between vestibular and other sensory inputs.
- Oculomotor nuclei. These mediate vestibulo-ocular reflexes: eye movements in the orbit are produced that are equal in amplitude and opposite in direction to head movements, so that gaze remains steady. Vestibular nystagmus (see below), a physical sign that often accompanies vertigo, is produced by a disturbance in this reflex system.
- Spinal cord. Projections to the spinal cord form the vestibulo-spinal tract, which mediates the vestibulo-spinal reflexes that assist in maintaining posture and balance, particularly on the muscle groups that act against gravity. The postural imbalance that often occurs in vestibular disease is caused by abnormal activation of these pathways.

Traditionally, the anatomical characteristics of the vestibular system have led to the distinction of peripheral (labyrinthine or vestibular nerve) from central (brainstem or vestibular connections) vertigo. The timing, context, and accompanying symptomatology usually lead to proper classification into one

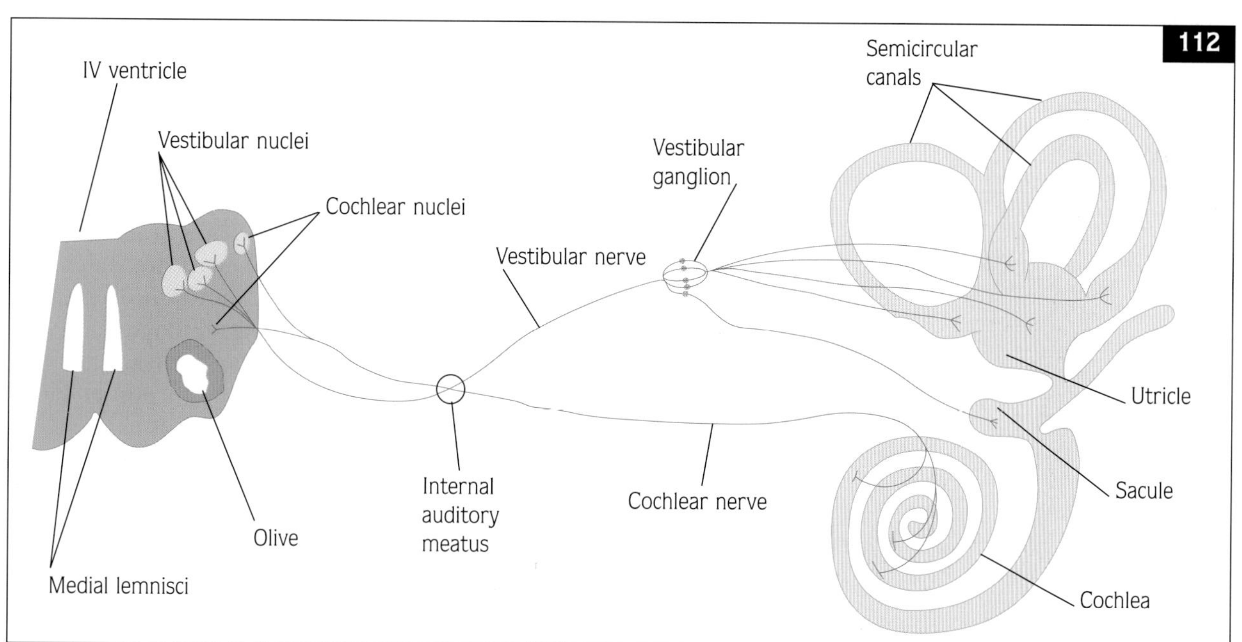

112 Diagram to show the central connections of the vestibular system. Information from the utricle, saccule, and semicircular canals is relayed to first-order vestibular neurones. The cochlea (acoustic) and vestibular divisions of cranial nerve VIII travel through the internal auditory meatus, and then pass through the subarachnoid space in the angle between the pons and cerebellum. Each enters the brainstem separately at the pontomedullary junction.

of these two categories, and to the correct diagnosis of the cause of the vertigo. The nature and direction (**113**) of the vertigo itself cannot be relied on absolutely to make this distinction, but generally peripheral rotational vertigo is in a yaw plane. Vertigo in other planes should raise the suspicion of a central disorder.

CLINICAL ASSESSMENT

Focused history taking

There are numerous potential causes of dizziness and vertigo, and the process of obtaining a history needs to be primarily one of listening and understanding the exact nature of each symptom. The standard pattern of localization followed by pathophysiology (beyond the distinction of central from peripheral above) tends to lead to mistakes.

Definition

The specific meaning of the terms vertigo, disequilibrium, and presyncope are described above. It is very important to determine which of these broad distinctions applies, since localization and pathological possibilities follow on from this. Nonspecific complaints ('dizziness', 'giddiness', 'woozy', 'light-headedness') should be explored. Direct and leading questions may be necessary, but should be viewed and recorded as such. Sometimes, despite the best attempts of the physician to classify the symptomatology more closely, it is impossible to determine the specific complaint; in this situation it is more sensible to enquire about the other features of the problem described below than to 'pigeonhole' the patient into a category that may lead to inappropriate investigations and treatments.

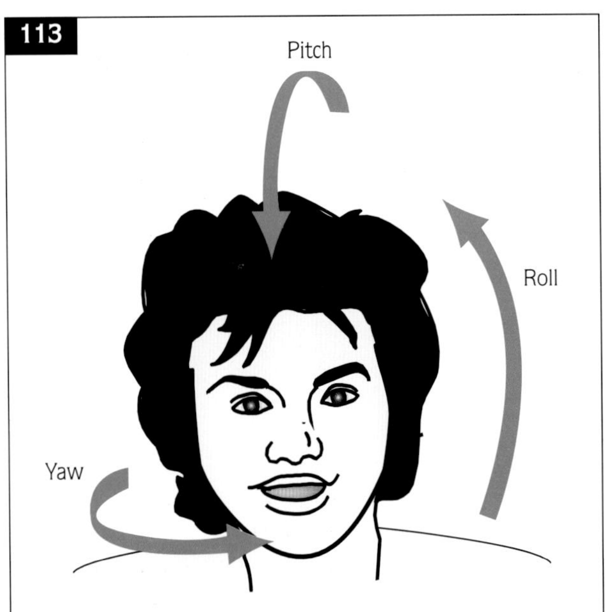

113 Diagram to illustrate the three planes of head movement. Yaw (horizontal about a vertical axis) is the common plane of rotation in peripheral vertigo. Pitch (flexion and extension about a vertical axis) and roll (lateral head tilt about a horizontal axis) are less common in peripheral vertigo.

Symptom complexes

Medical dizziness and vertigo often have specific situational features or present as part of a group of symptoms. It is useful to consider these 'symptom complexes' as an aid to reaching a differential diagnosis. The possibilities for each complex are shown in *Table 22*, along with other features specific to each diagnosis.

- *Acute severe vertigo* refers to sudden, usually very disabling, vertigo accompanied by nausea and often profound vomiting. Often there will be a history of such an attack in a patient who goes on to develop positional vertigo: such patients have partially compensated (adapted), but continue to have symptoms when the vestibular system is provoked.
- *Positional vertigo (bed spins).* Patients complain of brief spells of rotatory vertigo on changing position, typically when getting into or out of bed, or on rolling from one side to the other. Most patients with this symptom will have benign paroxysmal positional vertigo (BPPV).
- *Vertigo with headache.* The characteristics of the headache may give more clues to the diagnosis (for example vertebrobasilar migraine causing recurrent throbbing headache or Chiari malformation causing headache on stooping or coughing) than the vertigo.
- *Hydrops (hearing disturbance, vertigo, tinnitus).* Patients complain of recurrent periods of vertigo, tinnitus (ringing or roaring in the ears), and transient hearing loss, often preceded by a feeling of fullness in the ear. Most patients with this symptom complex will have Ménière's disease.
- *Medical dizziness.* A 'nonspecific' and generally acute presentation of giddiness, light-headedness, or presyncopal symptoms caused by low blood pressure, low blood glucose, and/or metabolic derangements associated with systemic infection or medications.

Table 22 Differential diagnosis of vertigo and dizziness symptom complexes

Symptom complex	Diagnostic possibilities	Other features
Acute severe vertigo	❑ Acute peripheral vestibulopathy (often referred to as labyrinthitis, vestibular neuronitis, or vestibular neuritis)	❑ Nausea, vomiting, ataxia, and nystagmus
	❑ Posterior circulation stroke	❑ Other symptoms of acute brainstem disease; focal brainstem signs
Positional vertigo	❑ BPPV	❑ Lack of other symptoms; short lived; vertigo induced by changing head position; Dix–Hallpike test
	❑ Vestibular decompensation	❑ History of acute event before positional symptoms
	❑ Central vertigo	❑ Other symptoms of brainstem disease; focal brainstem signs
	❑ Postural hypotension	❑ *Getting out* of bed, rather than turning in bed; systolic blood pressure drop of >20 mmHg (2.7 kPa) on standing
Vertigo or dizziness with headache	❑ Vertebro-basilar migraine	❑ Severe throbbing episodic headache; associated photophobia
	❑ Post-traumatic vertigo	❑ History of moderate to severe trauma; associated memory disturbance and ataxia
	❑ Chiari malformation	❑ Posterior headache with pressure features; down-beat nystagmus
	❑ Central vertigo	❑ Other symptoms of brainstem disease; focal brainstem signs
	❑ Anxiety	❑ Headache, often with tension features
Hydrops (hearing disturbance, vertigo, tinnitus)	❑ Ménière's disease	❑ Vertigo duration *usually* a few hours; low tone sensorineural hearing loss
	❑ Post-traumatic hydrops (Ménière's variant)	❑ Significant ear trauma
	❑ Syphilis	❑ Bilateral hearing loss; risk factors for syphilis
Medical dizziness	❑ Postural hypotension	❑ Occurs on standing; systolic blood pressure drop of >20 mmHg (2.7 kPa) on standing; may relate to medications
	❑ Cardiac arrhythmia	❑ Palpitations, breathlessness, chest pain, autonomic symptoms
	❑ Hypoglycaemia	❑ Osmotic symptoms; history of diabetes
	❑ Medication effect	❑ May also present with true vertigo; hypotensives, sedatives, antiepileptics, vestibular suppressants
	❑ Systemic infection	❑ Fever, malaise, myalgia, arthralgia
	❑ Hyperventilation	❑ Paraesthesiae around the mouth and in the fingers

BPPV: benign paroxysmal positional vertigo.

Timing and duration

Are the symptoms episodic or constant? If they are episodic, how long do they last? Many of the conditions causing vertigo will occur episodically (many times per day or week), and the duration of the symptomatology when it occurs is a key factor in reaching a diagnosis. Vertigo can occur suddenly or appear gradually, and once present can disappear quickly, resolve over minutes, hours, or days, remain static, or progress. Some illnesses may only occur once (monophasic), but their diagnosis may have major implications because the physician must concentrate on preventing further episodes (for example transient ischaemic attacks, or TIAs). If such problems become recurrent, perhaps occurring two or three times on specific occasions rather than the episodic pattern described above, accurate diagnosis becomes even more important. Progressive disequilibrium is likely to have a toxic cause (for example persistent treatment with intravenous gentamicin, which is oto- and vestibulo-toxic), and progressive vertigo is likely to occur in the context of other worsening brainstem neurology, raising the possibility of a neoplastic lesion. *Table 23* shows the diagnostic possibilities that are raised by each type of presentation.

Triggering or exacerbating factors
Dizziness on standing up suggests postural hypotension. Changes in the position of head or body often exacerbate vertigo (see positional vertigo symptom complex above). Walking in the dark will exacerbate vestibular disturbances, but dizziness or imbalance *only* in the dark suggests a problem with proprioceptive inputs (a sensory ataxia). Coughing, sneezing, bending down, or straining at stool raises intracranial pressure, and so may worsen symptoms from a posterior fossa mass lesion or malformation (for example Chiari malformation). Situations or times when vertigo occurs may lead to a pattern suggesting a relationship to certain foods or medications (for example alcohol) or to situational anxiety. Symptoms of dizziness and vertigo may cause acute anxiety and hyperventilation, but anxiety and hyperventilation can be the root of the problem itself, and should be enquired about sensitively.

Associated otologic history
Hearing loss and tinnitus generally imply peripheral dysfunction, usually involving the inner ear. It is important to enquire closely about the components of the hydrops symptom complex above. Acute peripheral vestibulopathy (often attributed, though without much evidence, to a viral infection of the vestibular nerve – so called vestibular neuritis) presents with vertigo, nausea, vomiting, ataxia, and nystagmus. When combined with tinnitus and/or hearing loss it is known as labyrinthitis. Tumours compressing the VIIIth nerve (the most common example being acoustic neuroma) generally produce progressive asymmetric hearing loss and mild ataxia rather than vertigo.

Associated general and neurological history
A history of diabetes raises the possibility of hypoglycaemia and a history of cardiac disease should alert the physician to the possibility of cardiac arrhythmia (see medical dizziness symptom complex above). Systemic infection may cause medical dizziness, and may be accompanied by either general (fever, malaise) or specific (diarrhoea, cough) signs of infection. Vascular risk factors (age, smoking, diabetes, hypertension, hyperlipidaemia) increase the likelihood of TIA or stroke as the cause of vertigo or dizziness. A history of previous focal neurological events raises the possibility of demyelination (multiple sclerosis, MS). A history of migraine is common in patients with Ménière's disease.

Any of the following 'brainstem' symptoms imply a central basis for vertigo: diplopia, facial numbness, dysarthria, dysphagia, lateralized limb weakness or numbness, and lateralized incoordination. Since facial (VII) nerve fibres travel in close proximity to the VIIIth nerve in the internal auditory canal, cerebellopontine angle and brainstem, complete facial nerve palsy can occur in conjunction with vertigo and this indicates disease of one of these structures.

Ataxia (unsteadiness of gait) is very commonly associated with both peripheral and central vertigo, is frequent with cerebellar disease and diseases causing loss of proprioceptive input, but is uncommon in medical dizziness. Nausea and vomiting accompany dizziness and vertigo in all contexts, but tend to be more marked and dramatic in peripheral vertigo than in central vertigo. Patients may experience oscillopsia, which is an awareness of jumping of the environment. This may occur as a consequence of rapid jerking eye movements (nystagmus) or because of failure of the vestibulo-ocular reflex. The complaint of unsteadiness and imbalance (disequilibrium) may be caused by vestibular dysfunction, but may also be secondary to cerebellar disease or impaired proprioception due to large fibre peripheral nerve or spinal cord posterior column dysfunction. Presyncope is often accompanied by visual dimming, palpitation, sweating and pallor, and suggests one of the causes of the medical dizziness symptom complex. Hyperventilation may be accompanied by paraesthesiae around the mouth and in the fingers. Enquiring about the symptoms of anxiety is mandatory in the dizzy patient, but is particularly useful in a patient who may be hyperventilating.

Age
Common causes of vertigo in the elderly include BPPV, acute peripheral vestibulopathy, trauma, medication (see below), and ischaemia of either the posterior (brainstem) circulation or the labyrinthine system. Common causes of vertigo in younger adults include Ménière's disease, acute peripheral vestibulopathy, head trauma, and medication. Causes of medical dizziness tend to occur more often in the older age group, since heart disease, prescription of antihypertensive medication, and diabetes are more common.

Family history
A family history of vascular disease or risk factors, Ménière's disease, autoimmune disease in a patient with Ménière's disease, or migraine may be obtained.

Medication history
Some medications are toxic to the vestibular nerve, the most common example being aminoglycoside antibiotics. Numerous medications can make patients feel dizzy and unsteady, including anticonvulsants (carbamazepine, phenytoin), antihypertensives (which can cause symptomatic hypotension and medical dizziness), antidepressants (which can have cardiovascular side-effects including postural hypotension), and sedatives (benzodiazepines, narcoleptics). Drugs can also cause ataxia, anticonvulsants being the most common example.

Substance abuse history
Alcohol causes dizziness and vertigo during acute ingestion. Heroin, benzodiazepines, and other sedatives can cause dizziness, as can amphetamine-based drugs and lysergic acid diethylamide (LSD). Chronic use of alcohol producing a cerebellar syndrome is the most common cause of ataxia in the United Kingdom.

Table 23 Differential diagnosis of dizziness and vertigo by timing and duration of symptoms

Presentation		***Course***			
Duration	**Onset**	**Episodic**	**Monophasic**	**Recurrent**	**Progressive**
<1 minute	Sudden	BPPV variants Vestibular decompensation Epilepsy	 Arrhythmia	 Arrhythmia	
Minutes to hours	Sudden	Orthostasis Vestibular decompensation	TIA	TIA	
	Gradual	Panic attacks and situational anxiety Hyperventilation			
Hours to days	Sudden		Posterior circulation stroke	Posterior circulation stroke	
	Gradual	Ménière's disease	Demyelination/ CNS inflammation Vertebro-basilar migraine	Demyelination/ CNS inflammation Vertebro-basilar migraine	
≥2 weeks	Sudden		Vertebro-basilar stroke		
	Gradual	Anxiety	Acute peripheral vestibulopathy	Acute peripheral vestibulopathy	Brainstem tumour
		Drug intoxication	Demyelination/ CNS inflammation	Demyelination/ CNS inflammation	Chiari malformation
			Bilateral vestibular paresis	Multisensory disequilibrium of the elderly	Bilateral vestibular paresis
			Drug intoxication	Drug intoxication	Multisensory disequilibrium of the elderly
				Chiari malformation	Drug intoxication

BPPV: benign paroxysmal positional vertigo; CNS: central nervous system; TIA: transient ischaemic attack.

Examinations

Focused examination

The focused physical examination of the dizzy or vertiginous patient is outlined in *Table 24*. The various components of the assessment are discussed below.

General examination

Presence of a tachy- or bradyarrhythmia raises the possibility that symptoms of medical dizziness are attributable to cerebral hypoxia as a consequence of reduced cardiac output and consequent hypotension. A fall in systolic blood pressure of >20 mmHg (2.7 kPa) on standing constitutes significant postural hypotension. The presence of a third or fourth heart sound may imply heart failure (leading to hypotension), or significant hypertension (increasing vascular risk), respectively. Heart murmurs can be caused by valvular disease, which may be an embolic source. Arterial bruits (carotid, subclavian, femoral) imply major vessel stenotic arterial disease, which increases the probability that symptoms are attributable to ischaemia, while not being directly implicated in the aetiology of the problem. Carotid sinus massage is useful if carotid sinus hypersensitivity is suspected.

Balance assessment

The gait pattern of particular importance in the assessment of dizziness and vertigo is the ataxic gait: wide-based, stumbling, and unstable. Any instability will be exaggerated by tandem walking (walking with one foot in front of the other 'as if on a tightrope'). Young, fit patients should be able to do this backwards as well as forwards. Ataxia can be caused by significant cerebellar disturbance, significant (particularly acute) vestibular disturbance, or significant (particularly acute) proprioceptive disturbance. Romberg's test (illustrated in **114**) should be performed with the eyes open and then with the eyes shut. Vision tends to compensate for chronic vestibular and especially proprioceptive deficit, so difficulty standing with the eyes closed (or a 'positive Romberg's test', **114**) specifically indicates a deficit in one or both of these systems.

Otologic examination

A brief assessment of hearing (for example rubbing the thumb and forefinger beside each ear) is useful as a screening test for hearing disturbance. Normally young persons should be able to perceive this at arm's length from their ear, and elderly patients should be able to perceive it at 15 cm (6 inches). An audiogram (see below) quantifies and characterizes the hearing loss, but simple clinical tests can be helpful. A distinction is made between conductive (related to disease or blockage in the external auditory meatus, eardrum, or ear ossicles) and sensorineural (cochlear, VIIIth nerve or brainstem) hearing loss. This distinction is made clinically using Rinne's and Weber's tests, illustrated in **115a, b**. During Rinne's test, a vibrating high frequency tuning fork (preferably 512 Hz) is held close to the ear, and the patient is asked to compare the volume of the sound

Table 24 Examination for vertigo and dizziness

Assessment	Examination
General	Pulse (rhythm, rate)
	Blood pressure lying and standing
	Cardiac auscultation
	Arterial bruits
	Carotid sinus massage
Balance	Gait
	Tandem walking
	Romberg's test
Otological	Hearing
	Rinne and Weber tests
	Tympanic membranes
Neurological	
Cranial nerves	Fundoscopy
	Eye movements
	Vestibulo-ocular reflexes
	Facial movement
	Facial sensation and corneal reflex
Motor system	Lateralized weakness
	Reflexes
	Plantar responses
Cerebellar system	Finger-to-nose testing
	Rapid alternating movement testing
	Heel-shin testing
Sensory system	Vibration and position sense testing
Nystagmus	Spontaneous nystagmus
	Gaze-evoked nystagmus
	Hallpike manoeuvre
	Head shake test
	Vestibulo-ocular system testing

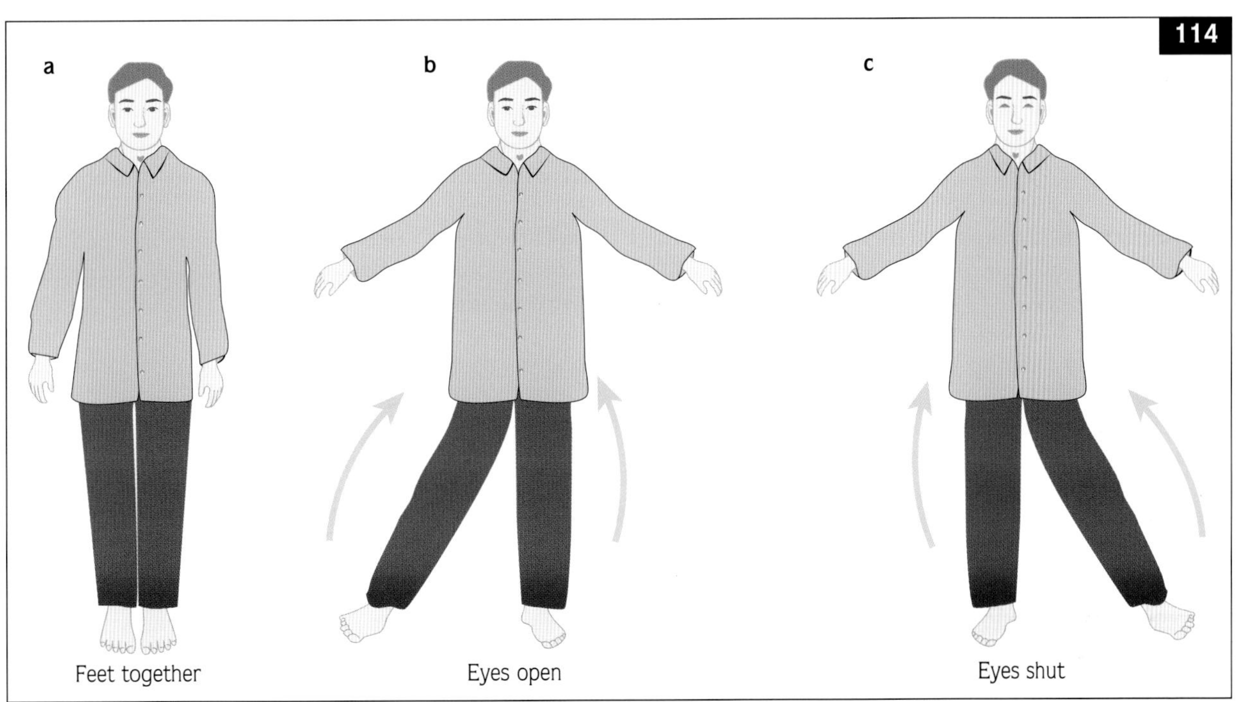

114 Diagram to illustrate Romberg's test. The patient should be asked to stand upright, with feet together and eyes open (**a**). Staggering and unsteadiness with the eyes open suggest a cerebellar lesion (**b**). The patient is then asked to shut their eyes; unsteadiness at this stage is strongly suggestive of a defect of joint position sense, but can also occur in patients with vestibular impairment (**c**).

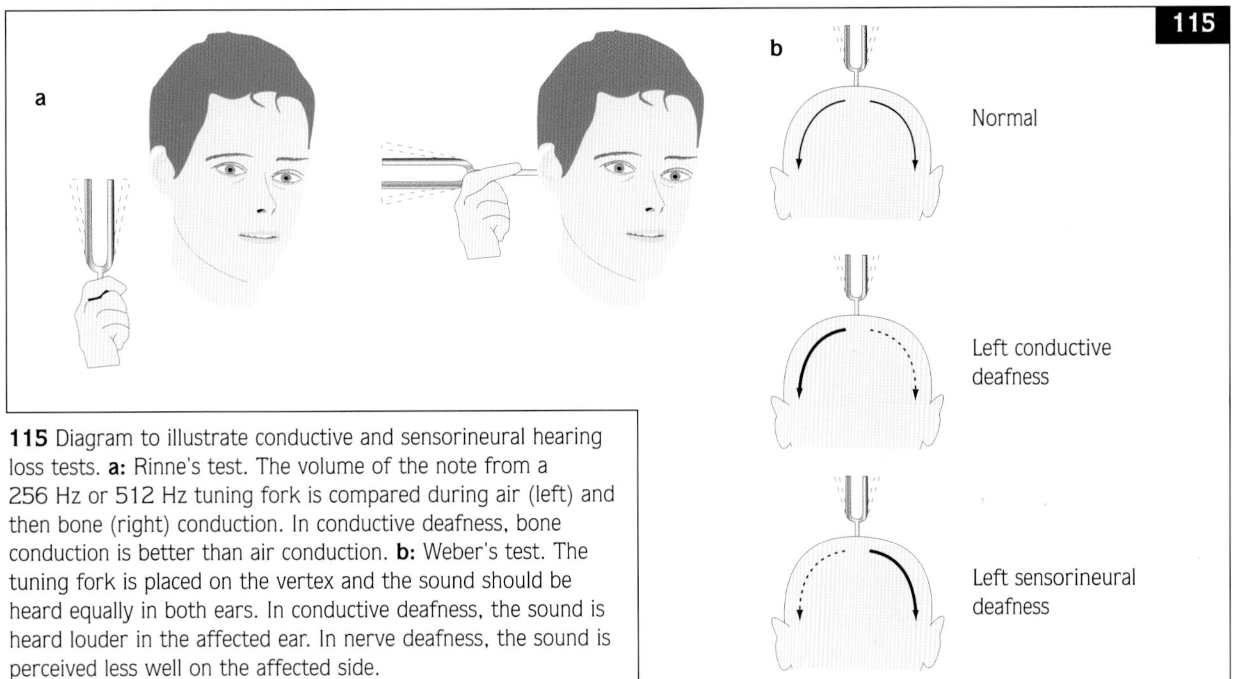

115 Diagram to illustrate conductive and sensorineural hearing loss tests. **a:** Rinne's test. The volume of the note from a 256 Hz or 512 Hz tuning fork is compared during air (left) and then bone (right) conduction. In conductive deafness, bone conduction is better than air conduction. **b:** Weber's test. The tuning fork is placed on the vertex and the sound should be heard equally in both ears. In conductive deafness, the sound is heard louder in the affected ear. In nerve deafness, the sound is perceived less well on the affected side.

heard with that perceived when the tuning fork is pressed against the mastoid bone. Normally air conduction of sound is more efficient than bone conduction, but when there is conductive deafness the reverse is the case. In Weber's test, the vibrating tuning fork is applied to the midline of the forehead and the patient is asked whether they hear the sound in the middle of their head, or in either ear.

> If a patient has sensorineural deafness in one ear the sound will appear to arise on the healthy side (in the good ear). Conversely, if there is conductive hearing loss on one side, the sound will appear to arise from the affected side (the bad ear): it is for this reason that Rinne's test must be performed first to exclude conductive hearing loss before proceeding to Weber's test.

Causes of hearing loss associated with vertigo tend to be sensorineural. Tympanic membranes should be inspected for wax, perforation, otitis, and mass lesions, particularly if conductive hearing loss is detected by Rinne's test.

Neurological examination

Cranial nerves

Fundoscopy should be performed to look for signs of raised intracranial pressure and vascular changes associated with diabetes and hypertension. Optic atrophy (seen as a pale optic disc) should be sought as evidence of previous, possibly subclinical, demyelination. Eye movements should be examined, firstly to look for nystagmus (see below), but also to seek evidence of gaze palsy, internuclear ophthalmoplegia, or III, IV, or VI cranial nerve palsy, any of which would indicate structural brainstem disease and a central cause of vertigo. Examination for these problems is discussed in more detail on pages 104–112. Facial nerve palsy accompanying vertigo indicates structural disease of the internal auditory canal, cerebellopontine angle, or brainstem. The fifth (V) cranial nerve may also be affected by lesions in the cerebellopontine angle, hence the importance of testing for facial numbness and absent corneal reflex. Generally, cerebellopontine angle lesions (common examples being acoustic neuroma, meningioma, and metastasis) present with hearing loss rather than vertigo.

Motor system (see page 148)

Testing for long tract motor signs (tone, power, and reflexes) is important to document any subclinical disease affecting the pyramidal tracts. This localizes the cause of vertigo or imbalance in the brainstem (for example in brainstem stroke or Arnold–Chiari malformation), or indicates pyramidal pathology elsewhere in the nervous system, which can occur in demyelination.

Cerebellar system (see page 176)

Cerebellar disease causes unsteadiness and ataxia, rather than the sensations of dizziness or vertigo, but because of the close interrelationship between the cerebellar and vestibular systems both functionally and neuroanatomically, it is mandatory to test for upper limb cerebellar signs (finger-nose-finger test and rapid alternating movements [dysdiadochokinesis]) and lower limb cerebellar signs (heel-shin test) in all dizzy and vertiginous patients. Abnormalities indicate disease of the cerebellum or its connections, and tend to occur ipsilateral to any cerebellar lesion.

Sensory system (see page 214)

Proprioception (joint and position sense), mediated by large fibre peripheral nerves and the posterior columns of the spinal cord, is fundamental to maintaining equilibrium. If reduced it will cause imbalance and unsteadiness; this may be initially apparent only in the dark because vision compensates for any deficiency. Minor reductions in proprioception, common as people age, may exacerbate dizziness from other causes.

Nystagmus assessment

Nystagmus is an involuntary oscillation of the eyes. Nystagmus may be pendular (equal velocity and amplitude in both directions of movement [sinusoidal]) or jerk (slow phase drift in one direction, then a corrective quick phase in the other). The fast phase of jerk nystagmus is used to define the direction of the nystagmus, though the pathological movement is the slow one. Nystagmus usually involves a to-and-fro oscillating movement of the eyes, but there may be torsional or rotatory components. Torsional movements (around the viewing axis of the eye) are seen with both end-organ and brainstem vestibular disturbance. Rotatory nystagmus (a variety of pendular nystagmus, but occurring in two planes) usually implies brainstem disease. A full discussion of nystagmus is beyond the scope of this chapter, but a distinction should be made between spontaneous nystagmus and that observed on provocative testing.

Spontaneous nystagmus. Nystagmus seen in the primary position is usually either congenital or due to an acquired vestibular disturbance. Vestibular nystagmus is typically brought out by the elimination of visual fixation (e.g. covering one eye while viewing the other with an ophthalmoscope), congenital the reverse. Nystagmus only seen on eccentric gaze is most often gaze-evoked nystagmus, and is commonly seen in drug intoxication and cerebellar disease.

Provocative testing. Dix–Hallpike's test for positional nystagmus is vital to diagnose BPPV (**116**). Headshake testing involves vigorously shaking the head from side to side some 20 times. It stimulates the vestibular system, and may 'bring out' a latent asymmetry of the vestibular apparatuses, manifest as a short-lived vestibular nystagmus.

The integrity of the vestibulo-ocular system can be assessed in a number of ways. In the Doll's eye manoeuvre, the head is oscillated vertically or horizontally, and normally a fully corrective movement of the eyes in the opposite direction is observed. This is particularly helpful in the unconscious patient (to demonstrate intact vestibulo-ocular reflexes) or when looking for supranuclear gaze disorders. The head thrust test involves a more rapid head movement with the eyes fixed on a point ahead. Abnormality of the reflex is demonstrated by lagging eye movements relative to the head shift. Dynamic visual acuity is an assessment of any alteration in visual acuity when the head is turned back and forth (at approximately 2 Hz). Normal subjects drop a maximum of one line of Snellen visual acuity with head movement.

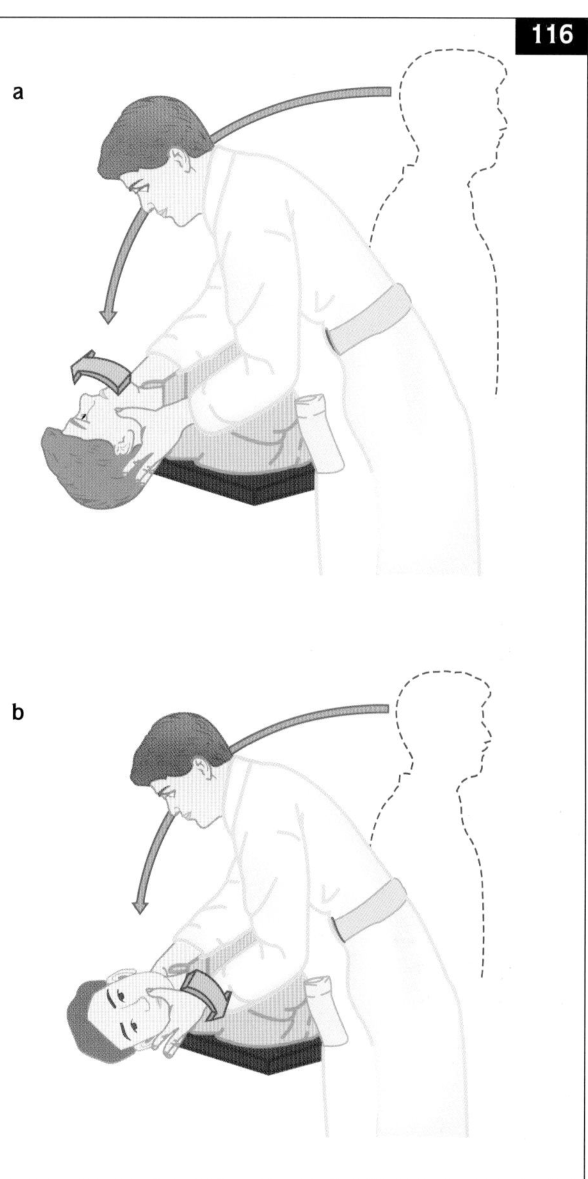

116 Diagram to illustrate the Dix–Hallpike positional test. The patient is positioned so that when lying flat, the head extends over the end of the table. With the patient sitting upright, the physician turns and holds the patient's head at 45° to the side (right or left). The patient is then rapidly laid down with the head extended over the edge of the table (**a, b**). The eyes are carefully observed for the development of positional nystagmus, which is usually not immediate. Severe vertiginous symptoms usually accompany a positive test. Finally, the patient should be sat upright and the eyes observed for nystagmus.

Investigations

These are guided by history and examination findings. Specific tests that are useful in different clinical situations are illustrated in *Table 25*.

SUMMARY

- ❑ Dizziness is a nonspecific term which should provoke further enquiry to establish what the patient means.
- ❑ Vertigo is an illusion of movement due to disturbance of the vestibular system or its connections.
- ❑ Normal balance requires inputs from the visual, proprioceptive, and vestibular systems; impairment of any can contribute to impaired balance. Assess all three.
- ❑ Brief episodes of rotatory vertigo lasting seconds are usually due to benign paroxysmal positional vertigo or vestibular decompensation.
- ❑ If the history suggests syncope or presyncope, a cardiovascular cause should be sought.
- ❑ Dizziness makes people fearful and anxious; anxiety and concern can make people feel dizzy. Sorting out the physical and emotional issues is a challenge for the physician.

Table 25 Clinical syndromes and their investigation

Acute severe vertigo	FBC, ESR, CRP, cholesterol, glucose ECG, echocardiogram MRI posterior fossa +/- gadolinium Audiogram (if hearing disturbance)
Positional vertigo	MRI posterior fossa +/- gadolinium Tilt table testing
Vertigo or dizziness with headache	MRI head +/- gadolinium Audiogram (if hearing disturbance)
Hydrops (hearing disturbance, vertigo, tinnitus)	Audiogram TFT, ESR VDRL / FTA
Medical dizziness	FBC, ESR, CRP, cholesterol, glucose ECG, echocardiogram 24-hr Holter monitor Tilt table testing Autonomic function tests

CRP: C-reactive protein; ECG: electrocardiogram; ESR: erythrocyte sedimentation rate; FBC: full blood count; MRI: magnetic resonance imaging; TFT: thyroid function test; VDRL/FTA: serological tests for syphilis.

CLINICAL SCENARIOS

CASE 1

A previously well 58-year-old female bank clerk was referred by her general practitioner (GP) to the hospital complaining of recurrent attacks of dizziness.

The nature of the problem is at present unclear. 'Dizziness' can mean many things and requires closer investigation.

Her problems had started 5 months previously when she developed an illness over days, consisting of a sensation that the room was moving around her, nausea, vomiting, and malaise. Her GP had seen her, told her that she had a viral infection, and had treated her with antibiotics and a vestibular sedative (betahistine). At the start she had been unable to move because it made her so dizzy. Her symptoms slowly improved over 2 weeks, and she was then able to return to work at the bank.

Careless questioning or very directed inquiry into the present problem may have missed this vital aspect of the history. The major symptom of this illness, which appears to have been monophasic, sounds like vertigo. It is difficult to be absolutely certain merely on the basis of this history whether the vestibular disturbance causing the vertigo was peripheral or central: histories recalled some time after the event are likely to be a little uncertain. The other symptoms of nausea, vomiting, and malaise can occur in both peripheral and central disturbances, but there are no specific brainstem features to suggest that she may have suffered a stroke, and the onset was not sudden. Her symptoms slowly resolved over 2 weeks, and the onset, timing, and nature of the illness seem most consistent with acute peripheral vestibulopathy, presumed secondary to viral infection.

Since that time she complained of recurring attacks of the room spinning around her in a horizontal (yaw) plane. This was happening on multiple occasions every day. Each attack lasted about 10 seconds and seemed to occur whenever she turned in bed, lay down, or sat up from the supine position.

This disorder is episodic, and the complaint is specifically one of vertigo. The problem is clearly positional, which immediately narrows the possibilities (for example cardiac arrhythmias are unlikely to be positional). It does not appear to be a postural problem (suggesting postural hypotension), because turning and lying down cause difficulties as much as standing up. The duration of each episode is extremely short, and this is very characteristic of BPPV. It can also occur in vestibular decompensation after acute events.

There were no other associated symptoms, including no visual symptoms, no numbness, and no weakness. Her general health was excellent in the past. She was a teetotal nonsmoker who exercised regularly and lived with her husband. She was taking no medication when seen.

These are important negatives: central disorders affecting vestibular tracts usually (but not always) cause other brainstem symptoms. The lack of past history and low vascular risk again make stroke unlikely as the cause of her initial illness.

She had equal and reactive pupils. Extraocular movements were full and there was no spontaneous nystagmus. Visual fields were full and fundoscopy was normal. There was no facial weakness or sensory disturbance and hearing was normal. Motor examination showed normal bulk, tone, and power throughout. There were no upper limb cerebellar signs and tandem gait was normal. Reflexes were symmetric and plantar responses were flexor.

These are all important negatives: standard neurological examination was normal. The symptoms, however, are clearly provoked by positional change, and so it is mandatory to perform positional manoeuvres.

A Dix–Hallpike manoeuvre performed with the head turned toward the right did not produce any nystagmus. On repetition with the head turned toward the left, she developed an up-beating torsional nystagmus after a period of 5 to 10 seconds. This subsided after an additional 10–15 seconds. Repetition of the manoeuvre resulted in identical symptoms of lesser severity.

(Continued overleaf)

CASE 1 *(continued)*

These findings on examination establish a diagnosis of BPPV referable to her left posterior semicircular canal.

After a single Epley repositioning procedure (a postural means of treating this condition), no more positional vertigo and nystagmus could be provoked and symptoms resolved.

It is important to realize that 50–80% of patients with BPPV are cured by a single Epley manoeuvre. If it is unsuccessful, the procedure should be immediately repeated, and this increases the success rate to approximately 90%.

CASE 2

A 51-year-old diabetic female developed episodes of dizziness and falling, and was referred to the hospital for investigation. She had been diabetic for 30 years, and had been treated with subcutaneous insulin for that time. She had a history of depression, and her diabetes had been poorly controlled for many years, in part due to poor compliance with medication. For the last 3 years she had been on peritoneal dialysis for end-stage renal disease, and she was awaiting a kidney transplant. She had hypertension and had developed numerous diabetic complications including retinopathy, peripheral vascular disease, and cerebrovascular disease. She had recently been in hospital after a right subcortical stroke that had caused a minor left hemiparesis.

It is often rewarding to enquire about complex medical histories such as these at the start of consultations, since this kind of background is likely to have such an important bearing on the interpretation of the current problem. Diabetic patients can become dizzy because of hypoglycaemia, and patients with renal disease (particularly those on dialysis which involves large fluid shifts) often have difficulties with blood pressure control. Retinopathy may affect the visual component of the sensory system, peripheral vascular disease may affect sensation from the feet, and diabetic patients often have peripheral neuropathy, which commonly affects joint position sense. The patient's recent stroke will have affected motor control, making her more prone to falls. Interpretation of the current problem is much more straightforward if it is considered in the context of the past medical history.

About 3 weeks previously, she had developed episodes of weakness, dizziness, and lightheadedness. Her symptoms were intermittent, unrelated to time of day or meal times, and variable in duration and severity. She felt that nearly all of the episodes had occurred when she was standing, and that a number had occurred shortly after she had stood up from sitting down. When she felt dizzy her vision had become blurred and dark on a number of occasions and friends had said she had been pale. She felt that she was unsteady and losing her balance, and said that when she was walking she veered from side to side. She had had a number of sudden and unexpected falls. Her blood glucose readings had been either normal or high.

She has a number of symptoms. She has symptoms of presyncope that seem to be postural, she has symptoms of disequilibrium, and her loss of balance and walking difficulty raise the possibility that she is ataxic. She does **not** *describe vertigo. The events are not occurring at particular times of the day, and monitoring of her glucose had not shown anything to suggest hypoglycaemia, so this seems unlikely. Because her medical history is so complex and could affect so many systems, it is very possible that a number of aetiologies are contributing to the clinical picture here.*

(Continued on page 145)

Case 2 *(continued)*

She was taking oral iron, multivitamins, an angiotensin-converting enzyme (ACE) inhibitor (enalapril 10 mg/day), subcutaneous insulin, and warfarin adjusted to her international normalized ratio (INR). This had been recently introduced because her subcortical stroke had occurred while she was taking aspirin and the physician in charge of her care wanted a stronger treatment to prevent further cerebrovascular events occurring. She had also been taking amitryptiline (100 mg) at night for depression, but had recently discontinued this on her own, having been concerned that this may be causing her to feel dizzy. This had improved her dizziness markedly, and she had had no further falls.

Often the patient will be an excellent judge of both the nature and cause of the problem: discontinuing the amitryptiline has helped her symptoms. This agent is known to cause postural hypotension, and probably caused more problems because she was also taking enalapril. Dialysis patients are more prone to postural hypotension, as mentioned above. The warfarin prescription is a concern. Patients who are prone to falls should only be prescribed warfarin after very careful consideration because it makes them more likely to have major haemorrhage if they sustain significant trauma.

She was in sinus rhythm. Blood pressure was 146/92 mmHg (19.5/12.3 kPa) supine, and 138/86 mmHg (18.4/11.5 kPa) when standing. There were no murmurs or bruits. Pulses in the legs were absent below the femoral. She was unable to tandem walk, and Romberg's test was positive. Corrected visual acuity was 6/24 on both sides. Fundoscopy revealed dot and blot haemorrhages and hard exudates around the macula. Eye movements were normal. She had a minor left facial weakness and mild left hemiparesis with the arm worse than the leg. Reflexes were absent at the ankles, but otherwise present with reinforcement. Her left plantar response was extensor. She had marked reduction in sensation to pin prick and temperature distally up to mid shin, and markedly decreased joint position sense loss and vibration sense loss in the feet.

There is no significant blood pressure fall on standing now, but this does not negate the history of postural events, and the symptomatic improvement on stopping amitryptiline. She has severe peripheral vascular disease, and retinopathy that appears to be affecting her macula and acuity. The left hemiparesis and extensor plantar response are consistent with the known history of recent right subcortical stroke. The new and pertinent finding is of signs consistent with a diabetic peripheral neuropathy.

A selective serotonin reuptake inhibitor (citalopram) was introduced for depression in place of amitryptiline. Anticoagulation was discontinued (there was no real indication for it, and it posed significant risk if falls recurred), and she was started on a statin and clopidogrel as vascular prophylaxis. She was assessed by a physiotherapist and provided with a stick.

Several factors contributed to the dizziness and falls in this case, including presyncope from orthostatic hypotension, motor disequilibrium related to her hemiparesis, and sensory disequilibrium related to her neuropathy and impaired proprioception.

Case 3

A 34-year-old female was referred for a neurological opinion because of persistent dizziness. She described a constant feeling of being dizzy with fluctuating severity over the past 6 months. The problem had begun while in a shopping centre when she felt very unwell, thought she would faint, became very frightened, and had to be helped to the car and driven home by her husband. Ever since she had been reluctant to go shopping on her own.

So far there is nothing in this history to suggest an obvious cause. As previously mentioned, patients who experience dizziness from whatever cause find the experience frightening, and anxious patients frequently complain of dizziness. One possibility is that this was an episode of presyncope but more information is needed.

On direct questioning, it was clear that she had never experienced vertigo either in relation to the present symptoms or in the past, had no symptoms to suggest middle or inner ear disease, and nothing to suggest a brainstem disorder. There was no history of cardiac arrhythmia and no previous faints or migraine.

Again, no history to give a clear pointer as to a cause for her dizziness. The medical interview should also involve an attempt to get to know a little about the patient as a person, what is happening in their lives, how they are feeling in themselves, and what their concerns are. It seems as if this may be particularly important here.

On gentle enquiry, it emerged that she was under great strain at the present time. She was a mother of three young children and also ran a preschool nursery. Her husband was a busy accountant, and she had to care for her elderly mother who lived nearby and who had become increasingly infirm. She prided herself on her ability to cope with all these pressures, but had recently begun to feel tired during the day and to have disturbed sleep. She had found the episode in the shopping mall very frightening, and specifically had thought she was going to die of a stroke like her father. When concern about this abated she became convinced that she had a serious disorder such as a tumour or MS.

The neurological and general medical examinations were normal. Specifically, there was no evidence of vestibular disorder, nothing to suggest other neurological disease, and the cardiac examination was unremarkable.

All of the above suggests that the complaint of dizziness is related to her life situation and not disease of the nervous system. The strict psychiatric terminology for her symptoms would require expert assessment and a great deal more information, but physical symptoms of 'stress' are very common, especially in patients who 'cope' with difficult and stressful lives. Such patients are often resistant to a psychological or stress-related interpretation of their symptoms, largely because they seem so real and serious. Terminology in this area is notoriously difficult. 'Somatization' refers to the process whereby mental distress is expressed in physical symptoms. 'Functional neurological symptoms' is a better term, implying a deficit of functioning of the nervous system, rather than a structural disorder of it. The brain can frequently produce physical symptoms that suggest a disorder of the body and hence cause illness without evident disease.

An explanation that there was no sign of serious disease as feared by the patient produced a degree of relief but the subsequent suggestion that the symptoms might be stress-related was met with considerable scepticism. Eventually normal investigations including cerebral imaging together with the support of her family and physician encouraged her to make alterations in her life that led to the ultimate resolution of her symptoms.

Revision questions

1 Which of the following statements are true?
  a Dizziness often coexists with vertigo, but is not the same as vertigo.
  b Dizziness always implies neurological disease.
  c The vestibular apparatus projects sensory information to the cerebellum and parieto-temporal cortex.
  d Peripheral vertigo is often rotational and in a yaw plane.
  e Vestibular sensory information is conveyed with sensory information from the cochlea (hearing) in the VIIIth cranial nerve.

2 Five 'symptom complexes' and five common 'disease processes' are shown below. Match each symptom complex with a disease process that is a common cause:

a Acute severe vertigo.	1 Migraine with aura.
b Positional vertigo.	2 Ménière's disease.
c Vertigo with headache.	3 Postural hypotension.
d Hydrops (hearing disturbance, vertigo, tinnitus).	4 Acute peripheral vestibulopathy.
e Medical dizziness.	5 Benign paroxysmal positional vertigo.

3 Which of the following statements about the assessment of a patient complaining of dizziness are true?
  a Cardiovascular examination may be omitted if there is no history of altered consciousness.
  b Weber's test lateralizes to the right in a patient with conductive hearing loss on the right.
  c In a patient with benign paroxysmal positional vertigo, Hallpike's test usually reproduces the symptoms.
  d A history of imbalance in the dark is suggestive of a proprioceptive (joint position sense) deficit.
  e Sudden severe vertigo in combination with diplopia is most likely to be caused by acute peripheral vestibulopathy.

Answers

1 a, c, d, e

2 a with 4
b with 5
c with 1
d with 2
e with 3

3 b, c, d

Disorders of motility

WEAKNESS

Richard Petty

INTRODUCTION

The assessment of a complaint of weakness is critically dependent on the correct interpretation of patients' subjective symptoms. The term weakness means a reduction in strength but is rarely used in this medical sense (*Table 26*); it is more often used to describe a feeling of fatigue. The most important step with complaints of weakness is to be certain to understand what the patient is trying to describe. A complaint of weakness and malaise is common but disorders producing weakness are relatively uncommon; motor neurone disease (MND) has a prevalence of 1:20,000 and Duchenne muscular dystrophy (DMD), the commonest muscular dystrophy, is present in 1:3,500 male births. Non-neurological disease may also result in complaints of weakness and fatigue (*Table 27*). *Table 28* indicates the range of symptoms arising from weakness in differing distributions. Asking specifically about these abilities will help to clarify the clinical problem.

Table 26 Symptoms giving rise to complaints of 'weakness'

- ❑ Fatigue
- ❑ Feelings of tiredness/sleep disorders
- ❑ Depressive illness
- ❑ Numbness leading to motor dysfunction
- ❑ Incoordination
- ❑ Stiffness in Parkinson's disease

Table 27 Non-neurological causes of complaints of weakness and fatigue

Cardiac disease	Ischaemic cardiac disease: angina pectoris Low-output cardiac failure, congestive cardiomyopathies Low output secondary to obstruction: aortic stenosis
Pulmonary disease	Gas exchange failure: pulmonary fibrosis Bellows failure (diaphragm or intercostals weakness) may be a neuromuscular cause
Systemic disease	Anaemia Cachexia in malignancy Depression with complaints of weakness

Table 28 Symptoms resulting from weakness in differing distributions

Distal upper limb	Unable to open door handles Difficulty with zips and buttons Unable to carry shopping Deterioration in handwriting
Proximal upper limb	Cannot put on shirt/jacket Unable to lift objects down from a high shelf Difficulty in combing hair
Distal lower limb	Easy tripping if ankle dorsiflexors are weak Inability to run if ankle plantarflexors are weak Instability over rough ground
Proximal lower limb	Difficulty in rising from a low chair or bath Difficulty ascending the stairs (glutei) Difficulty descending the stairs (quadriceps) Waddling gait

Functional anatomy and physiology

The motor unit comprises the anterior horn cell or motor neurone, its axon, and the muscle fibres innervated by that axon (**117**). The number of muscle fibres supplied by a single motor neurone is variable and is dependent on the function of the muscle. Large muscles such as the quadriceps have motor units comprising many hundreds of muscle fibres, whereas in the facial muscles there may be single numbers. The movement of interdigitating filaments of myosin and actin generate muscle contraction (**118**). The interaction of actin with myosin is triggered by the

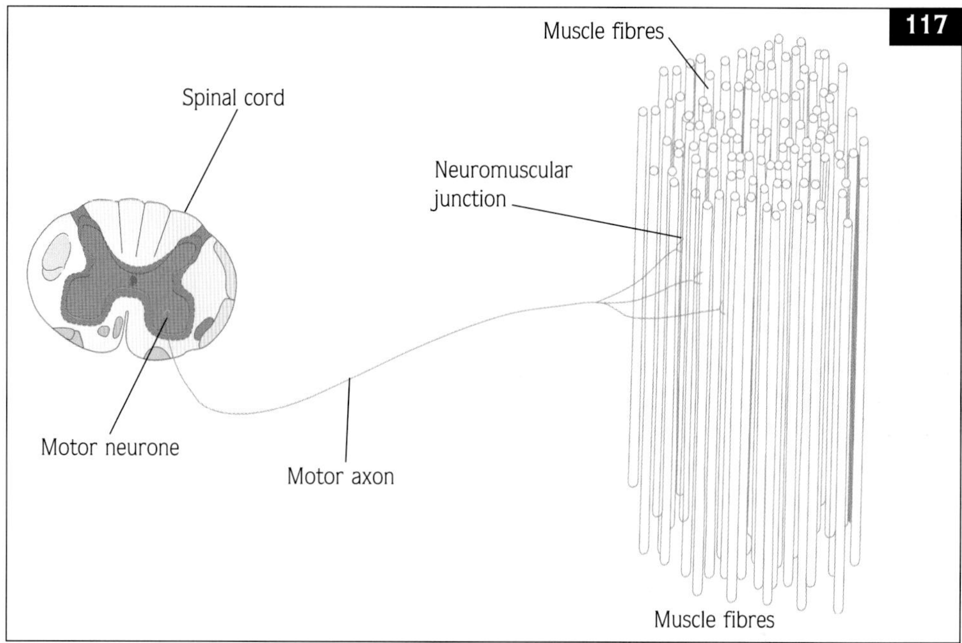

117 Diagram of a motor unit showing axon supplying many muscle fibres.

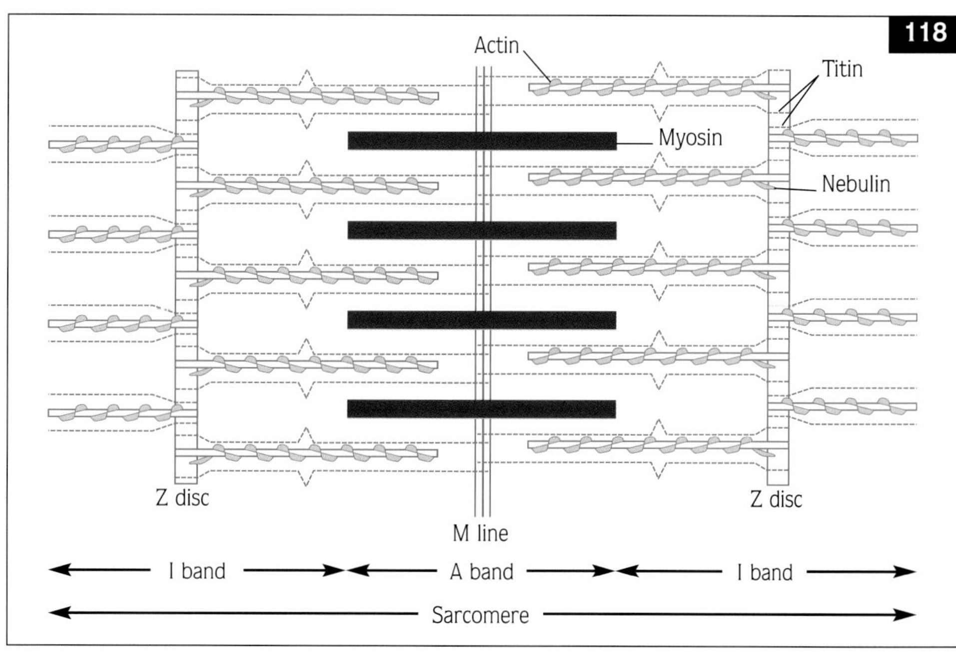

118 Diagram of a sarcomere with subcomponents.

release of calcium from the specialized endoplasmic reticulum termed the sarcoplasmic reticulum (**119**). This calcium release is triggered by the passage of an electrical impulse along the muscle membrane. Neuromuscular transmission is a complex process involving influx of calcium into the terminal motor axon, which then triggers the release of acetylcholine stored in presynaptic vesicles. Acetylcholine diffuses across the synaptic cleft, activates the acetylcholine receptor on the muscle membrane to allow ingress of sodium, and sets off the electrical impulse in the muscle fibre. The energy for muscle contraction is generated by glycolysis (the breakdown of glucose) occurring in the sarcoplasm and by oxidative phosphorylation taking place in the mitochondria.

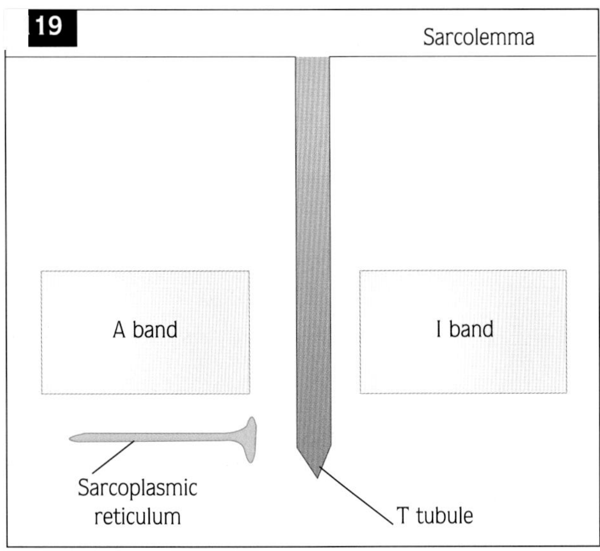

119 Diagram of the sarcoplasmic reticulum.

The pattern of innervation determines many physiological and biochemical characteristics of the muscle fibre. The major division is between fast twitch, glycolysis-dependent fibres and slow twitch, fatigue-resistant, oxidative fibres. Disease or dysfunction of any component may result in weakness and it can be hard in practice to distinguish between weaknesses due to the individual components. Many systems determine the activity of the motor unit, and dysfunction of these systems may also give rise to weakness (**120**).

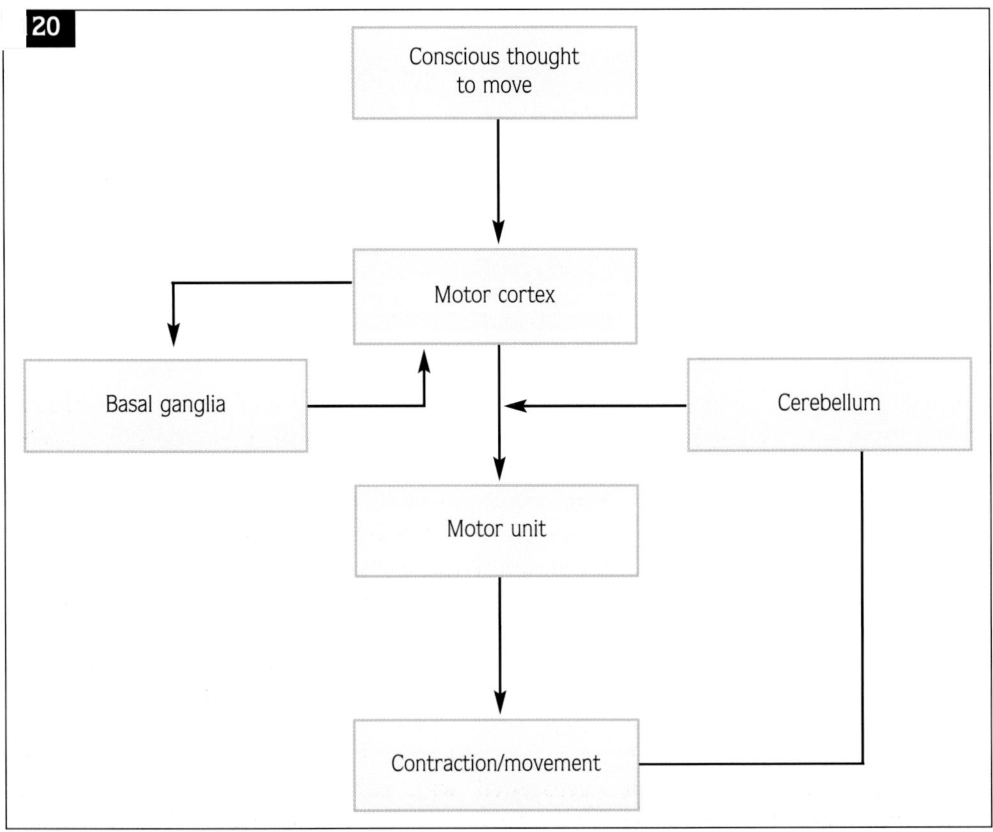

120 Diagram to show the anatomy of motor control.

> A critical distinction that has to be made is between weakness resulting from a motor unit (lower motor neurone [LMN]) weakness and from the upper motor neurone (UMN).

The distinction rests on aspects of the examination and the presence or absence of additional features (*Table 28*; see Introduction).

The following terms are used to describe the localization of weakness and reflect important anatomical distinctions:

- Intracranial; remember the cranial nerve nuclei are within the skull.
- Spinal; taken to mean the process is localized below the foramen magnum but with no better localization.
- Disorders of the motor neurone itself are referred to as motor neuronopathies.
- Disorders of the emerging motor axons (for example disc protrusions) within the spinal canal are referred to as root lesions or radiculopathies.
- A plexus lesion (often infiltrative) is due to damage to all or part of the brachial or lumbosacral plexus.
- Peripheral nerve disorders are classified according to whether a single nerve is involved: a mononeuropathy (often mechanical); many individual nerves at discrete sites (mononeuritis multiplex, seen in inflammatory diseases); or, if all nerves are involved, a diffuse peripheral neuropathy (as in diabetes mellitus). Further refinements in description refer to the involvement of sensory, motor, or autonomic fibres. On occasion it is also possible to describe whether the axon or myelin sheath is the site of pathology, axonal or demyelinating neuropathies.
- The neuromuscular junction is a potential site of pathology.
- A myopathy is any disease where the muscle cells are the primary site of pathology. A muscular dystrophy is a genetically determined, progressive disorder of muscle characterized by muscle fibre necrosis.

Clinical assessment

Focused history taking

History taking from a patient with a complaint of weakness must start by characterizing the severity and pattern of the weakness. The problems shown in *Table 28* offer a guide, but patients should be encouraged to elaborate on the difficulties they have. It is also critical in formulating a diagnosis to be certain about the timing of onset of symptoms and the pattern of evolution. Questions should be asked of early development (of parents if necessary) and abilities at games at school. Lost skills or abilities noted either by the patient or other family member will give an index of the rate of evolution of the illness. In addition, the specific aspects described below should be covered.

Pain

Pain arising as a direct consequence of primary muscle disease is usually precisely localized by the patient to muscle. They know it is muscle pain and not joint or nonspecific deep pain. In metabolic defects such as McArdle's disease (a disorder of glycogen breakdown), it is clearly related to exercise: severe pain with contracture develops often within 1 minute of ischaemic exercise and affects the exercising muscle only.

Cramp

Muscle cramps are universal and normal and are most often felt in the calf muscles. They are associated with high frequency, irregular bursts of muscle fibre activity and originate in distal motor axons. Fasciculations are the spontaneous discharge of all the muscle fibres in a motor unit and are common in motor unit diseases such as amyotrophic lateral sclerosis (i.e. MND). Patients may be aware of this spontaneous activity. Painful cramps on exercise are a feature of some metabolic myopathies and, if cramps are complained of, the relationship to exercise should be clarified.

Fatiguability

This is another term rarely used in the medical sense of an excessive failure of strength on repeated contraction. It is more often used in the context of systemic disorders such as anaemia or nonspecific feelings of exhaustion. True fatigue is a feature of neuromuscular transmission disorders and is also a major feature of disorders of energy metabolism (such as mitochondrial disorders), where it is often associated with malaise, headache or nausea and (sometimes) vomiting, reflecting an exercise-induced lactic acidosis. The word is also often used to describe the exercise limitation occurring in disorders associated with cardiomyopathies or respiratory muscle weakness (which may exist without clinically obvious limb muscle involvement) such as myotonic dystrophy or acid maltase deficiency.

It is also important to then ask about any possible symptoms of weakness elsewhere that the patient may not recognize as due to weakness, or may not have recognized as important.

Complaints of double vision occur when control of eye movement is lost. This can be as a result of brainstem disease, a lesion affecting the oculomotor nerves, a neuromuscular transmission disorder, or a primary myopathy. Changes in the quality of speech have been discussed in the Introduction, but it is often helpful to ask the patient to talk for a period of time if weakness of the bulbar muscles is suspected. Relatives may also comment on a change not noted by the patient. Changes in swallowing, like double vision, can be due to problems at many sites but it is important to ask directly whether the patient has noted change. Questions concerning family history, drug history, and social history are also critical:

- Family history. Inherited disorders of peripheral nerve and muscle are among the most common inherited disorders. It is important when taking a history to ask about other family members. Some disorders are mild and it may be necessary to examine other family members to establish the diagnosis of an inherited disorder.
- Drug history. Drug toxicities are a major cause of peripheral nerve disease. Some cytotoxic drugs used in cancer treatment will almost invariably cause some damage to peripheral nerves. A full current and recent past drug history must be taken. Steroid drugs are a common cause of a proximal muscle weakness although muscle toxicity is an unusual drug side-effect.
- Occupational history. This is important not only in establishing prior levels of physical ability but will also determine the impact of a particular deficit on an individual. Questions should also be asked of current domestic circumstances and how people are managing daily tasks within the home.

Questioning should then return to the presenting complaint and should involve direct questions pertinent to the possible localization of the problem. Such questions might include:

- Cortical: lateralized weakness may be due to a cortical lesion where questions about headache or focal seizures are important. A frontal lesion may give rise to anosmia.
- Hemisphere: movement disorder if basal ganglia are involved, headache if a mass lesion is suspected.
- Brainstem: many possible features including diplopia, dysarthria, dysphagia, facial sensory abnormalities, vertigo, and disequilibrium.
- Spinal cord: the important observation is that symptoms can be localized to a level; there will be no symptoms or signs referable above and the problems can be accounted for by disease at one level. Problems may include sensory loss (which may be dissociated, see below) and bladder dysfunction (see below).
- Nerve root: symptoms and signs may involve a sensory disturbance in the territory of the affected root (**121**) and discomfort in the innervated myotome, i.e. the muscles innervated by that root (*Table 29*). The reflex arc subserved by that root may be depressed or absent as the process affects both afferent and efferent pathways (**122**).

Table 29 Myotomes of importance

C5	Deltoid, biceps
C6	Biceps, brachio-radialis
C7	Triceps
C8	Finger flexors
T1	All intrinsic hand muscles
L1, 2	Hip flexion
L3	Knee extension
L4	Knee extension, hip flexion, ankle dorsiflexion
L5	Ankle dorsiflexion and eversion, hip extension, knee flexion
S1	Ankle plantarflexion

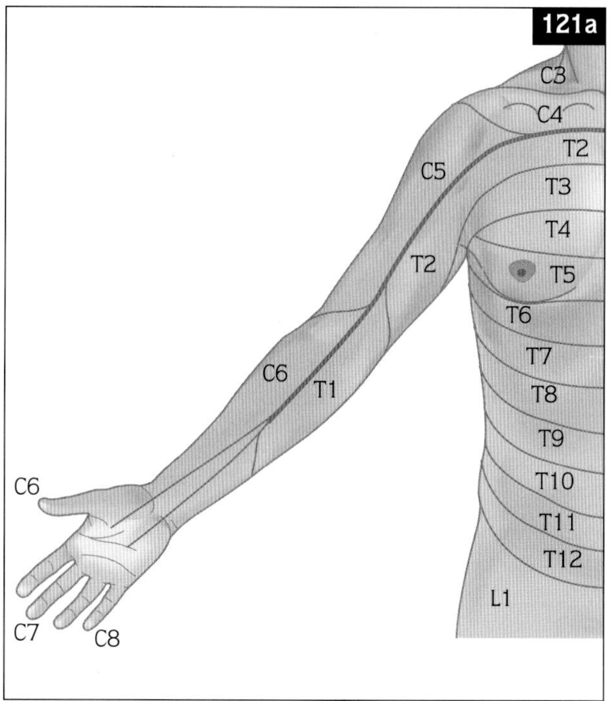

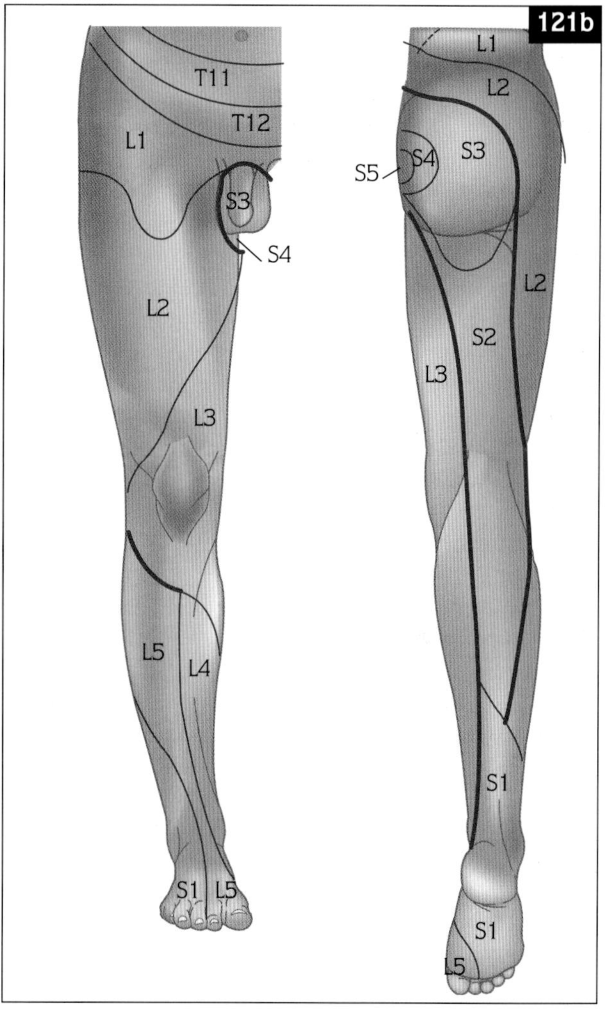

121 Diagram to show the dermatomal supply of the upper (**a**) and lower (**b**) limbs.

122 Diagram to show the anatomy of the spinal cord.

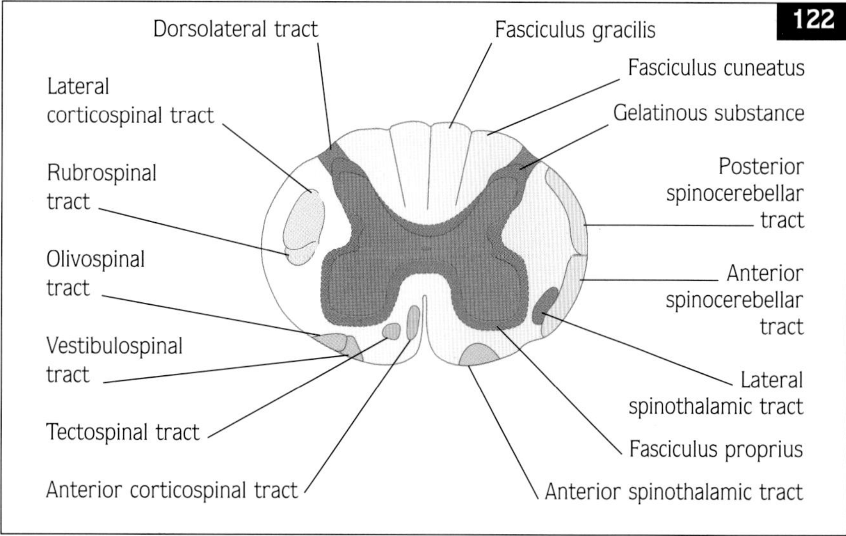

- Peripheral nerve: symptoms and signs will be restricted to the distribution of the affected nerve. Again, motor and sensory function will be affected (*Table 30*, **123**).
- Neuromuscular junction: symptoms and signs will be purely motor. Fatiguability, if sought, is usually a prominent feature. These disorders, despite affecting all muscles, may present with very focal symptoms. Reflexes are usually preserved.
- Muscle: problems will be purely motor. Weakness and wasting are prominent features. Reflexes are usually unaffected; there is no damage to the reflex arc. The distribution of the weakness will be critical in making a diagnosis: is it proximal, distal, or selective?

Focused examination

Observation

It is important to watch someone walking. This may show the scissoring gait of spasticity, reveal a foot drop gait, or the slow initiation and turning of a movement disorder such as Parkinson's disease. If specific tasks are described as difficult then the patient should be asked to perform them if possible, and any difficulty observed. It is also critical to examine for muscle wasting; the upper limbs should be first examined from behind the shoulders so that the periscapular muscles can be seen. The arms, forearms, and hands are then looked at. These muscles are usually larger in the dominant arm. The hands should be held supinated to look at the forearm flexor muscles. The first dorsal interosseus and thenar eminence should be examined with care; wasting is easily missed. The limbs should be examined for any evidence of joint contracture.

Palpation

This is less important in the assessment of weakness, though inflammatory disorders may cause induration and muscle tenderness.

Power

Table 31 lists the muscles that should be routinely tested. This allows the major roots and peripheral nerves to be included in the assessment. It is important to recognize that the lower limb muscles are, in the normal situation, much stronger than the examiner's upper limb muscles, and mild weakness will not be detectable when testing strength on the couch. In this situation, other tests are needed. Asking the patient to rise from a crouch tests hip extensors and knee extensors; to stand on tiptoes tests ankle plantarflexion; to walk on the heels tests dorsiflexion.

Table 30 Patterns of deficit in major peripheral nerve lesions

Radial nerve in radial groove on humerus
- Weakness of wrist extension
- Weakness of finger extension
- Loss of sensation in anatomical snuffbox

Ulnar nerve at elbow
- Weakness of flexor digitorum profundus III, IV
- Weakness of interossei in hand
- Sensory loss as shown (**123**)

Median nerve at wrist
- Weakness of abductor pollicis brevis
- Sensory loss as shown (**123**)

Lateral popliteal nerve at knee
- Weakness of ankle dorsiflexion
- Weakness of eversion

Table 31 Movements to be routinely tested

Movement	Muscle(s)	Peripheral nerve(s)	Root(s)
Shoulder abduction	Deltoid	Axillary	C5
Elbow flexion	Biceps	Musculocutaneous	C5,6
	Brachioradialis	Radial	
Elbow extension	Triceps	Radial	C7
Finger flexion	Long flexors	Anterior interosseus	C8
		Ulnar	
Finger abduction	Interossei	Ulnar	T1
Thumb abduction	Abductor pollicis brevis	Median	T1
Hip flexion	Iliopsoas		L1,2
Hip extension	Gluteus maximus	Sciatic	L5,S1
Knee flexion	Hamstrings	Sciatic	S1
Knee extension	Quadriceps	Femoral	L3,4
Ankle dorsiflexion	Tibialis anterior	Deep peroneal	L4,5
Ankle plantarflexion	Gastrocnemius Soleus	Tibial	S1,2

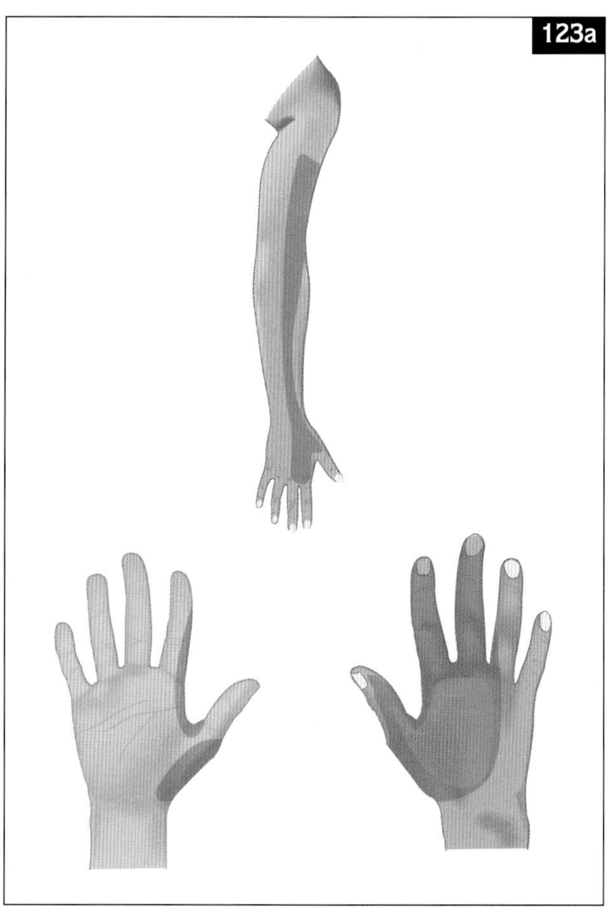

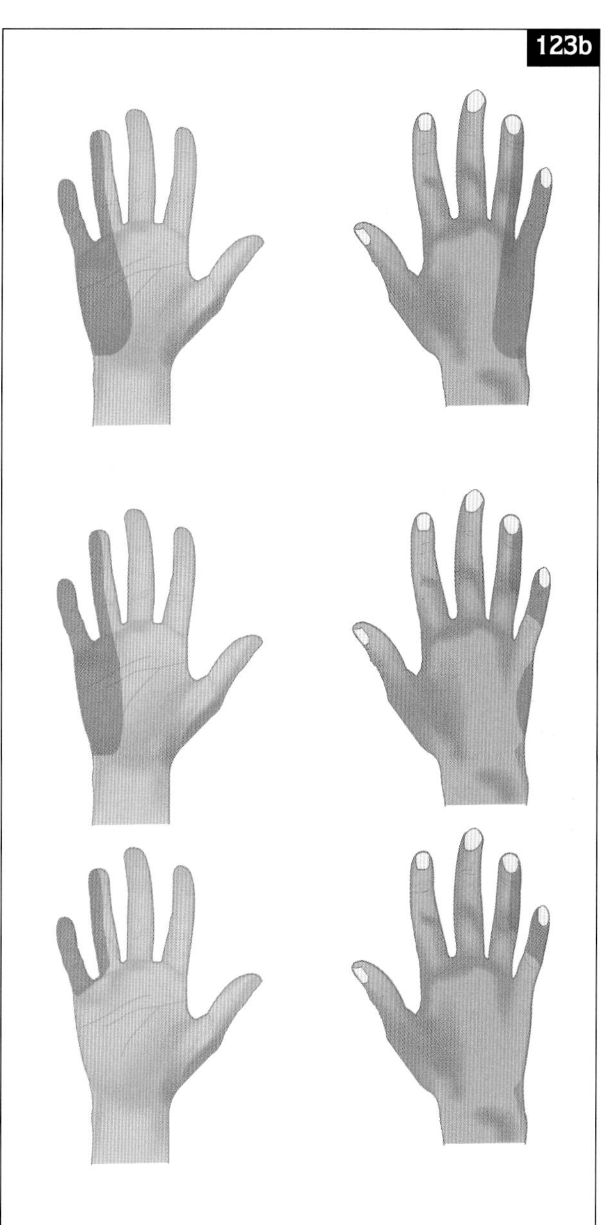

123 Diagram to show the sensory loss in lesions to the radial (**a**), ulnar (**b**), and median (**c**) nerves.

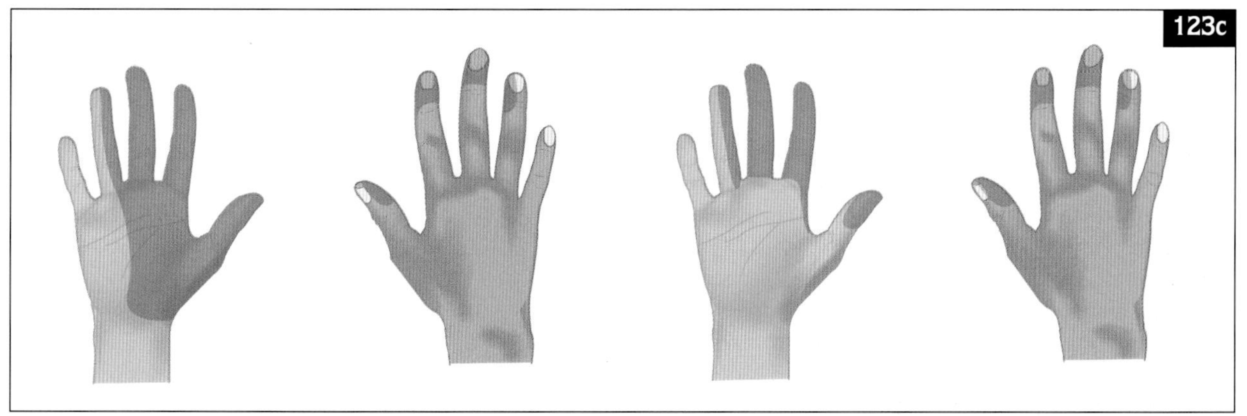

Tone, coordination, reflexes, and plantar responses
Muscle tone should assessed at the elbow, knee, and ankles. The assessment of coordination is usually regarded as part of the assessment of the motor system. It is important to remember, however, that coordination depends on an intact sensory system, brainstem, and cerebellum as much as on muscle power. Coordination can appear impaired if there is severe weakness. The reflexes that should always be assessed are shown in *Table 32* with the localization of the reflex arc.

The investigation of complaints of weakness is clearly critically dependent on accurate anatomical localization. It is usually possible to make a distinction between upper and lower motor neurone patterns (*Table 33*). Furthermore, careful history taking and examination should allow a judgement to be made as to whether a purely motor disorder is present or one involving sensory or autonomic function. If an anatomical localization is possible and a structural lesion is suspected, then imaging can be directed to that area. If muscle is thought to be the site of pathology the investigations described below may be considered.

Serum creatine kinase
Creatine kinase (CK) is an enzyme localized to the muscle sarcoplasm. A process leading to a loss of integrity of the muscle cell membrane will allow leakage of CK. CK levels can be measured in blood; however, it is important to recognize that the normal distribution in the population is skewed and although normal ranges are often quoted as 170 IU/l, many normal individuals will have levels between 200 and 300 IU/l. It is also a very sensitive test. Unaccustomed exercise can provoke a rise from normal to upwards of 1000 IU/l. This means that an isolated elevation must be interpreted with caution. Indeed, the changes in muscle arising from loss of the nerve supply (denervation) can be associated with rises of CK to 500–1000 IU/l.

Electromyography and nerve conduction studies
These neurophysiological studies address different questions. Electromyography (EMG) detects the electrical activity of muscle fibres using a needle inserted into resting and active muscle. The pattern of activity changes if there is ongoing denervation, damage to muscle membranes, or abnormally small muscle fibres. It also allows the detection of the large motor units seen in disorders where denervation is followed by reinnervation by surviving motor axons (**124**). Nerve conduction studies (NCS) use electrodes to record from both motor and sensory nerves. In usual practice, only myelinated axons are studied. Information is gathered on conduction velocity and the amplitude of the nerve impulse under study. The findings often allow a distinction to be made between disorders affecting the axon and those affecting the myelin sheath. They also allow motor and sensory fibre populations to be studied independently.

Muscle biopsy
Pathological examination of muscle is used if a primary disorder of muscle is suspected. It allows the specific diagnosis of some metabolic disorders and muscular dystrophies and is also important in the diagnosis of inflammatory muscle disease. The biopsy can be obtained by use of a wide bore needle (needle biopsy) or under direct vision (open biopsy).

Table 32 Reflexes routinely assessed

Reflex	Nerve root level
Biceps	C5, 6
Triceps	C7
Finger jerks	C8
Knee jerk	L3,4
Ankle jerk	S1,2

Table 33 Clinical features of upper and lower motor neurone weakness

	Upper motor neurone	Lower motor neurone
Power	Weakness of extensor muscles in the upper limbs and flexors in the lower limbs	Weakness restricted to muscles innervated by affected lower motor neurone(s)
Tone	Increased with spastic quality	Normal or reduced if marked wasting is present
Reflexes	Increased	May be reduced or absent
Plantar responses	Extensor	Flexor
Bulk	Normal	Wasting

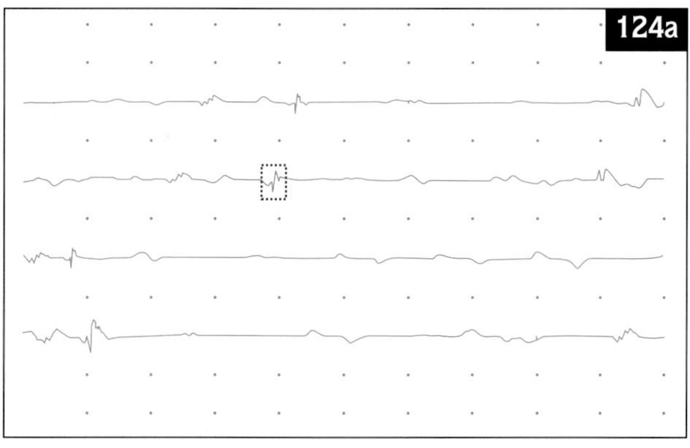

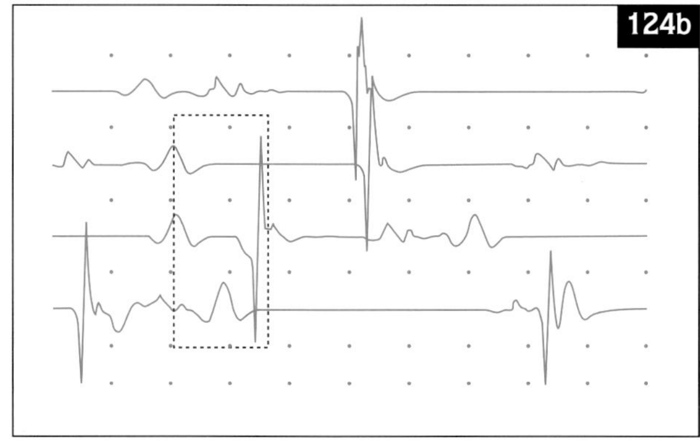

124 Electromyography studies in myopathy, showing myopathic potentials (**a**) and large neurogenic potentials (**b**).

SUMMARY

- ❏ Time must be given to listen to and understand the quality of the symptoms the patient is describing.
- ❏ The rate of evolution and date of onset of symptoms must be carefully documented; it may be longer than at first apparent.
- ❏ Any family history should be documented.
- ❏ The distinction between upper and lower motor neurone weakness is critical to accurate diagnosis.
- ❏ Fatiguable disorders kept in the waiting area prior to seeing the clinician may return to normal.
- ❏ A diagnosis should be formulated and localized prior to requesting imaging or neurophysiological studies.
- ❏ The motor unit is the functional lower motor component; differentiating neurogenic from myopathic weakness can be very difficult.
- ❏ It is necessary to remember that the spinal cord terminates at the level of L1 or L2; lumbar disease cannot produce upper motor neurone signs in the legs.
- ❏ The patient should be observed walking.
- ❏ The shoulder and periscapular muscles should always be examined from behind.

CLINICAL SCENARIOS

The following case histories illustrate how this approach allows localization and diagnosis in neurological practice.

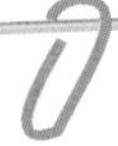

Case 1

A 56-year-old female seeks advice because of a 3-year slowly worsening problem with her legs. She says 'they won't go'. Friends have told her she is dragging her legs and looks as if she is limping. Things feel worse on the right than the left and she has decided to ask for help as she has begun to trip up over her right ankle.

This history gives some useful information. It sounds like an acquired disorder, coming on in mid life and progressing. There is involvement of both lower limbs, and the right is more affected than the left. The problem cannot be localized at present but further questioning reveals more information.

She does not think her arms are weak but has had some discomfort between her shoulder blades for the past 6 months. This is worse at night and feels like a band around her chest going to the right hand side. When asked to describe what is wrong with her legs she says they don't feel right, they are 'stiff, like tree trunks. I am walking like a robot'. Further questioning reveals she cannot feel the temperature of the bath water properly; it feels suddenly very hot when she puts her hands in, having previously tested it with her left foot. She is sure her upper limbs are normal, she has had no symptoms referable to her cranial nerves, and there is no history of headache.

The words she uses to describe her problems suggest an increase in muscle tone. The sensory story is striking and suggests that the process is involving both motor and sensory systems. This implies an upper motor neurone (UMN) disturbance and that the problem also affects sensory pathways. There are no associated features to suggest that the UMN pathway (the pathway from the motor cortex to the anterior horn cell) is being affected within the head, and the upper limbs are normal. The history of chest pain is interesting as a lesion in the thoracic cord at that level could involve the UMN pathway to the lower motor neurones as it traverses the thoracic cord.

The examination confirmed a gait abnormality and she walked with a scissoring motion, tending to scuff her right toe on the ground. The cranial nerves and upper limbs were normal.

A spastic gait disorder has been confirmed and no abnormalities have been found to imply disease above the site of her pain.

Examination of her trunk showed that pinprick sensation was felt normally above the level of T7 (**121**) but below this level was felt only as a prod on her left-hand side. Examination of her legs showed no wasting. She had a spastic increase in tone more marked on the left than the right and there was clonus elicitable at both ankles, which was sustained on the right. She had weakness diffusely in both legs, more marked on the right with relative sparing of antigravity muscles.

A UMN problem is being confirmed. The pattern of weakness is also typical of involvement of the UMN.

The reflexes were all brisk and both plantar responses were extensor. Sensory examination showed she had reduced joint position sensation at the right great toe, with reduced vibration sensation.

(Continued on page 159)

Case 1 *(continued)*

Bilateral disease has been confirmed and a pattern of sensory loss demonstrated that can be explained on the basis of a lesion affecting the spinal cord. A mass lesion compressing the spinal cord from the right side would be expected to:

- *Damage the UMN pathways more on the right than left.*
- *Damage the ipsilateral ascending posterior columns, which contain fibres subserving joint position sensation and proprioception.*
- *Damage ascending but crossed pain fibres in the lateral spinothalamic tract.*
- *Damage descending fibres controlling bladder function.*

All of these findings have been demonstrated, a pattern referred to as a Brown-Séquard syndrome. **Figures 125** and **126** show the MRI scans demonstrating a neurofibroma at T6 compressing the cord from the right.

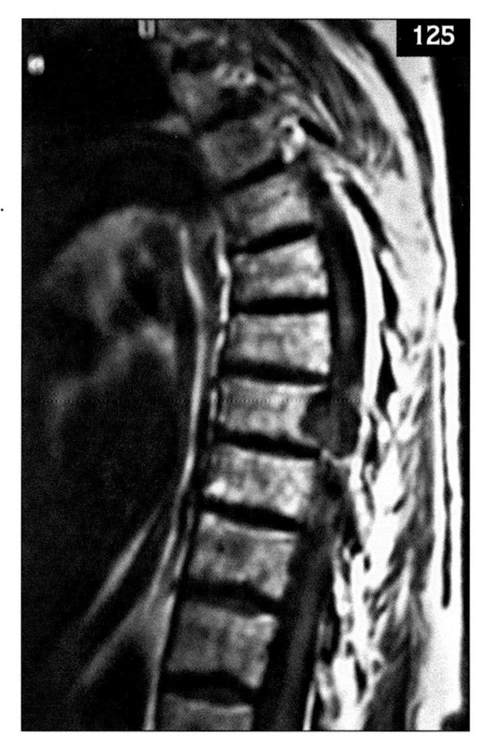

125 Sagittal magnetic resonance image showing thoracic neurofibroma.

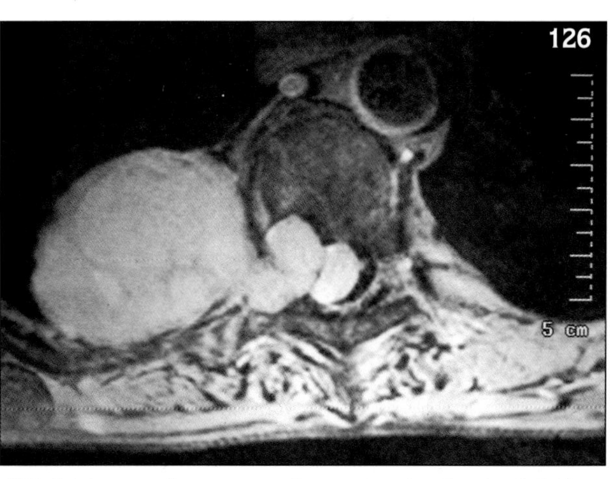

126 Axial magnetic resonance image showing the dumb-bell appearance of thoracic neurofibroma.

Case 2

A 65-year-old male smoker presents with a 2-month history of soreness in his right arm and a poor grip. He had sought help because he could no longer turn his car key in the lock. Further questions revealed a story of a 1-stone (6 kg) weight loss over the previous 4 months. He had also felt nonspecifically unwell. He gave no story of weakness elsewhere, but on direct questioning remarked that sensation on the inner side of his right arm was odd.

The story with weight loss is, in this context, suggestive of an underlying neoplasm. The story is progressive and localized to the right arm. The pain implies the involvement of either sensory pathways or non-neurological structures.

General examination was normal other than some tenderness in the right supraclavicular region. The left arm and lower limbs were normal. Cranial nerve examination was normal with the exception of a right-sided mild and partial ptosis and the right pupil was smaller than the left. Both reacted to light and accommodation. The right arm had weakness and wasting involving all the small hand muscles. The forearm muscles were of normal bulk and power. The biceps, triceps, and supinator reflexes were normal. There was loss of sensation to pinprick over the medial right arm and forearm.

The weakness and wasting of the hand muscles indicate a lower motor neurone (LMN) problem. This is localized and while a combined median and ulnar nerve problem peripherally could account for this, the sensory loss corresponds to a T1 distribution. Note that the dermatome of T1 (the skin area corresponding to the sensory fibres entering the spinal cord at T1) does not overlie the myotome (the muscles innervated by the T1 motor fibres). The T1 root supplies all the intrinsic muscles of the hand so there may be localization. The ptosis on the right can be explained. The eyelid is maintained in position by the action of levator palpebrae superioris (innervated by the IIIrd cranial nerve). The sympathetic nerves also innervate fibres within this muscle. These fibres also act as pupil-dilating. The consequence of damage to the sympathetic nerve fibres going to the eye is thus partial ptosis and miosis. Additional effects of damage to these fibres include a lack of sweating over the face and enophthalmos, but these are less often clinically apparent. These sympathetic fibres reach the orbit having exited the spinal cord at the T1 root. They synapse in the stellate ganglion and reach the orbit by travelling in the sheath of the internal carotid and ophthalmic arteries. Thus a lesion involving the T1 root could account for this clinical picture.

The tenderness in the right supraclavicular region corresponds to the erosion of this area by a lung tumour arising at the apex of the right lung, as was seen on chest X-ray and MRI (127, 128). This complex of symptoms and signs is referred to as a 'Pancoast' tumour.

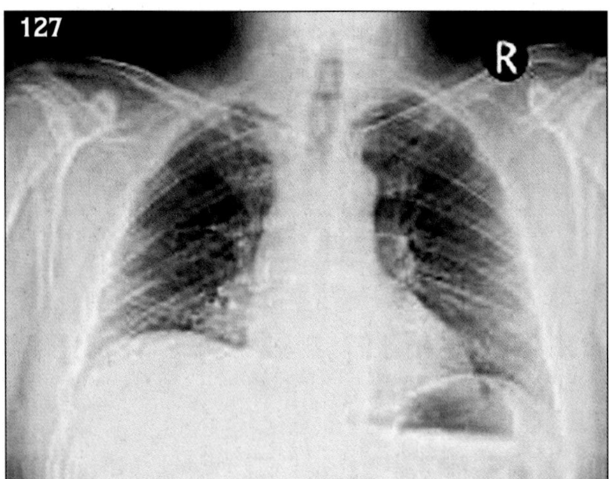

127 Chest X-ray showing right apical opacity due to a Pancoast tumour, with partially destroyed second and third ribs.

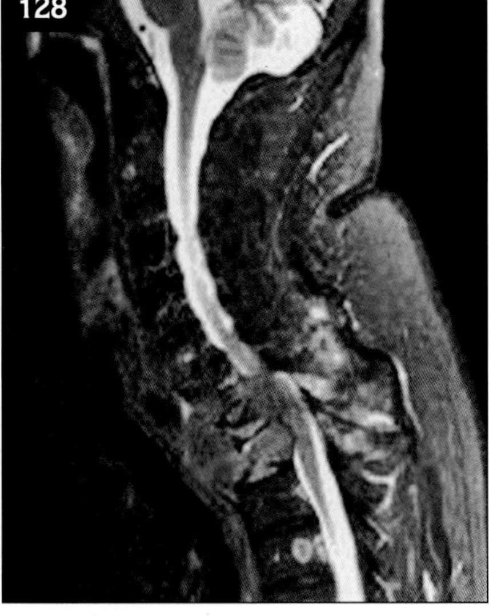

128 T2 magnetic resonance image showing soft tissue mass involving C7, T1, and T2 with vertebral collapse and moderate cord compression.

Case 3

A 57-year-old female who has been well in the past gives a 6-month story of a problem with her left foot. She says it won't work and she has begun to trip over on it. It is becoming a little more troublesome but she has only attended at her relative's insistence. She denies any weakness elsewhere and is not aware of any sensory problems or change in bladder control.

This sounds like a purely motor problem so far and it seems to be localized but there is very little else to help make the diagnosis. Tripping up usually means weakness of the ankle dorsiflexors, but these muscles will become weak in the context of an evolving UMN lesion as well as with L5 root disease or a lesion of the lateral popliteal nerve.

There is no story of pain and she is otherwise medically well and on no drug therapy. She does, however, say that she has noticed a lot of cramps recently, not only in her calf but also in both thighs and across her shoulders. Examination of the cranial nerves is normal. In the limbs there are widespread twitching movements visible. These have the appearance of fasciculations. She does have mild proximal weakness diffusely in the arms. The legs show weakness of plantar and dorsiflexion on the left. There is wasting of all the muscles below the knee of the left leg and again widespread twitching is visible. The reflexes are all intact including the left ankle jerk where the wasting is most clearly seen. Both plantar responses are extensor. Sensation is normal.

This is a slightly confusing array of signs. The wasting and weakness imply LMN pathology. The fasciculations also may be due to anterior horn cell disease; more extensive abnormalities are present that cannot be explained on the basis of either an L5 root or lateral popliteal nerve lesion. Abnormalities are present in both upper and lower limbs so a focal lesion is impossible. A disease process involving the spinal cord from the cervical region to the lumbar expansion could produce such widespread LMN signs, but some sensory features or bladder disturbance might be expected. The reflexes, however, are brisk and the plantar responses extensor, implying UMN pathology.

The investigating physicians were concerned that the spinal cord may be diseased along its length but images and examination of cerebrospinal fluid were normal. EMG studies were arranged to identify the extent of LMN involvement and she also underwent NCS to examine motor nerve function. EMG demonstrated evidence of ongoing denervation in the muscles of her neck, arms, and legs. This was present in all sites and on right and left. NCS showed normal sensory function and no evidence of damage to the myelin sheath of the motor fibres, but did show evidence of motor axonal loss.

This clinical scenario is of a woman with motor neurone disease (MND). This is a degenerative process involving the upper and lower motor neurones. It is progressive and incurable leading to slowly increasing weakness of all striated muscle. It will be important when speaking to her about the diagnosis to recall her lack of initial concern; the giving of bad news when unanticipated requires great tact and delicacy.

Revision questions

1 A lesion of the left S1 root would be expected to reduce or abolish the left ankle jerk reflex.
2 Muscle wasting is a characteristic feature of lower motor neurone weakness.
3 An elevation of serum creatine kinase activity to twice the upper limit of normal invariably indicates neuromuscular disease.
4 Extensor plantar responses are not a feature of upper motor neurone weakness.
5 A motor nerve always innervates a single muscle fibre.
6 A defect in oxidative muscle metabolism would be expected to produce limitation of sustained exercise rather than brief intense exercise.
7 Disorders of neuromuscular transmission may be associated with fatigue.
8 Cramps may be a prominent feature of motor neurone disease.
9 A lesion of the right C5 sensory root would be expected to be associated with sensory loss in the axilla.
10 A lesion in the spinal cord may produce both upper and lower motor neurone features.
11 It is appropriate to image the lumbar spine of a patient with spastic leg weakness and numbness involving the legs and up to just below the umbilicus.
12 Transection of the ulnar nerve at the elbow will cause weakness of all the intrinsic hand muscles.
13 Diseases of the motor unit would be expected to give rise to sensory symptoms.
14 Some inherited neuromuscular disorders are so mild affected individuals may never seek medical advice.
15 Steroid administration may cause muscle weakness.

Answers

1 True.
2 True.
3 False.
4 False.
5 False.
6 True.
7 True.
8 True.
9 False.
10 True.
11 False.
12 False.
13 False.
14 True.
15 True.

TREMOR AND OTHER INVOLUNTARY MOVEMENTS

Vicky Marshall, Donald Grosset

INTRODUCTION

Disruption of the basal ganglia and extrapyramidal system causes abnormal involuntary movements that are either reduced (hypokinetic) or increased and excessive (hyperkinetic). The general lack of movement seen in Parkinson's disease (PD) is an example of a hypokinetic disorder. Chorea is an example of a hyperkinetic movement disorder, characterized by excessive involuntary movements.

This chapter covers clinical aspects of involuntary movements, and how to use the clinical examination to differentiate between the different types of movement disorder. It provides anatomical and physiological insights into the mechanisms of control of movement, and therefore disturbance of movement. Tremor disorders will be considered in the main, but information on the taxonomy of other involuntary movements will be provided.

TREMOR

Tremor, as defined by the Movement Disorder Society, is a rhythmical, involuntary, oscillatory movement of a body part. It is the rhythm that distinguishes tremor from other abnormal involuntary movements. Usually the differentiation of types of tremor is straightforward based on history and examination, although difficulties may be met particularly in the early stages of tremor.

Tremor classification

Tremors are most commonly classified according to causes or clinical characteristics, but as the aetiology of many tremors is not fully understood and needs to be continuously updated, use of the clinical characteristics tends to be favoured and is more clinically useful. *Table 34* defines each tremor type (rest and action, postural and kinetic) and details the main conditions in which these tremors commonly occur. It should be recognized that different tremor conditions may be 'mixed' comprising more than the main tremor type

Table 34 Tremor classification

Characteristics	*Disorder*
Rest Occurs when a body part is not voluntarily activated and is fully supported against gravity, e.g. arms and hands resting in the lap	Parkinson's disease: may also have postural and intention components but usually rest tremor is more prominent Drug-induced parkinsonism (dopamine antagonists, e.g. neuroleptics) Drug-induced tremor Palatal tremor Seldom occurs in other conditions
Action Any tremor occurring during voluntary contraction of muscle. Includes postural, kinetic (which includes intention), and isometric tremor	
Postural, present while maintaining position against gravity, e.g. arms maintaining outstretched position	Enhanced physiological tremor Essential tremor Drug-induced tremor Orthostatic tremor Neuropathic tremor syndrome Dystonic tremor Psychogenic tremor
Kinetic, present during any voluntary movement; target (intention tremor) or nontarget directed movement	
Intention tremor, e.g. finger–nose test	(Disturbances of cerebellar pathways) Cerebellar tremor Drug-induced tremor Holmes tremor Dystonic tremor
Task-specific kinetic tremor	Primary writing tremor

characteristic for that condition. For example, although a rest tremor is characteristic for PD, action components to the tremor can coexist.

Specialist anatomy and physiology

The basal ganglion is a term which refers to four main subcortical nuclei that regulate and coordinate movement: the striatum (comprising the putamen and caudate), globus pallidus, subthalamic nucleus, and the substantia nigra (**129, 130**). These grey matter nuclei maintain muscle tone needed to stabilize joint positions or inhibit muscle tone during initiation of movement. PD is a neurodegenerative disease of unknown aetiology, in which degeneration of dopaminergic neurones projecting from the substantia nigra pars compacta to the striatum occurs, resulting in deficiency of dopamine within the striatum. The degeneration of the neurones within the substantia nigra causes loss of the characteristic black ('nigra') pigmentation. Clinical symptoms occur when there is depletion of 50–70% of striatal dopamine.

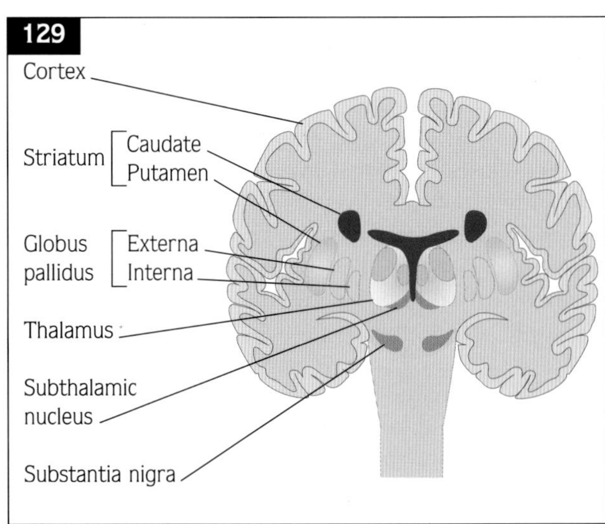

129 Neuroanatomical schematic diagram of extrapyramidal structures.

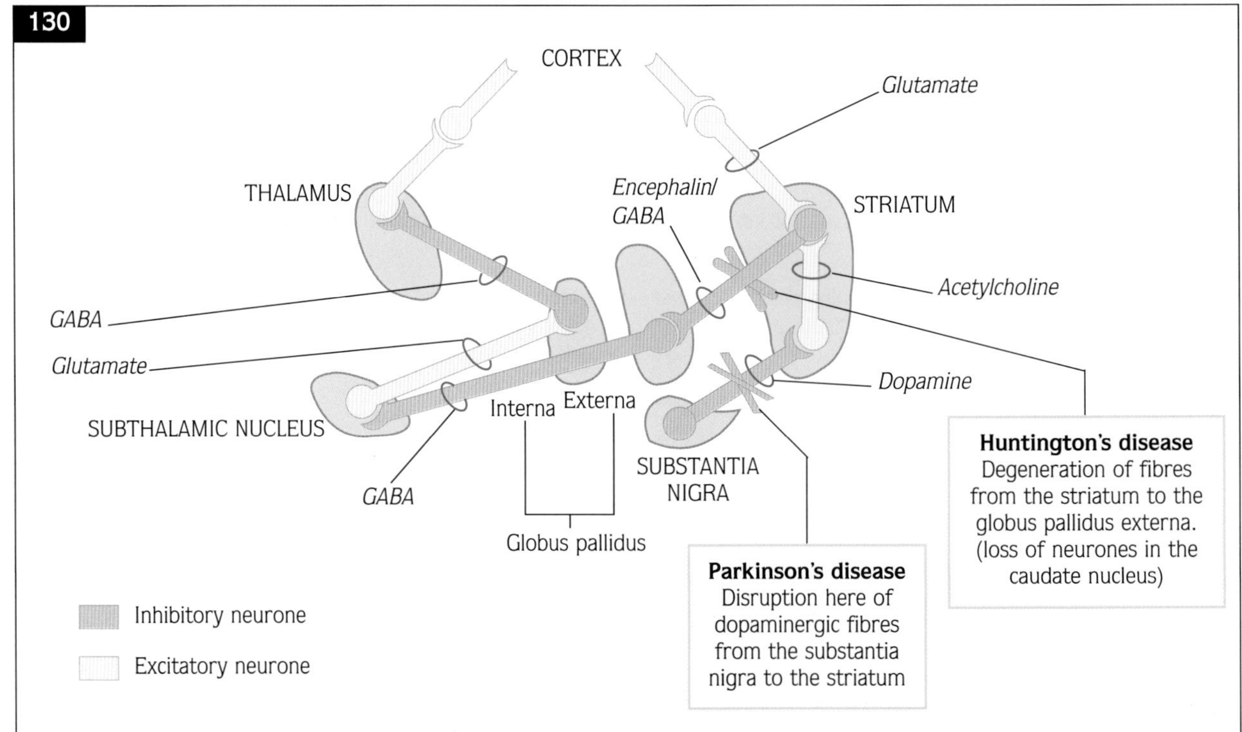

130 Schematic representation of the interaction between basal ganglia, thalamus, and cortex. GABA: gamma amino-butyric acid.

SPECIFIC TREMOR DISORDERS

Parkinson's disease and 'Parkinson's plus' disorders

PD has a prevalence of approximately 1% in those over 65 years, but occasionally has younger onset as low as 30 years (juvenile PD). In early disease, patients may describe small handwriting (micrographia), rest tremor, or stiffness of a limb. Relatives may note a reduced facial expression, diminished blinking, or an arm that does not swing on walking. Some patients may notice a reduction in sense of smell. Features are typically asymmetrical and include bradykinesia, rigidity, tremor, and postural instability (*Table 35*). Tremor is the first symptom in up to 75% of patients with PD, but 20% of patients never develop tremor. Up to 25% of patients diagnosed with PD in life have an incorrect diagnosis.

The characteristic tremor usually has a frequency of 4–6 Hz, starting in an arm and spreading to the leg on the same side then to the contralateral limbs. It is also called a 'pill-rolling' tremor on account of it being a back-and-forth motion of the thumb and index finger occurring at rest. It becomes less during posture holding and intention (movement). Sometimes tremor is the most prominent feature with little in the way of other features, and this is referred to as benign tremulous PD. In other cases, where tremor is absent, the patient is described as having the akinetic-rigid form of PD. Primitive reflexes may be present. Patients may be stooped. Walking may be affected; patients may stop in mid stride with difficulty in restarting movement, called 'freezing'. When a patient walks with small steps as if hurrying forward to keep balance it is known as festination.

Patients may have reduced facial expression causing some people to think they are depressed, and a soft voice. Other symptoms that patients may complain of are depression, emotional changes and memory loss, constipation and urinary problems, sexual difficulties, and sleep difficulties. As the disease progresses, some patients may have trouble swallowing or chewing and may develop dementia, hallucinations, or delusions (caused by a combination of medication and disease). Involuntary choreiform movement of trunk, limbs, or head usually occurs after many years of drug treatment, and is referred to as dyskinesia.

'Parkinson's plus' disorders consist of parkinsonism plus additional features, which result from neuronal degeneration outwith the basal ganglia. 'Parkinson's plus' should be considered a concept rather than a diagnosis. These conditions only respond to antiparkinson drugs in the first few years, unlike PD where a long-term treatment response is maintained. Progressive supranuclear palsy (PSP), previously known as Steele–Richardson–Olszewski syndrome, is characterized by axial rigidity (particularly neck rigidity), ophthalmoplegia (the supranuclear palsy component of the name) with reduced vertical eye movements (reduced downward gaze is more specific), and early and frequent falls. Multiple system atrophy (MSA) is classified according to whether patients demonstrate primarily parkinsonism (MSA-P) or cerebellar (MSA-C) features, in which speech and limb movements become ataxic. Autonomic features (e.g. postural dizziness, bladder and sexual dysfunction) may be prominent in either. Corticobasal degeneration (CBD) may have limb dystonia, myoclonus, apraxias, and the 'alien limb' phenomenon in addition to parkinsonism. All the Parkinson's plus disorders are less common than PD and all have unique neuropathological findings.

Drug-induced parkinsonism

The signs of PD may be mimicked by the use of medications that cause dopamine depletion. These include some antipsychotics (although the newer atypical antipsychotics are less likely to cause the same problems) and antiemetics such as metoclopramide and prochlorperazine. The signs are reversible on drug withdrawal and usually take weeks to a couple of months to resolve. Occasionally, the use of dopamine-depleting drugs may 'unmask' PD in patients with preclinical disease (when clinical signs were not present prior to drug treatment).

Table 35 Cardinal criteria for parkinsonian syndrome

- ❑ Bradykinesia
- ❑ And at least one of the following:
  - – Muscular rigidity
  - – 4–6 Hz rest tremor

Many additional conditions can have parkinsonian signs associated with them: cerebrovascular disease affecting the subcortical areas (causing lower body parkinsonism which, as the name suggests, affects legs more than arms, while PD is the other way around), hydrocephalus (a classical triad of gait disorder, urinary incontinence, and dementia), encephalitis, hypoxic brain injury; and toxin exposure (e.g. carbon monoxide).

Table 36 Criteria for classic essential tremor

Inclusion criteria

- ❑ Bilateral, largely symmetrical postural or kinetic tremor, involving hands and forearms that is visible and persistent
- ❑ Additional or isolated tremor of the head may occur but in the absence of abnormal posturing

Exclusion criteria

- ❑ Other abnormal neurological signs, especially dystonia
- ❑ Presence of known causes of enhanced physiologic tremor
- ❑ History or evidence of psychogenic tremor
- ❑ Convincing evidence of sudden onset or evidence of stepwise deterioration
- ❑ Primary orthostatic tremor
- ❑ Isolated voice tremor
- ❑ Isolated position-specific or task-specific tremors
- ❑ Isolated tongue or chin tremor
- ❑ Isolated leg tremor

Essential tremor

Essential tremor is at least 2–3 times commoner than PD, though only about 10% of patients with essential tremor seek medical advice. It is often a hereditary disorder; autosomal dominance is common but many cases are sporadic. Typically, there is a symmetrical tremor of the upper limbs, with insidious onset and slow progression. The tremor is worse on posture holding and intention, and is rarely prominent at rest. Patients may describe difficulty in holding a cup without spilling it and are often embarrassed by the tremor. The head, chin, jaw, and lips may be affected and occasionally the legs, but never in isolation (*Table 36*). The tremor may be transiently improved with alcohol. Parkinsonian signs are typically absent, but in the older population a degree of age or arthritis-related slowing may cause difficulty in distinguishing this from parkinsonian disorders (*Table 37*).

OTHER TREMORS (131)

Physiological tremor occurs in every normal subject around every joint that is free to move. It is of low amplitude and of high frequency in the fingers and hand (just visible to the naked eye) and low in proximal joints, and is enhanced by muscular fatigue and anxiety. It is called enhanced physiological tremor when it is easily seen by the eye, usually postural and of high frequency, and is reversible if a cause is found (such as thyrotoxicosis, phaechromocytoma, drug withdrawal states, caffeine excess, and alcohol intoxication).

Table 37 Typical features which aid differentiation between Parkinson's disease and essential tremor

	Parkinson's disease	Essential tremor
Tremor character	Rest; 4–6 Hz	Postural, kinetic; 6–12 Hz
Site	Hands, legs	Hands, head, voice
Onset	Unilateral	Bilateral
Other features	Bradykinesia Rigidity	Postural instability
Family history	Usually negative	Positive 50%
Alcohol	No effect	Marked reduction in tremor
Beta-blocker	May reduce tremor	Effective
Levodopa	Effective	No effect

Cerebellar tremor syndromes include intention tremor and titubation. Many medications may cause **drug-induced tremor**, e.g. amiodarone, lithium, sodium valproate, prednisolone, and selective serotonin reuptake inhibitors (SSRIs). A clear causal relationship with onset of medication is sought but not always found as tremor onset may be delayed. These tremors are usually kinetic in nature. Drug-induced parkinsonism has already been mentioned above.

Holmes tremor was previously labelled as rubral, thalamic, and midbrain tremor and is caused by a lesion of the brainstem/cerebellum and thalamus. It is a slow (<4.5 Hz) rest and intention tremor which may not be as rhythmic as other tremors. There may be some delay between lesion (for example stroke) and tremor onset. **Orthostatic tremor** may present with a feeling of unsteadiness and is a fine fast tremor of the thighs on standing. Electromyography is required to confirm the typical 13–18 Hz frequencies.

Neuropathic tremor may occur in patients with many peripheral neuropathies but most frequently occurs in demyelinating and dysgammaglobulinaemic neuropathies. Most often these are postural and kinetic tremors. **Dystonic tremor** is tremor in a body part that is affected by dystonia, e.g. a head tremor in cervical dystonia. **Psychogenic tremor** is still mostly a diagnosis of exclusion as there are no definite clinical characteristics that are specific to a psychogenic tremor. Many patients may have a variability of tremor frequency or reduction of frequency or amplitude by distraction, an unusual combination of rest/ kinetic tremors, somatization in past history, or appearance of other unrelated neurological signs. Tremors may be of acute onset with remissions. The 'coactivation' sign may be present: a resistance to passive movements around a joint, due to voluntarily increased tone necessary to continue the tremor, which disappears when the patient completely relaxes.

Wilson's disease

Wilson's disease is a rare, autosomal recessive inherited disorder of copper metabolism with copper accumulation. The liver is not capable of biliary excretion of copper. It usually presents in early adulthood (but may be later) with hepatic dysfunction (leads to cirrhosis if untreated), neurological dysfunction, or psychiatric dysfunction. Patients may show a rest tremor of parkinsonian type, usually mixed with action tremor (bat's wing tremor) and other extrapyramidal signs (dysarthria, dystonia, rigidity, chorea). Slit-lamp examination may reveal corneal copper deposition (Kayser–Fleischer rings) and serum caeruloplasmin level is low, with elevated urinary copper. Copper-chelating drugs can be used to prevent copper deposits.

TAXONOMY OF OTHER INVOLUNTARY MOVEMENTS

Chorea, athetosis, ballism, dystonia, and motor tics are all hyperkinetic disorders associated with basal ganglia dysfunction. These involuntary movements characteristically disappear during sleep. **Chorea** is derived from the Greek word for 'dance'. Chorea is a

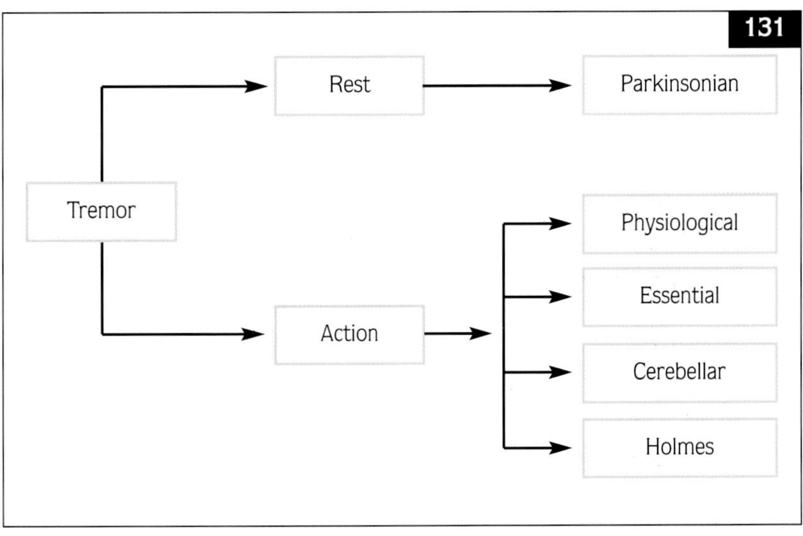

131 Tremor flow diagram: action tremor encompasses postural and kinetic tremors (*Table 35*).

nonrhythmic, involuntary, purposeless motion which primarily involves the face or extremities and may flow from one body part to another. Movements may be jerky and relatively rapid. If several choreic movements are present, they may appear slow and writhing, resembling athetosis (choreoathetoid). Some causes of chorea are listed in *Table 38*.

Huntington's disease

Huntington's disease (HD) is a progressive disorder characterized by chorea and dementia. It is due to an expanded and unstable trinucleotide repeat (CAG) on chromosome 4, which is inherited in an autosomal dominant manner. Mean age of onset is 40 years old and survival time 15–18 years after onset. This disease is characterized neuropathologically by striatal degeneration. It manifests with problems of voluntary and involuntary movements (typically choreiform), emotional control, and cognitive ability. Patients describe clumsiness with motor speed; fine motor control and gait are affected. Choreiform movements may be of distal muscles such as quick jerking movements of the fingers resembling cigarette flicking; later they may become slower and continuous (choreoathetoid) or flinging movements resembling ballism. Other involuntary movements such as bradykinesia, rigidity, and dystonia can occur with advancing disease duration. Speech problems occur early and swallowing difficulties later in disease duration. Death usually occurs as result of infectious complications of immobility. HD can usually be distinguished from other diseases causing chorea based on family history, course of disease, and associated findings.

Table 38 Causes of chorea

- Sydenham's chorea: sporadic, postinfectious chorea associated with rheumatic fever
- Chorea gravidarum (chorea of pregnancy)
- Drug-induced (e.g. contraceptives, levodopa, neuroleptics)
- Structural lesions of subthalamic nucleus (e.g. cerebrovascular accident)
- Systemic lupus erythematosus
- Metabolic disorders: thyrotoxicosis, Wilson's disease
- Huntington's disease
- Neuroacanthocytosis

Other basal ganglia dysfunctional disorders

Athetosis (derived from the Greek word 'without position') is characterized by slow, writhing, continuous movements of the distal parts of the extremities. It is often associated with chorea (choreoathetosis). **Ballism** (derived from the Greek word for 'jump or throw') demonstrates abrupt, flailing, and violent involuntary movements of proximal muscles. Movements are often unilateral (hemiballismus), contralateral to a lesion within the subthalamic nucleus.

Involuntary and inappropriate muscle contractions of agonist/antagonist muscles when changing or maintaining posture cause a twisting movement with abnormal posture that may be painful, **dystonia.** An example is cervical dystonia. Movements are usually slow but may be more rapid and repetitive. **Motor tics** are abrupt and rapid purposeless involuntary movements that are repetitive and irregular. Examples are eye blinking or shoulder shrugging. They may be suggestible, worsened with anxiety, and partially suppressible. Most are benign. A chronic and severe type of motor and vocal tics (including involuntary swearing) associated with behavioural disturbance is Tourette's syndrome.

Other involuntary movements

Clonus, asterixis, and myoclonus are all involuntary movements whose primary pathology is not disease within the basal ganglia and are sometimes mistaken for tremor. **Clonus** is rhythmic movement elicited though the stretch reflex around a joint and is most often looked for around the ankle by sharp dorsiflexion of the foot, the presence of which signifies an upper motor neurone (UMN) lesion. It is usually associated with increased muscle tone. **Asterixis** may resemble an irregular tremor. Asterixis may be unilateral (caused by focal hemispheric lesions) or bilateral (endocrine, metabolic dysfunction [e.g. hepatic encephalopathy], intoxication, or focal brainstem disease). It has a characteristic flapping pattern during tonic contraction (noted for example with dorsiflexion of the wrist), due to sudden lapses of innervation. Patients may have other physical signs such as those associated with liver failure. **Myoclonus** is an intermittent, sudden, abrupt, brief muscle jerk which may be irregular or rhythmic and of slow frequency arising from the central nervous system.

Clinical assessment

Focused history taking

Initial history taking should concentrate on onset of involuntary movement (sudden or gradual), duration, location and spread, and whether the condition is progressive or intermittent. Family or friends may be able to report if the disorder was present prior to the patient noticing it. A family history is important as many movement disorders have a familial tendency, e.g. tremor of early adult onset suggests essential tremor; a family history of chorea (and mental impairment) suggests Huntington's disease. Medication and illicit drug history is necessary, as is noting a response to alcohol (essential tremor improves with alcohol; the tremor of PD does not). History should be focused according to tremor type, e.g. a patient with a fine, symmetrical, postural tremor should be questioned about symptoms of thyrotoxicosis. History taking has been covered in previous chapters of this book and so this chapter concentrates on clinical aspects of involuntary movements, especially using clinical examination to differentiate between movement disorders.

Examination of tremor

While taking the medical history, the clinician should watch for tremor unobtrusively, as the characteristics of tremor may change if the patient is aware of being scrutinized. An affected limb should be watched while fully supported against gravity (at rest), while maintaining a position against gravity (postural), and during target directed movements (intention) (*Table 34*). When writing a sentence, micrographia may be noted in a patient with PD, while in patients with essential tremor the writing will be tremulous but not small (**132**). Alternative measures to assess essential tremor are by copying a spiral, which can be used to assess progression or therapy response at intervals (**133**). If appropriate from the history, an attempt to bring on the tremor in a task-specific manner, e.g. writing or in a standing position for orthostatic tremor should be made. For any tremor, neurological examination should look particularly for the following signs:

Bradykinesia (slowness of movement). Assessment is made of repeated finger and heel taps, watching particularly for reduction in amplitude or

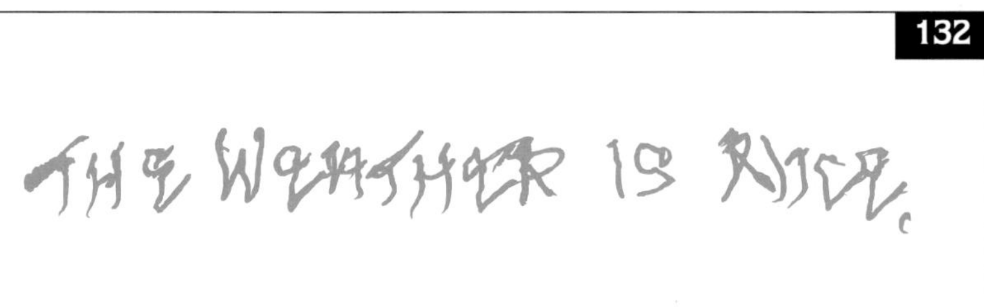

132 Tremulous writing in a patient with essential tremor.

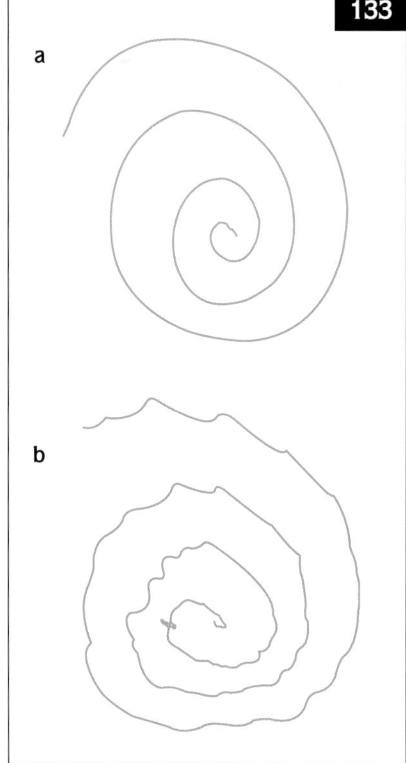

133 Normal Archimedes spiral (**a**) and abnormal tremulous spiral in a patient with essential tremor (**b**).

hesitation, and reduced arm swing on walking. Bradykinesia may occur to an extent in elderly patients due to coexistent disease such as arthritis.

Rigidity. Assessment is made of passive movements around joints. The patient should be as relaxed as possible. Cogwheeling is a rhythmic brief increase in resistance during passive movement. Froment's sign is increased tone felt during voluntary movement of the other limb. Voluntary resistance to passive movements may be found in psychogenic tremors.

Postural instability. Typically found in PD, impaired balance may cause patients to fall easily or develop a forward or backward lean. If pulled gently by the shoulders from behind and told to try to keep their balance (the 'pull' test), patients with PD have a tendency to step backwards (retropulsion) or fall (the test must be fully explained to the patient and the clinician must be ready to catch if necessary).

Gait. A shuffling gait with short steps and difficulty turning corners or going through doorways is seen in PD.

Bradykinesia, rest tremor, rigidity, and postural instability are features of PD and atypical parkinsonian disorders (MSA, PSP, CBD) and in other disorders such as dementia with Lewy bodies. Medication use with dopamine depletors (e.g. antipsychotics or some antiemetics) may mimic PD.

Cerebellar signs. Essential tremor often has an intention component to the tremor. The presence of other cerebellar signs, e.g. dysdiadochokinesis, poor coordination on heel–shin testing, nystagmus, cerebellar speech disturbance, raises the possibility of a structural disorder and suggests neuroimaging and other investigations. Cerebellar features may represent MSA in the presence of parkinsonian signs.

Pyramidal signs. These may raise the possibility of cerebral disorders of many aetiologies and should prompt further investigation, such as structural brain imaging. Pyramidal signs (e.g. brisk reflexes or extensor plantar responses), in the context of a parkinsonian disorder may be due to MSA.

Primitive reflexes. While no primitive reflex is specific, the presence of them adds weight to a diagnosis of PD in a patient with a tremor disorder. The glabellar tap, pout, and palmomental reflexes should be assessed.

Evidence for neuropathy, such as chronic demyelinating neuropathies, polyneuropathies (diabetes, uraemia), should be sought.

General examination. Signs of metabolic upset (e.g. hyperthyroidism, hypocalcaemia, alcoholism, and hepatic disturbance) should be looked for.

Investigations

Blood tests and structural brain imaging (CT or MRI) are often needed to exclude metabolic disorders or structural brain disease as a cause of tremor or other involuntary movement. Functional neuroimaging may be used to assess the integrity of the pre- or postsynaptic dopaminergic neurone with SPECT or PET. Nerve conduction studies or electromyography may be required in some cases to clarify the diagnosis.

Summary

- ❏ History taking in movement disorders should include rate of onset, position, precipitants and relievers, and full drug and family history.
- ❏ A full neurological examination is important to perform in patients with tremor, for evidence of other extrapyramidal signs, cerebellar features, and pyramidal signs for instance.
- ❏ Tremor should be described in terms of site and type (rest or action [postural and kinetic]) and amplitude of movements.
- ❏ PD is due to degeneration of the dopamine neurones from the substantia nigra in the midbrain to the striatum. The aetiology is unknown.
- ❏ PD is typically of unilateral onset spreading to become bilateral and most patients will present with resting tremor.
- ❏ The cardinal features of PD are bradykinesia, tremor, rigidity, and postural instability.
- ❏ Mimics of PD include Parkinson's plus disorders, drug-induced parkinsonism, and vascular parkinsonism.
- ❏ Essential tremor presents with postural and intention tremor and often shows transient improvement with beta-blockers or alcohol.
- ❏ Movement disorders presenting in early adulthood should prompt a screen for Wilson's disease.
- ❏ Chorea may be due to metabolic disturbances, structural lesions, inflammatory disorders, medications, and neurodegenerative disorders.
- ❏ Huntington's disease presents with chorea and dementia and is an autosomal dominant disorder.

CLINICAL SCENARIOS

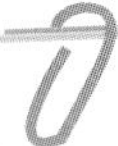

Case 1

A 72-year-old female is referred by her GP having noticed a tremor of insidious onset in her right (dominant) hand over the previous year. Within the last 4 months it has begun to affect the left hand as well. Initially it was intermittent but now it is continuous, and interfering with her ability to cook and write. Tremor is more apparent when she is sitting watching television and is worse with anxiety. She notices a general slowing that she puts down to 'age' but denies any stiffness. She has had no falls. Handwriting is shaky but no smaller than usual. Past medical history includes osteoarthritis of shoulders, elbows, and hips with a left hip replacement. She takes negligible alcohol and is an ex-smoker. Currently she takes an anti-inflammatory painkiller for joint ache. Previously she tried a beta-blocker for the tremor without any benefit. Family history is negative for any tremor disorders.

Tremor had an asymmetrical onset and is worse at rest, both suggesting PD. Anxiety worsens tremor regardless of cause. Essential tremor often improves with beta-blockers but the nonresponse does not exclude the diagnosis, neither does the lack of family history. There is no information on response to alcohol. Slowing may represent bradykinesia but may also be found in an older patient, to which arthritis may contribute.

As the patient walked into the room a reduction in arm swing on the right was apparent. She was slightly stooped, which may have been normal for her age. Walking was slow with small steps, with no freezing, shuffling, or festination. Facial expression was a little reduced. General examination was normal. While sitting with her hands fully supported on her lap, there was no tremor initially but when she was asked to count down from 20, a bilateral rest tremor was present, more obvious in the right arm. It was a coarse tremor with a rubbing action between the thumb and index finger but also involved other fingers. On passive movement around her right wrist no rigidity was noted unless she performed voluntary movement in the left arm (Froment's sign). Mild rigidity was present around the right knee and ankle joints. Bradykinesia was noted in the right arm as assessed by finger taps; although initial taps were quick and with good amplitude they quickly fatigued with some hesitation. There was no rigidity or bradykinesia in the left arm or leg. The 'pull' test was performed and retropulsion was apparent. There was a positive glabellar tap and positive palmomental reflexes bilaterally. Limb power, sensation, and reflexes were all normal. There were no cerebellar signs.

The diagnosis is likely to be PD. Examination reveals a very asymmetrical pattern with all the cardinal signs present: rest tremor, bradykinesia, rigidity, and postural instability. Abnormal primitive reflexes lend weight to the diagnosis.

Patients with PD often interpret their initial slowness as being due to age. Tremor became more apparent as she concentrated upon subtracting numbers, a technique that can be used to make tremor more apparent. (Tremor may also be noted in a hand and arm when walking.)

(Continued overleaf)

Case 1 *(continued)*

*When there is clinical uncertainty over the presence of parkinsonian features a FP-CIT SPECT brain scan shows presynaptic dopamine deficit in PD and Parkinson plus disorders, and is normal in essential tremor (**134**). Structural imaging (CT or MRI) is usually not performed unless there are atypical clinical features. As PD is functionally interfering with her life, treatment should be offered with, for example, levodopa (Sinemet or Madopar) or a dopamine agonist (Pramipexole or Ropinirole). A significant improvement in symptoms was noted after starting treatment (in keeping with idiopathic PD) with resulting improved quality of life.*

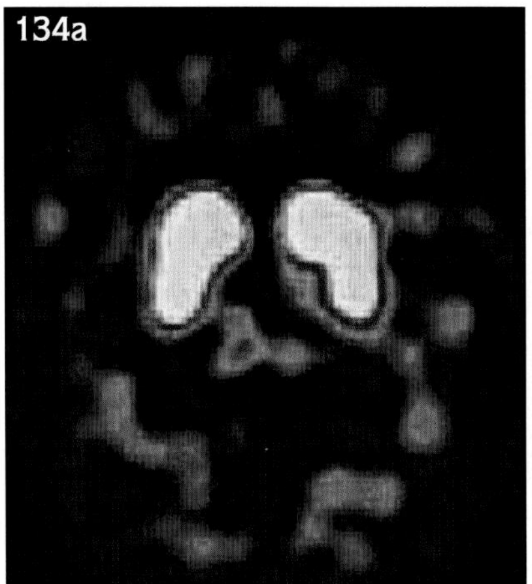

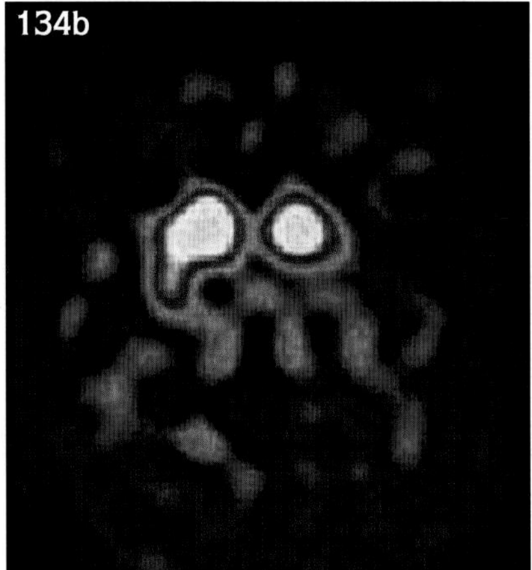

134 Dopamine transporter imaging (presynaptic): FP-CIT single photon emission computed tomography scans. **a:** normal uptake of ligand with bright signal in caudate (anteriorly) and putamen (posteriorly). Uptake is normal in essential tremor, drug-induced parkinsonism, and vascular parkinsonism (unless there is a focal infarction within the striatum which then shows a 'punched out' lesion atypical of true parkinsonian syndrome); **b:** abnormal with reduced uptake bilaterally in caudate and putamen, but more reduced in left than right putamen. Asymmetrical finding is typical of Parkinson's disease as dopaminergic neurones are lost in the putamen before the caudate and on the side contralateral before ipsilateral to the affected side. Abnormal uptake is also found in Parkinson's plus disorders thus this imaging technique will not differentiate between Parkinson's and Parkinson's plus disorders.

CASE 2

The pregnant daughter of a 46-year-old male raised concerns about his abnormal movements with the GP. These movements had occurred gradually over 5 months and were becoming more noticeable. They consisted of quick involuntary movements of his fingers and hands that she felt he tried to disguise, incorporating some of these movements into purposeful activity, such as tidying his hair. He was unaware of any involuntary movements. Facial grimacing had been noted. He had attended a psychiatrist with depression, anxiety, and irritability over the last 2 years with one recent episode of psychosis for which he was taking a neuroleptic drug. Adopted at birth, his family history was unknown.

HD is a possibility in the context of psychiatric disturbance and involuntary movements that sound choreiform in the extremities. Some patients may show no awareness of involuntary movements. The presence of a positive family history would have been helpful confirmatory information, but no family history is available in this case. Tardive dyskinesia, a condition which can be caused by neuroleptic medication, manifests as involuntary facial movements, with grimacing, lipsmacking, and chewing movements and can occasionally be accompanied by choreoathetoid movements of the trunk, arms, and legs. Other possibilities include Wilson's disease. A rare autosomal dominant condition known as neuroacanthocytosis may present with chorea and dementia, and should be considered if evidence of muscle wasting and neuropathy is present; it can be diagnosed by finding acanthocytes (derived from the Greek word 'acantha' meaning thorn) which are abnormally shaped red blood cells with finger-like projections due to membrane instability, in a thick, wet, blood film smear. Thyrotoxicosis needs to be excluded which can also present with chorea and may account for his anxiety and irritability; associated findings in history (diarrhoea, weight loss, heat intolerance) and examination (postural tremor, tachycardia) should be apparent.

Positive findings on examination were intermittent choreiform movements of the fingers and hands. Facial grimacing was present but without the stereotyped movements typical of tardive dyskinesia. Reflexes were generally brisk. He scored poorly on cognitive tests and had no insight into this. MRI of brain showed bilateral atrophy of caudate and putamen. Tests of copper metabolism and thyroid function were normal and no acanthocytes were found.

*This man should be referred for counselling prior to genetic testing for HD. DNA-based testing is currently 98.8% sensitive for HD and detects the CAG repeat length. His test was positive. The daughter was referred for counselling as she has a 50% chance of having inherited the gene and her unborn baby 25%. She opted not to have the test (**135**).*

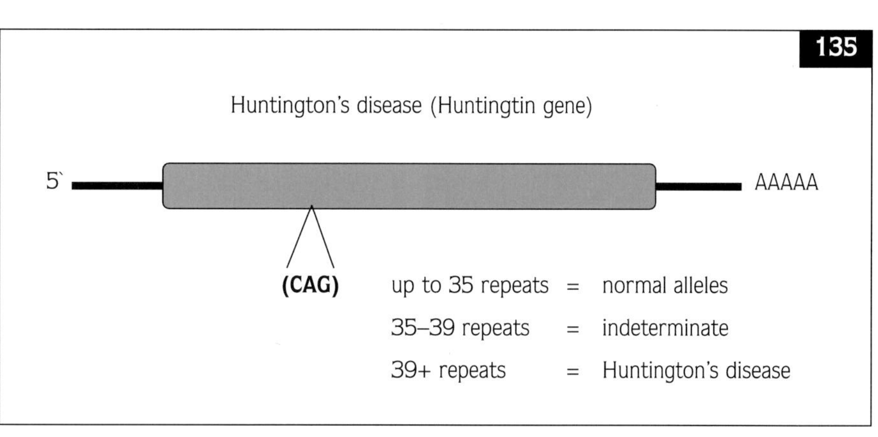

135 Schematic diagram of the trinucleotide cytosine-adenine-guanine (CAG) repeat in the short arm of chromosome 4, which encodes the protein Huntingtin. The repeat is present in normal alleles with up to 35 repeats. Patients with >39 repeats will develop Huntington's disease; those with 35–39 repeats are 'indeterminate' and may or may not develop the disease. The length of the repeats determines the age of onset.

Case 3

A 65-year-old male presented with stiffness and slowness of movement coming on gradually over 9 months in all limbs. This was particularly noticed on walking; his wife noticed he took slow shuffling steps and had reduced arm swing bilaterally. He reported no tremor. He had experienced several falls. He noticed lightheadedness over the same time period on standing from a sitting position and this contributed to his falls. He had urinary symptoms of dribbling incontinence and frequency. His GP had started a levodopa preparation as she found features of parkinsonism; the initial benefit to motor movements was mild and short-lived and the treatment worsened his lightheadedness. He had hypertension and was a smoker. He has been on aspirin and an ACE inhibitor for 4 years.

The lack of good response to levodopa, absence of tremor, and bilateral onset of symptoms suggest that PD is unlikely and one of the 'Parkinson's plus' disorders is more likely. The early autonomic (dizziness and bladder) symptoms suggest the autonomic variant of MSA rather than a drug side-effect, as the onset did not coincide with drug initiation. A pseudoparkinsonian state may be caused by cerebrovascular disease. Both MSA and vascular parkinsonism may have a partial response to levodopa.

On examination he had parkinsonian facies with positive frontal reflexes; moderately severe bradykinesia and rigidity were found symmetrically in all limbs but not the neck. He was stooped with a shuffling gait and postural instability. There was no tremor; he had normal reflexes and no cerebellar features. Eye movements were normal. There was evidence of postural hypotension with a lying blood pressure of 110/60 mmHg (14.7/8.0 kPa) and a standing blood pressure of 80/50 mmHg (10.7/6.7 kPa) from which he was symptomatic. MRI brain was normal.

*The autonomic variant of MSA is the likeliest diagnosis. Vascular parkinsonism is typically lower body which is not the pattern seen here and the MRI brain showed no evidence of ischaemic lesions. Antihypertensive drugs are likely to be aggravating his hypotension and should be phased out. A D2 SPECT brain scan that reflects the integrity of postsynaptic dopaminergic neurones is abnormal in 'Parkinson's plus' disorders and normal in PD and may be used if there is difficulty distinguishing the disorders clinically (**136**). Use of antiparkinsonian drugs was avoided because of the poor response and worsening of hypotension. Deterioration in his condition occurred over 4 years with gait disorder and falls contributed to by his postural hypotension.*

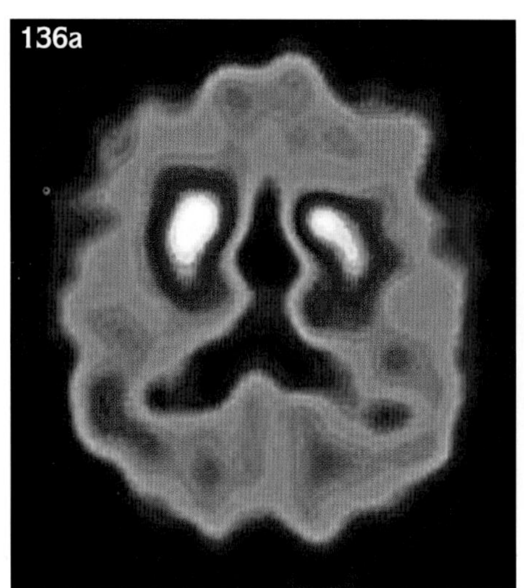

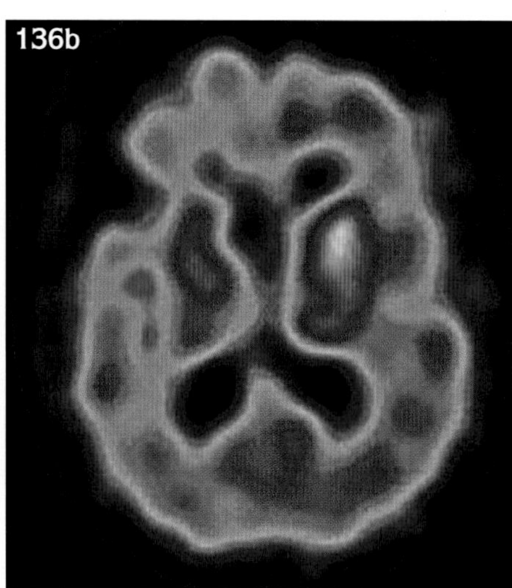

136 Dopamine 2 receptor imaging (postsynaptic): iodobenzamide (IBZM) single photon emission computed tomography scans. **a:** normal uptake of ligand as seen in Parkinson's disease; **b:** bilaterally reduced uptake compatible with multiple system atrophy (and other Parkinson's plus syndromes).

Revision questions

1 Parkinson's disease typically presents with unilateral postural arm tremor.
2 Essential tremor typically presents with bilateral postural arm tremor.
3 Huntington's disease is inherited in an autosomal recessive manner.
4 Wilson's disease often presents in patients aged over 50 years.
5 A fine bilateral postural arm tremor can be caused by sodium valproate.
6 An ischaemic lesion in the subthalamic nucleus could be the cause of acute onset hemiballism.
7 Imaging of the presynaptic dopaminergic neurone is expected to be abnormal in essential tremor.
8 Everybody with chorea should undergo genetic testing for Huntington's disease.
9 Thyroid function tests are indicated in a patient presenting with bilateral postural tremor and weight loss.
10 Structural brain imaging is not indicated when pyramidal signs (e.g. hyper-reflexia and extensor plantars) are found in conjunction with parkinsonian signs.
11 Antiemetic medications may cause parkinsonism.
12 Dopamine-depleting medications may cause Huntington's disease.
13 Beta-blockers may cause tremor.
14 Lithium may cause tremor.
15 Essential tremor responds to levodopa.

Answers

1 False.
2 True.
3 False.
4 False.
5 True.
6 True.
7 False.
8 False.
9 True.
10 False.
11 True.
12 False.
13 False.
14 True.
15 False.

POOR COORDINATION

Abhijit Chaudhuri

INTRODUCTION

Coordination is an essential requirement for any purposeful, goal-directed, motor movements. Poor coordination or loss of coordination is known as ataxia, which literally means 'without order'. Patients recognize ataxia as clumsiness of movement or poor balance that is distinct from weakness. In clinical practice, it is usual to restrict the term ataxia to describe movements characterized by 'motor error', i.e. an inaccuracy of movements and gait in the absence of obvious paralysis, involuntary movements of the limb, or visual impairment. A patient with a weak arm from a corticospinal lesion or with athetoid arm movements will appear clumsy, but these should not be termed ataxia. Similarly, disturbed vision due to blindness or squint will limit one's ability to target motor activities because of an inability to appreciate the position of an object in space. As a corollary, ataxia is always made worse under conditions of visual deprivation and this is often an important clinical observation in ataxia caused by the loss of proprioceptive input (sensory ataxia).

> Ataxia due to cerebellar lesions (cerebellar ataxia), unlike that due to the involvement of the sensory pathway, is always present even when the eyes are open.

After weakness and tremors, poor coordination is the next most common symptom of disorders that affect the motor system. In a number of common neurological conditions, ataxia is the dominant symptom. Ataxia may also be the consequence of a general medical disorder or a medication side-effect. Alcohol misuse is the commonest toxic cause of ataxia.

Classification

Disorders of the cerebellum or its connections and proprioceptive sensory pathway are not the only causes of poor coordination. Some authors have described an additional type of ataxia in **frontal lobe disorders**, characterized by disturbed standing and walking. This has been termed gait ataxia, but it is probably more appropriate to consider it as an apraxia of gait rather than a true ataxia. **Middle ear diseases** affecting vestibular function may also cause problems of balance. Destruction of the hair cells of the vestibular labyrinth from advanced Ménière's disease or after prolonged administration of aminoglycoside antibiotics results in vestibular ataxia. Patients with vestibulopathy due to these and other causes are unsteady while standing and walking and usually find it very difficult to climb down the stairs without holding the bannister. Frequently, they complain of a sense of imbalance even when lying or standing still and are liable to be dismissed as hysterical. However, just like patients with cerebellar and sensory ataxia, their staggering and unsteadiness increase in the dark, occasionally to the point of actual falling. This type of ataxia is caused by the loss of vestibular input necessary for ocular fixation and is a not uncommon problem in the elderly. For the remainder of this chapter, however, only cerebellar and sensory ataxias will be discussed, as these are most common in neurological practice.

Pathophysiology

Cerebellar anatomy and physiology

The cerebellum regulates movement, posture, and gait. It does so indirectly by influencing the output of the descending motor tracts (e.g. corticospinal tract) that are directly involved in voluntary movements. Cerebellar lesions do not cause motor weakness (paralysis) but disrupt the smooth execution of normal movements. This leads to poor coordination of limb, eye, and trunk movements, impaired balance, and unsteady gait. A simple way to understand the function of the cerebellum is to consider it as an integrator that corrects errors in voluntary movement by constantly comparing intended action with the actual performance (**137**).

Anatomically, the cerebellum occupies most of the posterior cranial fossa. It has an outer mantle of grey matter (cerebellar cortex), internal white matter, and a set of deep nuclei. There are two cerebellar hemispheres connected by a midline strip termed the cerebellar vermis. The part of the hemisphere closest to the vermis is called the intermediate region and the rest of the hemisphere comprises the lateral region. The cerebellum receives input from all levels of the central nervous system, mostly by way of two pairs of large fibre tracts known as inferior and middle cerebellar peduncles. The paired superior cerebellar peduncles comprise the major cerebellar outflow tracts to the motor regions of the cerebral cortex and brainstem. These fibres originate in the deep cerebellar and vestibular nuclei before relaying through the Purkinje cells.

The cerebellum receives its blood supply from the posterior circulation. The vertebral and basilar arteries give rise to three paired branches: the superior (SCA), the anterior inferior (AICA) and the posterior inferior cerebellar arteries (PICA). These are interconnected by extensive arterial anastomoses.

There is a topical representation of individual body parts within the cerebellum (the cerebellar homunculus), and certain cerebellar regions are correlated with distinct function. This may have some significance in localizing lesions in cerebellar ataxia. Midline cerebellar lesions affect stance, gait, and truncal posture. Lesions in the lateral part produce ipsilateral limb ataxia (this occurs because of a double crossing effect of the superior cerebellar peduncle and the corticospinal tracts respectively). Cerebellar signs by themselves do not distinguish lesions in the cerebellar hemispheres from lesions in any of the cerebellar pathways; however, most severe cerebellar dysfunction is often seen in the lesions affecting the cerebellar outflow (deep cerebellar nuclei and the superior cerebellar peduncle).

Proprioceptive sensory pathway

Position and vibration sensations comprise the two most important proprioceptive inputs. Proprioception is carried by the large, myelinated, fast-conducting sensory fibres in the peripheral nerves. These afferent fibres comprise the axons of the bipolar nerve cells located in the dorsal root ganglia outside the spinal cord. In the spinal cord, proprioceptive fibres collect into a bundle in the posterior part of the cord (dorsal column) ipsilaterally and ascend to the lower medulla, where they synapse into the second order neurones (within the nuclei gracilis and cuneatus). Axons from these nuclei cross over to the other side as arcuate fibres and ascend to the thalamus as a large fibre bundle known as the medial lemniscus. Third order sensory neurones from the thalamus then pass through the posterior limb of the internal capsule before reaching the primary sensory (parietal) cortex (**138**).

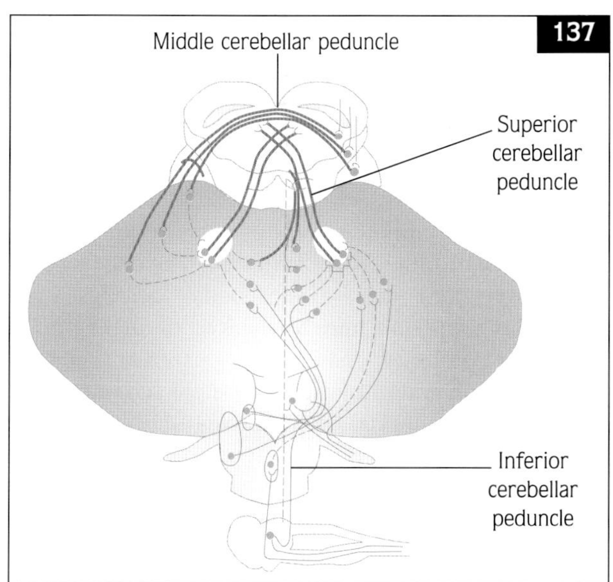

137 A schematic diagram of the anatomy of the cerebellar peduncles that carry the afferent and efferent fibres. The inferior peduncle mostly contains all afferents, e.g. from the vestibular system and the spinal cord. The middle peduncle contains only afferents from the pontine motor nuclei, and the superior peduncle contains mostly efferent fibres. Because both the entering fibres (in the inferior and middle peduncle) and the exiting fibres (in the superior peduncle) cross to the other side, the cerebellar output control is ipsilateral due to the double decussation.

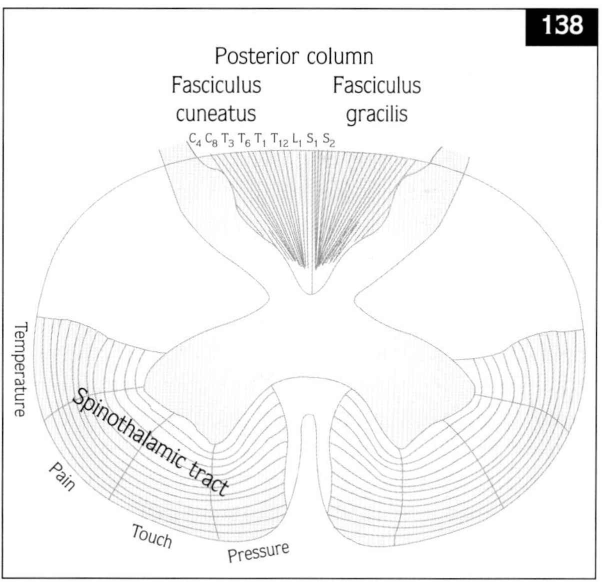

138 A schematic diagram showing lamination of the ascending sensory fibres in the posterior column of the spinal cord. C: cervical; L: lumbar; T: thoracic; S: sacral nerve roots. The sensations of temperature, pain and nondiscriminatory touch are carried in the anterolateral system (spinothalamic tract).

A lesion in the peripheral nerve, dorsal root ganglia, the dorsal column within the spinal cord, medulla, medial lemniscus, thalamus, or parietal cortex may cause a similar sensory ataxia. Essentially, the symptoms are due to loss of position sense and can be compensated by normal visual input with information informing on the position of the body in space.

It is only in the absence of the visual input on body position that sensory ataxia becomes obvious.

Differential diagnosis of ataxia

Ataxia needs to be distinguished from loss of dexterity due to motor weakness (paralysis), restricted movement due to pain, involuntary movements, and from lack of cooperation due to cognitive or behavioural problems. The nature of ataxia (cerebellar, sensory, or vestibular) can usually be identified from the history and neurological examination. Poor coordination is only a symptom and is not a syndrome or disease in itself. It is the underlying problem or disease that needs to be identified and the symptom of ataxia only provides a clue in this exercise.

CLINICAL ASSESSMENT

Focused history taking

The onset, natural history, and the associated symptoms of ataxia are of diagnostic relevance. In particular, the effect of eye closure on ataxia must be determined. Motor symptoms such as dysarthria (see page 163) are invariably associated with cerebellar ataxia and symptoms of peripheral sensory disturbance (burning hands and feet, numbness) are common with sensory ataxia. Age of onset and family history are very important in slowly progressive cerebellar ataxia as so many of these rare syndromes have a hereditary basis. Cerebellar ataxia may be acute, subacute, or chronic and a list of possible causes is provided (*Table 39*). Rarely, patients may experience symptoms of an intermittent ataxia, appearing normal in between attacks (episodic ataxia). Sensory ataxia may be acute (e.g. brainstem stroke or demyelination), subacute (e.g. vitamin B_{12} deficiency, paraneoplastic neuropathy) or part of a chronic progressive myelopathy (e.g. tabes dorsalis, demyelination) or neuropathy (e.g. demyelinating peripheral neuropathy). Common causes of sensory ataxia are listed (*Table 40*).

Examination

Focused examination

The examination of the ataxic patient should be part of a general medical and neurological examination. At the outset, it is important to emphasise that tests for coordination are only meaningful in the presence of retained power (MRC grade 4 or above). Ataxia may be most obvious to the patient when he/she tries to button or unbutton their shirt, fasten clothes, or use a knife and a fork or, in the case of sensory ataxia, in the dark or when the eyes are closed.

A general medical examination is important because it may aid in the aetiological diagnosis of ataxia. Some examples are middle ear disease (with or without cerebellar abscess), bradycardia (hypothyroidism or raised intracranial pressure), papilloedema (posterior fossa tumours), short neck, low hair line, and related dysmorphic features (developmental anomalies of the craniocervical junction such as Chiari malformation), pes cavus (Friedreich's ataxia and hereditary neuropathy), scoliosis (Friedreich's ataxia, syringomyelia, and neurofibromatosis), cutaneous telangiectasia (ataxia-telangiectasia) and dermatitis herpetiformis (associated with coeliac disease).

Neurological examination

This includes special attention to the testing of speech, external eye movements, upper and lower limb coordination, assessment of involuntary movements, and observation of gait. The anatomical localization of ataxia is only possible by means of a thorough neurological examination. The degenerative hereditary and familial cerebellar ataxias have cerebellar signs that may be marked or slight but, in addition, patients also show posterior column, corticospinal, and/or neuropathic signs (characteristic of Friedreich's ataxia). Thrombosis of the posterior inferior cerebellar artery due to vertebral occlusion is the commonest vascular lesion of the cerebellum, and presents with acute vertigo and distinctive medullary signs (cranial nerve IX/X palsy, Horner's syndrome, impairment of facial and contralateral pain and temperature sensations). These features occur in addition to more obvious cerebellar features of nystagmus and limb ataxia. The same artery also supplies the lateral part of the medulla.

Cerebellar dysarthria

There are two types of cerebellar dysarthria, one characterized by 'explosive' speech as if the patient was speaking with his mouth full of marbles. The

Table 39 Presentations of cerebellar ataxia

Acute (over hours to days)	
Acute, reversible	Viral and postinfective cerebellitis (Case 1)
Acute, relapsing	Episodic ataxias Multiple sclerosis Metabolic encephalopathies (hyperammonaemias) Toxic (alcohol, phenytoin, barbiturates)
Acute, persistent	Cerebellar infarcts Cerebellar haemorrhage (e.g. hypertensive), abscess, or metastases Wernicke–Korsakoff syndrome Hyperthermia Opsoclonus-myoclonus
Subacute (over days to weeks) or chronic (months)	
Pure cerebellar syndrome	Paraneoplastic (associated with gynaecological or small-cell lung tumours) Alcohol–nutritional Toxic (lithium, mercury, gasoline, glue, cytotoxics)
Cerebellar syndrome associated with additional signs or symptoms	Posterior fossa tumours (medulloblastoma, astrocytoma, haemangioblastoma, acoustic Schwannoma) Chronic subdural haematoma Multiple sclerosis Hypothyroidism Hashimoto's encephalomyelitis Lyme disease Coeliac disease Superficial siderosis
Cerebellar syndrome with dementia	Creutzfeldt–Jakob disease
Chronic (months to years)	
Childhood or early-onset	Congenital cerebellar ataxia Heredofamilial (e.g. Friedreich's ataxia) Ataxia-telangiectasia Ataxia associated with hereditary metabolic diseases Cerebellar syndrome with myoclonic epilepsy (e.g. Lafora body disease, Unverricht–Lundborg syndrome)
Adulthood or late-onset	Sporadic (olivopontocerebellar atrophy and inherited spinocerebellar degeneration spinocerebellar ataxia 1,2,3 etc.) Multiple system atrophy
Any age	Craniocervical junction anomalies (Chiari malformation, Dandy–Walker syndrome)

Table 40 Causes of sensory ataxia

Demyelinating peripheral neuropathies ('sensory ataxic neuropathy'):
- ❏ Chronic inflammatory demyelinating neuropathy
- ❏ Inherited neuropathy (Charcot–Marie–Tooth disease)
- ❏ Paraproteinaemic neuropathy
- ❏ Sarcoidosis

Dorsal root ganglionopathy
- ❏ Infective (syphilis, Lyme disease)
- ❏ Toxic (e.g. pyridoxine)
- ❏ Paraneoplastic (subacute sensory neuropathy)
- ❏ Sjögren's syndrome

Lesions affecting dorsal column in the spinal cord
- ❏ Compression of the cervical or thoracic spinal cord (e.g. meningioma)
- ❏ Inherited spinocerebellar degeneration (e.g. Friedreich's ataxia)
- ❏ Multiple sclerosis
- ❏ Syphilis
- ❏ Vitamin B_{12} deficiency

Lesions affecting medial lemniscus or its central projection
- ❏ Multiple sclerosis
- ❏ Vascular (infarct)
- ❏ Tumours

other type of speech is much slower with undue separation of the syllables, known as staccato or scanning speech (from a resemblance to the scanning of the Greek verse). The former is more characteristic of an acquired cerebellar problem (e.g. multiple sclerosis) and occurs because the patient attempts to speak normally but suffers from poor coordination of the muscles of articulation of speech and control of breathing. Scanning speech is relatively more common in either a developmental cerebellar disease (congenital or the early-onset type of heredofamilial ataxia) or a lesion acquired early in childhood. Cerebellar disease is often associated with distinctive eye movement abnormalities and nystagmus; these are discussed elsewhere (page 104).

Cerebellar ataxia is associated with reduced muscle tone and this, together with the errors imposed in the direction, range, speed, and force of movements, results in a characteristic set of clinical signs. A failure to integrate conjugate eye movements produces nystagmus. Heel-to-knee and finger-to-nose tests are the usual ways to demonstrate cerebellar incoordination in the lower and upper limbs respectively (Chapter 1). Sometimes, however, more delicate movements are necessary to unmask the impaired coordination, such as asking the patient to make imaginary finger movements as if playing the piano. Other examples include asking the patient to bring the tip of each finger rapidly in turn to touch the thumb of his own hand, or to pat the dorsum of his clenched fist first with the palmar aspect and then the dorsal aspect of his opposite hand with increasing speed, repeating the manoeuvre with the other hand.

A number of terms have been used in the literature to qualify cerebellar incoordination. These include **dyssynergia** (a lack of synergy or coordinated movements of synergistic muscles), **dysmetria** (an ineffectual range of movement, often resulting in target overshooting or hypermetria ['past-pointing']), **dysdiadochokinesia** (inability to perform complex repetitive movements smoothly and rapidly such as supination and pronation of forearms) and **rebound phenomenon** (a failure to brake movement smoothly, for example, when the external resistance to the forearm kept flexed at 90° is suddenly released, a patient with cerebellar disturbance may fail to check the unopposed flexion movement and may be hit by his own arm).

In mid-line cerebellar lesions, the trunk muscles are more severely affected than the limbs and the ataxia becomes obvious when the patient is asked to walk. With a cerebellar lesion, the patient walks with a broad base in order to maintain his balance. Often this is best demonstrable when a patient is asked to turn suddenly, when they tend to sway, reel to either side, or fall backwards. This is especially so with lesions in the cerebellar vermis. In less severe cases, as the patient turns on a wide base they abduct their lower limbs excessively to compensate for hypotonicity and then replace the foot on the ground away from the intended position (due to dysmetria). This results in the typical decomposition of gait seen in cerebellar disorders. Because such clumsiness is not corrected by vision (unlike the patient with a posterior column disease), a patient with cerebellar ataxia does not look to the ground while walking but instead looks straight ahead. In pure cerebellar lesions uncomplicated by central nervous system involvement at other sites, reflexes are not overtly affected but the tendon jerks may be mildly affected qualitatively. When the knee jerk is tested with the patient sitting at the edge of the bed, the knee may swing back and forth three times or more due to a combination of muscle hypotonia and rebound phenomenon. This is known as a pendular knee jerk and must not be interpreted as a sign of pathological hyperreflexia associated with corticospinal lesions.

Testing for joint position sense and vibration is covered elsewhere in the book (Chapter 1). Patients with sensory ataxia may have muscle hypotonia and diminished reflexes when the pathological process is at the level of the peripheral nerves, dorsal root ganglia or, rarely, in the posterior column without extending into the corticospinal tracts. In uncomplicated sensory ataxia, the patient walks on a broad base in order to maintain their centre of gravity. Limbs are lifted abnormally high due to the inability to appreciate the normal range of movements at the joints as a result of lack of proprioception. For the same reason, the heels are slammed back to the ground with excessive force, resulting in a 'stamping' gait, originally described with tabes dorsalis (literally meaning wasting of the posterior column), a form of neurosyphilis. A combination of proprioceptive loss, painless joint deformity (Charcot joints), and perforating ulcers of the lower limbs was virtually diagnostic of the locomotor ataxia of neurosyphilis, a condition that is now seldom seen but contributed a great deal to the understanding of sensory ataxia. In patients with sensory ataxia, the heels of the shoes tend to get worn more quickly as this part of the foot strikes the ground with so much force.

A positive Romberg's test refers to the situation where a patient is completely steady when standing on a normal base with eyes open and the feet drawn together but becomes unsteady as soon as the eyes are closed.

> Obviously, Romberg's test cannot be performed (or is meaningless even if performed) in a patient with cerebellar ataxia who is unsteady even with his eyes open.

In the upper limbs, sensory ataxia is best demonstrated by asking the patient to shut their eyes while keeping their pronated arms outstretched in the forward position. Since in sensory ataxia one cannot appreciate the limb position if the eyes are closed, the patient's forearms will drift away from the original position in an athetoid movement (**pseudoathetosis or sensory limb ataxia**). This swaying of the sensory ataxic arms must be distinguished from the sideways drift seen in the presence of motor weakness in corticospinal lesions (pronator drift sign).

Investigations

As a general rule, all patients with progressive cerebellar ataxia must be considered for imaging (preferably magnetic resonance imaging [MRI]) scans of the posterior fossa and the craniocervical junction (*Table 41*). Computed tomography (CT) scan of brain is particularly useful in an acute setting when patients present with increasing signs of ataxia due to cerebellar infarction with oedema, cerebellar haemorrhage, posterior fossa subdural haematoma, obstructive hydrocephalus, cerebellar tumours, and metastases.

The utilization of more specific investigations for cerebellar ataxia depends on the age of symptom onset, positive family history, additional neurological signs, and the potential differential diagnosis. A slowly progressive cerebellar syndrome with bilateral symmetrical involvement suggests a biochemical (metabolic), toxic, or inherited cause. Genetic tests are currently available for Friedreich's ataxia and a number of inherited spinocerebellar ataxias (SCA mutations) and should only be considered after a careful review of the family history with appropriate pretest counselling. Chronic gait ataxia of months' or years' duration usually suggests a metabolic or inherited ataxia; hypothyroidism should also be excluded in cases with a shorter history. Multiple sclerosis may present with cerebellar and/or sensory ataxia and the diagnosis is usually confirmed by MRI scans (brain and cervical spinal cord) and, if required, cerebrospinal fluid (CSF) examination and evoked response studies. In a patient over the age of 40 years who develops a subacute and progressive cerebellar ataxia and has negative family history, a normal MRI scan and normal CSF, and if alcohol and toxic causes have been excluded, underlying malignancy requires consideration. Paraneoplastic cerebellar degeneration is a recognized presentation of breast and ovarian carcinoma and in such cases serum samples should be tested for paraneoplastic antibodies (anti-Yo antibody). These are named after index cases. Another paraneoplastic (or occasionally, postinfectious) syndrome, opsoclonus-myoclonus, is associated with incapacitating gait ataxia. Folic acid, vitamin B_{12} and B_1 concentrations in the blood should be measured in patients in whom alcohol or a nutritional cause of ataxia is suspected. The electroencephalogram (EEG)

Table 41 Initial investigations of an ataxic patient

Cerebellar ataxia

All cases:
- ❏ Cranial CT and/or MRI of head
- ❏ Thyroid function test

Selected cases:
- ❏ CSF
- ❏ Genetic tests
- ❏ Toxicology or metabolic screen
- ❏ Paraneoplastic antibody (anti-Yo)
- ❏ Serology for coeliac disease
- ❏ Vitamin B_1
- ❏ EEG

Sensory ataxia

All cases:
- ❏ Vitamin B_{12} and folic acid levels
- ❏ Syphilis serology

Selected cases:
- ❏ MRI (head and/or spinal cord)
- ❏ Nerve conduction studies
- ❏ CSF
- ❏ Paraneoplastic antibody (anti-Hu)

Serology for Sjögren's syndrome, Lyme disease

CSF: cerebrospinal fluid; CT: computed tomography; EEG: electroencephalogram; MRI: magnetic resonance imaging.

is a valuable investigation in patients with myoclonus and cerebellar ataxia (mitochondrial encephalopathies, inherited myoclonic epilepsies, and Creutzfeldt–Jakob disease).

Nerve conduction studies and CSF examination are indicated in patients with peripheral neuropathy and sensory ataxia; these patients have absent or diminished tendon reflexes (areflexic ataxia). Conversely, sensory ataxia with hyperreflexia requires MRI scanning of the spinal cord or lower brainstem (medulla and the region of foramen magnum) depending on the anatomical localization, often based on the level of concomitant sensory loss. Rarely, sensory ataxia produces lateralized imbalance that involves one side of the body only. In such cases, symptoms can be caused by lesions in the parietal lobe or thalamus but alternatively may also be due to unilateral posterior column disease affecting the spinal cord as seen in Brown-Séquard syndrome (see page 148). Patients with sensory ataxia without a structural lesion in the brain and spinal cord should have blood samples tested for folic acid and vitamin B_{12}, serum protein electrophoresis, markers for Sjögren's syndrome, syphilis, and Lyme serology. Adult patients with a smoking history and a progressive ataxic neuropathy (Denny–Brown sensory neuropathy) will require screening for small-cell lung tumour and serum paraneoplastic antibody (anti-Hu antibody).

Summary

- The patient's symptoms of poor coordination should be interpreted as part of a wider neurological or medical problem.
- While specific attention should be given to identifying the nature of ataxia, a complete neurological examination is essential for the clinical diagnosis of the ataxic patient.
- Type of ataxia (i.e. sensory or cerebellar) as well as its possible anatomical localization is important in choosing the right investigation in a given patient.
- In rare cases (Case 3), cerebellar and sensory ataxia may coexist in the same patient.
- The treatment is directed to the underlying cause rather than to the ataxia itself.

CLINICAL SCENARIOS

Case 1

A 12-year-old female presented with an abrupt onset of limb and gait ataxia over a period of 24 hours. She was well and attending her classes 2 weeks previously when she had developed a mild fever with generalized skin rash. This was diagnosed to be chicken pox and she was kept at home. Her fever settled within a day or two and she did not have any other problem due to her chicken pox. She did not have any symptoms of double vision, lower cranial nerve symptoms, or vomiting but did have a mild headache with her ataxia. She had fallen twice while trying to go to the toilet since her balance became poor. She was also unable to hold a cup without spilling its contents. She also required assistance with feeding because of her inability to coordinate her hand movements by using a fork and a knife.

She was born full-term, normal delivery, and her developmental milestones were normal. She was an intelligent girl and did not have any other significant past medical history. She was not on any regular medications. She has two brothers (aged 9 and 16 years) who are healthy. There is no family history of cerebellar ataxia.

On examination, she was afebrile. Her general physical examination showed healed skin marks of chicken pox with one or two lesions where the scabs were still present. She appeared cheerful but had cerebellar dysarthria as she spoke. Her optic discs were normal and pupils were equal as well as reactive. External ocular movements showed bilateral jerk nystagmus in the horizontal plane. Her lower cranial nerves were intact. Motor examination showed normal limb tone, brisk reflexes, and flexor plantar responses. She had ataxia of both her arms and legs with quite marked ataxia of gait.

(Continued on page 183)

Case 1 *(continued)*

Clinically, a diagnosis of acute ataxia of childhood was made. This was considered to be due to an acute cerebellitis that is well recognized after chicken pox in children.

To exclude other possibilities such as a cerebellar tumour (medulloblastoma) and demyelination, MRI brain scan was advised. This was found to be entirely normal. She also had CSF examination by lumbar puncture for inflammatory causes of her ataxia. Her CSF showed 20 lymphocytes (normally less than 5)/mm^3 with a protein of 0.65 g/l. CSF polymerase chain reaction (PCR) was negative for Varicella zoster virus.

The patient and her parents were told that her ataxia was not due to a tumour, infection or brain injury and was probably caused by local inflammation in her cerebellum as a reaction to her recent viral exanthem (chicken pox). They were also told that she was expected to make a slow but full recovery spontaneously and she did so in 6 months' time. In a child who presents with acute cerebellar ataxia, the first concern is to exclude a structural lesion (tumour or an abscess) in the posterior fossa or cerebellum.

Case 2

A 52-year-old businessman of Indian origin presented with a 10-week history of frequent falls, poor balance, fatigue, and impaired short-term memory. For about 6 months prior to these symptoms he was experiencing painful sensations affecting his feet and, to a lesser extent, his arms. He was also known to be mildly diabetic for the past 2 years and was managed on diet alone. It was thought that his sensory symptoms were due to diabetes. He was advised to lose weight and do more physical activities. However, he discovered that he fell easily on a treadmill if he did not look down and had great difficulty in taking a walk because of poor balance. There was no other medical history of importance. He had no history of bowel surgery. He had a family history of diabetes. He was a strict vegetarian because of his faith for a number of years. He did not smoke or drink alcohol.

Clinical examination showed normal cranial nerves, pupils, and optic discs. Motor examination showed increased tone in his legs with normal power, absent ankle jerks, but brisk knee jerks bilaterally. Both his plantar responses were extensor. Sensory examination showed marked hyperalgesia of feet, proprioceptive loss to the level of his hips, and a strongly positive Romberg's test. His upper limb motor and sensory examinations were normal and he did not have any cerebellar signs.

A diagnosis of subacute combined degeneration of the spinal cord due to dietary vitamin B_{12} deficiency was considered.

This was confirmed by low levels of serum vitamin B_{12} (110 pmol/l), and supported by increased mean cell volume (105 fl), macrocytosis, and hypersegmented neutrophils in the peripheral blood smear. MRI of his spinal cord showed an area of patchily increased signal within the cervical segment of the cord. His CSF was normal and peripheral electrophysiology (nerve conduction studies) could not demonstrate any abnormality. He was found to be weakly positive for antiparietal cell antibody.

The patient was commenced immediately on intramuscular vitamin B_{12} injections and his sensory symptoms, fatigue, and poor concentration resolved rapidly. He made a good recovery from his sensory ataxia by 3 months. Vitamin B_{12} deficiency is not uncommon in the setting of a strict vegetarian diet or in patients with bowel problems (chronic gastritis or Crohn's disease). Neurological symptoms of vitamin B_{12} deficiency may appear before any haematological changes.

Case 3

A 35-year-old female was seen in the neurology outpatient clinic because of her history of poor coordination affecting her right arm, developing over the past 6–8 hours. She realized this as she was trying to brush her teeth. She was unable to appreciate what she was holding with her right hand unless she had looked at it. Three years previously, she had an acute attack of cerebellar ataxia from which she had made a good recovery with some residual symptoms in her left arm and left leg. She was treated with large doses of intravenous steroids at that time. About 10 years before the present episode, she had sudden loss of vision in her right eye but had made a full recovery without any treatment. When she was investigated on the last occasion, her MRI brain scans were found to be abnormal and the observed changes were consistent with a diagnosis of multiple sclerosis (MS). This diagnosis was further supported by additional tests. Visual evoked response from her right eye was delayed and her CSF was positive for oligoclonal bands.

On this occasion, the patient was concerned that she might have had a relapse of her MS. She was also feeling increasingly tired. As a single mother, she was finding it increasingly difficult to cope with her household work, full-time job as a receptionist, and also to look after her 5-year-old daughter.

She admitted that she was under 'a lot of stress' in the recent weeks. She took simple analgesics for pain relief but otherwise was not on any regular medication. There was no other contributory past or family medical history. She did not smoke and took alcohol only on rare social occasions.

Neurological examination showed some reduction of visual acuity in her right eye, a relative afferent right pupillary defect, jerk nystagmus of the abducting eyes in the horizontal plane bilaterally, and brisk jaw jerk. Motor examination showed minimally increased tone in the legs with reduced tone in the arms, normal power, brisk reflexes (arms and legs), ankle clonus, and extensor plantar response bilaterally. Her left heel–knee test was abnormal and she had past pointing with her left arm. In addition, she had marked proprioceptive loss in her right arm with pseudoathetosis.

The present problem was attributed to the sensory ataxia of her right arm due to a new demyelinating event. Her neurological examination also showed features of previous optic neuritis in the right eye, bilateral internuclear ophthalmoplegia, and left-sided cerebellar hemiataxia.

MRI scans of her cervical cord and lower brainstem revealed an area of demyelination involving the upper two segments of the cervical cord and extending to the right side of the medulla in its lower half (**139**).

This lesion was considered adequate to explain the sensory ataxia in the right arm. She was treated with a short course of intravenous steroid injections for her relapsing MS symptoms. She was advised to take time off her work and part-time child care for her daughter was arranged. She made a reasonable recovery from her upper limb sensory ataxia and was able to return to work 4 months later. Unilateral or upper limb sensory ataxia without lower limb involvement is suggestive of a lesion in the central nervous system. A patient may have symptoms of both cerebellar and sensory ataxia.

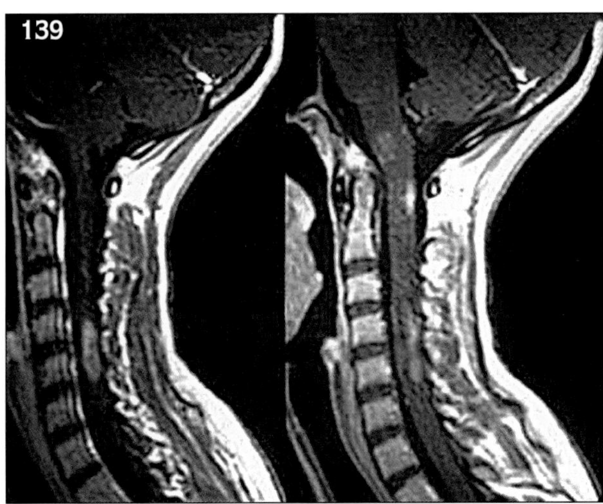

139 Magnetic resonance image of spinal cord of a patient with multiple sclerosis similar to Case 3, showing plaques in the cervical spinal cord and medulla.

Revision questions

1 The final common pathway in the cerebellar output involves:
  a Red nucleus.
  b Purkinje cell.
  c Dentate nucleus.
  d Granule cell.

2 Ataxia on eye closure but not with open eyes is suggestive of:
  a Cerebellar ataxia.
  b Sensory ataxia.
  c A positive Romberg's test.
  d Middle ear disease.

3 Neurological symptoms of vitamin B_{12} deficiency may present:
  a As noncompressive myelopathy, i.e. spinal cord disease.
  b With symptoms of burning feet.
  c Without haematological changes of megaloblastic anaemia.
  d With cerebellar symptoms.

4 Paraneoplastic neurological diseases affecting coordination may manifest as:
  a Weakness of neuromuscular junction (antivoltage gated calcium channel antibody).
  b Subacute sensory neuropathy (anti-Hu antibody).
  c Opsoclonus, truncal ataxia (anti-Ri antibody).
  d Cerebellar ataxia (anti-Yo antibody).

5 Blood supply of the cerebellum is derived from the branches of:
  a Carotid artery.
  b Vertebral artery.
  c Basilar artery.
  d All of the above.

6 Within the spinal cord, fibres carrying proprioception are located in the:
  a Spinocerebellar tract.
  b Spinothalamic tract.
  c Posterior column.
  d None of the above.

7 Ataxic hemiparesis refers to:
a Ipsilateral corticospinal weakness and contralateral ataxia.
b Corticospinal weakness and ataxia on the same side.
c Neither (a) nor (b).
d Both (a) and (b).

8 Sudden dizziness and vomiting, along with marked truncal ataxia in a hypertensive patient who is unable to stand upright, suggest a diagnosis of:
a Ménière's disease.
b Cerebellar haemorrhage.
c Internal capsular haemorrhage.
d Subarachnoid haemorrhage.

9 Ataxic neuropathies may be associated with:
a Monoclonal or polyclonal gammopathy.
b Paraneoplastic antibody.
c Sjögren's syndrome.
d Inflammatory demyelinating neuropathy.

10 Cerebellar features present in conjunction with a rapidly deteriorating level of consciousness is suggestive of:
a Expanding posterior fossa mass.
b Posterior inferior cerebellar artery infarct.
c Anterior inferior cerebellar artery infarct.
d Viral encephalitis.

11 The following clinical signs would suggest a diagnosis of acoustic neuroma (vestibular Schwannoma):
a Hearing loss.
b Cerebellar ataxia.
c Nystagmus.
d Decreased facial sensation.

12 Cerebellar ataxia is inherited as an autosomal recessive disorder in:
a Hypothyroidism.
b Friedreich's ataxia.
c Spinocerebellar ataxia.
d Ataxia-telangiectasia.

13 A combination of cerebellar and sensory ataxia may be seen in:
a Coeliac disease.
b Alcohol abuse.
c Lyme disease.
d B-vitamin deficiency.

14 Vertigo is a side-effect of toxicity from:
a Phenytoin.
b Aminoglycoside antibiotics.
c Salicylates.
d Alcohol.

15 The preferred neuroimaging for acute cerebellar ataxia is:
a MRI.
b CT.
c CT followed by MRI.
d Plain X-ray of the skull base.

Answers
1 b
2 b, c
3 a, b, c
4 b, c, d
5 b, c
6 a, b, c
7 b
8 b
9 a, b, c, d
10 a
11 a, b, c, d
12 b, d
13 a, c
14 a, b, c, d
15 c

Disorders of sensation

HEADACHE

Stewart Webb

INTRODUCTION

Headache is a common disorder, with 70% of the population having at least one episode every month. For most it is a benign self-limiting symptom, which does not cause concern. However, it may be a disabling complaint and, for a few, an indication of potentially life-threatening disease. The question for every doctor at some time is when to reassure, treat, and investigate. This chapter will discuss the clinical approach to patients with insidious worsening headache who commonly present to the outpatient clinic, and patients with acute onset headache who require urgent hospital admission and assessment to exclude potentially life-threatening conditions. A useful division of headache is into primary and secondary types (*Tables 42* and *43*).

Classification

The International Headache Society have classified and produced diagnostic criteria for both primary and secondary headache disorders. Although these

Table 42 Primary headache disorders

Lasting >4 hours	Lasting <4 hours
Tension type headache (69%)	Cluster headache (2%)
Migraine (16%)	Chronic paroxysmal hemicrania
	SUNCT
	Hypnic headache
	Idiopathic stabbing
	Exertional headache (0.1%)

SUNCT: shortlasting, unilateral neuralgiform headache attacks with conjunctival injection and tearing

Table 43 Secondary headache disorders

Systemic infection	(63%)	
Head injury	(4%)	
Medications and toxins	(3%)	Chronic analgesia abuse Acute alcohol abuse or withdrawal
Vascular disorders	(1%)	SAH Venous sinus thrombosis Vertebral or carotid dissection stroke
Brain tumours	(0.1%)	
Infection		Chronic CNS infection
Inflammation		Giant cell arteritis
CSF obstruction		Intraventricular tumour Aqueductal stenosis
Raised CSF protein		Post meningitis GBS Spinal cord tumours
Cerebral oedema		Post head injury Post cerebral anoxia Benign intracranial hypertension
Others		Malignant hypertension Hypercapnia Metabolic disorders Cervical spine Acute glaucoma

CNS: central nervous system; CSF: cerebrospinal fluid; GBS: Guillain–Barré syndrome; SAH: subarachnoid heamorrhage.

can be helpful in clinical practice, they are mainly used for clinical trials (*Table 44*) and represent work in progress rather then criteria that are written in stone.

Anatomy and pathophysiology of headache

Pain of both primary and secondary type headaches originates from either extra- or intracranial structures. The brain itself has no pain receptors and therefore lesions within brain parenchyma do not produce headache unless they directly or indirectly stretch or compress surrounding pain sensitive structures (*Table 45*).

Clinical assessment

History taking

The history is the most important part of the assessment process (*Table 46*), as there are no diagnostic tests for the primary headache disorders and it is impractical, unwise, and anxiety provoking to investigate all patients.

Persons may have more then one type of headache (mixed) and, although it is reasonable to concentrate on the most troublesome, it is important to get a clear description of each type. It is crucial, in patients who report a recent onset of headache, to determine if the headache is new, or whether it is an

Table 44 Abbreviated International Headache Society criteria for common primary headaches

Episodic tension type headache

- <15 headaches a month
- Headache lasts from 30 minutes to 7 days
- At least two of the following pain characteristics:
  - pressing/tightening (nonpulsating)
  - mild to moderate intensity
  - bilateral location
  - not aggravated by routine physical activity
- Both:
  - no nausea or vomiting
  - may have photophobia or phonophobia but not both

Chronic tension type headache

- ≥15 headaches a month for ≥6 months
- At least two of the following pain characteristics:
  - pressing/tightening (nonpulsating)
  - mild to moderate intensity
  - bilateral location
  - not aggravated by routine physical activity
- Both:
  - no vomiting
  - no more than one of nausea, photophobia, or phonophobia

Migraine without aura

- Headaches last 4–72 hours
- At least two of the following pain characteristics:
  - unilateral location
  - pulsating quality
  - moderate or severe intensity
  - aggravated by routine physical activity
- At least one of the following with the headache:
  - nausea and/or vomiting
  - photophobia and phonophobia

Migraine with aura

- At least three of the following:
  - reversible aura indicating focal cortical and/or brainstem dysfunction
  - aura develops over at least 4 minutes, or two symptoms occur in succession
  - no aura lasting >60 minutes
  - headache follows aura within 60 minutes (the headache may also begin before or with the aura)

Familial hemiplegic migraine

- Fulfils the criteria for migraine with aura
- Aura includes some degree of hemiparesis and may be prolonged
- At least one first degree relative with identical attacks

Basilar migraine

- Fulfils the criteria for migraine with aura
- Two or more aura symptoms of the following type:
  - visual symptoms in both the temporal and nasal fields of both eyes
  - dysarthria
  - vertigo
  - tinnitus
  - decreased hearing
  - double vision
  - ataxia
  - bilateral paraesthesia
  - bilateral pareses
  - decreased level of consciousness

In all criteria secondary causes must be excluded; this is usually on clinical grounds but where indicated, follows investigations.

existing headache which has become more frequent or severe. Patients may consider some headache as normal and fail to mention their 'sinus headache', which has been present for several years. The possibility of having a serious cause does not increase in proportion to the severity, frequency, or duration of the headache. Severe headache may be due to migraine, while patients with tumours rarely present with headache alone and then only occasionally complain of having a dull or muzzy head on direct questioning. Patients should be asked about the onset, progression, frequency, and duration of each headache (it may be useful for the patient to keep a diary). The site and spread of the headache should be established, its quality (e.g. dull, sharp, throbbing, or pressure) and intensity (is the patient's activity or function limited?). Patients should be asked about any associated features, in particular the presence or absence of nausea, vomiting, visual disturbance, photophobia, phonophobia, dysarthria, or ataxia and should also report any precipitating, aggravating, or relieving factors (e.g. lying, standing, movement, coughing, stooping, or straining). Medication history should be described, i.e. which drug(s) has been or is being used, in what dose, frequency and duration, and effect. It is also useful to enquire about occupation, family history, level of stress and depression, and any concerns or anxieties the patient may have about the headache.

Table 45 Pain sensitive structures of the head

Intracranial

- ❑ Dura at the base of the brain
- ❑ Venous sinuses
- ❑ Arteries (including): proximal part of anterior and middle cerebral arteries
  intracranial segment of the internal carotid artery
- ❑ Middle meningeal artery
- ❑ Cranial nerves:

Optic	(II)
Oculomotor	(III)
Trigeminal	(V)
Glossopharyngeal	(IX)
Vagus	(X)

Extracranial

- ❑ Skin and subcutaneous tissue
- ❑ Muscle
- ❑ Extracranial arteries
- ❑ Periosteum of the skull
- ❑ First three cervical nerves
- ❑ Eyes
- ❑ Ears
- ❑ Nasal cavities
- ❑ Sinuses

Table 46 Questions to ask the patient with headache

- ❑ Onset of headache
- ❑ Frequency and progression of headache
- ❑ Duration of headache
- ❑ Site and radiation
- ❑ Quality of headache
- ❑ Associated features
- ❑ Precipitating factors
- ❑ Aggravating factors
- ❑ Relieving factors
- ❑ Drug history
- ❑ Occupation
- ❑ Family history
- ❑ Level of stress and depression
- ❑ Concerns or anxieties

Examination

A thorough, thoughtful examination is essential to reassure patients with primary headache, eliminate secondary causes, and identify comorbid disease such as infection, hypertension, and depression (*Table 47*). After taking the history the examiner should be in a position to decide if the headache is of primary or secondary type and, if secondary, if the underlying pathology is likely to be intra- or extracranial or systemic. Decisions made will then help in directing a more focused neurological examination. In all patients, blood pressure should be recorded. The optic discs should be examined for evidence of papilloedema. The pupils should be noted to be equal and reactive to light. Eye movements should be full with no evidence of nystagmus or diplopia. Upper and lower limbs should be assessed for focal weakness and ataxia, asymmetry of reflexes, and plantar responses. Both gait and tandem walking should be assessed. Further examination will depend on the patient's symptoms and may include assessment of neck movements, pain and stiffness, local pain and tenderness (neck, occiput, scalp, temporal arteries, sinuses, eyes, temporomandibular joint), infection, and inflammation (meninges, eyes, ears, nose, throat, teeth).

Table 47 Minimum examination in patients with headache

	Possible abnormal findings
Cranial nerves	
Fundoscopy	Papilloedema
Visual fields (to confrontation)	Visual field defects
Pupils	Equal and reactive to light
Eye movements	Nystagmus Diplopia Abnormal pursuit movements
Facial movements	Asymmetrical weakness
Limbs	
Reflexes	Brisk/asymmetry
Finger–nose test	Ataxia
Plantars	Extensor plantar response
Gait	Spasticity/ataxia
Tandem gait	Ataxia
Scalp	
Temporal arteries	In patient >50 years Tenderness and absent pulsation
Additional examination depending on history	
Scalp	Tenderness
Cervical spine	Tenderness Restricted neck movements
Temporomandibular joint	Tenderness Click
Sinus	Tenderness Nasal obstruction
Ears	Deafness Infection
Teeth	Poor dentition Wear

Investigations

Patients in whom a diagnosis of primary headache is certain do not require investigation (*Table 48*). The history and examination should identify those patients with 'red flag' symptoms and signs (*Table 49*) who need investigation.

Table 48 Investigation of headache

	Comment
Bloods	
ESR	Temporal arteritis
Thyroid function	Thyroid disease
24 hour VMA	Phaeochromocytoma
Imaging	
CT	Compared to MRI it is poor in visualizing the posterior fossa, base of skull and foramen magnum. It cannot exclude subarachnoid haemorrhage completely
CT with contrast	Suspected mass lesion on plain CT
MRI	Availability limited
CT/MRI venography	Venous sinus thrombosis
CT/MRI angiography	Cerebral vasculitis or vascular malformations
Lumbar puncture	To exclude meningitis and to measure CSF pressure

CSF: cerebrospinal fluid; CT: computed tomography; ESR: erythrocyte sedimentation rate; MRI: magnetic resonance imaging; VMA: Vanillyl-mandelic acid.

INSIDIOUS WORSENING HEADACHE

Both primary and secondary headache disorders may present to the clinician with insidious worsening headache.

Primary headache disorders

Tension type headache

This is the commonest type of primary headache (lifetime prevalence 78%). Starting at any age, it can continue throughout life. It is separated into episodic and chronic forms, depending on whether patients have periods of freedom. The headache is nonpulsating and is described as a bilateral pressure or tight sensation of mild to moderate severity that may inhibit but not prohibit daily activities. Physical activity does not aggravate the headache and there is no associated vomiting. However, mild nausea, photophobia, or phonophobia may occur. Patients may also complain of being giddy, light-headed, and have difficulty concentrating. In the episodic form it may develop during, after, or in anticipation of stress, and tends to last <24 hours.

In the chronic form, patients may awaken with headache, which then persists throughout the day regardless of activity or stress. Four different varieties maybe distinguished. **Chronic daily headache** is tension type headache, which has become daily often as a result of analgesia overuse or depression. **Transformed migraine** applies to those patients with typical migraine headaches that increase in frequency until they are occurring daily, but still retain some of the features of migraine such as unilaterality or nausea. **New daily persistent headache** (*Table 50*) applies to patients who were previously headache free but who develop headache without any obvious physical or psychological factor to account for the headache. In this situation secondary causes (*Table 43*) need to be ruled out. **Hemicrania continuum** is a constant unilateral headache of uncertain cause responsive to indomethacin.

Migraine

Migraine headache affects between 10 and 20% of the population and is more common in females. Problems with diagnosis often arise because typical features are absent or atypical migraine features are present. Migraine may be associated with changes in mood (irritability, depression, or elation), alertness (drowsiness, yawning) and appetite (craving for sweet foods), which may precede the onset of headache by up to 24 hours.

Table 49 Red flag symptoms/signs

Symptoms

- Increased or new-onset vomiting
- Posture related headache or vomiting
- Visual obscurations
- Pronounced change in the character or timing of the headache
- Unusually abrupt onset
- Persistent headache especially beyond 72 hours
- Late onset >55 years
- Developing after head injury

Signs

- Fever
- Neck stiffness
- Papilloedema
- Drowsiness
- Neurological deficit (e.g. weakness, ataxia, cognitive dysfunction)
- Local tenderness (e.g. temporal artery tenderness)

Table 50 Causes of new daily persistent headache

Primary	Migraine
	Tension type
Secondary	SAH
	Low CSF volume headache
	High CSF volume headache
	Post traumatic headache
	Chronic meningitis

CSF: cerebrospinal fluid; SAH: subarachnoid haemorrhage.

Classical migraine is unilateral, fronto-temporal and ocular in site and throbbing in nature. It builds up over 1–2 hours, often progressing posteriorly and becoming diffuse and typically lasts >4 hours or subsides with sleep. However, migraine may also present with a pressure-type pain deep behind the eyes (orbital migraine), which can radiate backwards to the occiput, neck, or shoulders or it may start as a dull ache in the neck and radiate forward behind the eyes (occipital-orbital migraine). With both these patterns the pain is often bilateral. The pain can also affect the face (facial migraine) involving the nostrils, cheek, gums, and teeth. Rarely, it may affect the upper and lower limbs on the side of the headache, suggesting thalamic involvement. Attacks commonly occur during the day but may wake the patient from sleep or be present on wakening. Movement normally aggravates the pain and patients prefer to lie quietly. This is in contrast to tension headache, which is usually mild enough for patients to carry on their normal activities, or cluster headache where patients are usually restless.

As migraine without aura ('common migraine') is at least three times as common as migraine with aura ('classical migraine'), visual disturbance is not a feature in all. Visual aura generally arises in the occipital lobe and is therefore hemianopic and consists of hallucinations (fortification spectra, zig-zag lines, incomplete jagged circles, unformed flashes of light) or scotomas (holes in central vision). The hallucinations are white more often than coloured, and commonly shimmer or jitter as they gradually enlarge leaving behind an area of impaired vision (scintillating scotoma). These visual symptoms usually evolve over 5–10 minutes and clear gradually after 20–30 minutes. Less frequently, the aura may arise from other areas of the cortex or brainstem and produce symptoms such as dysphasia with unilateral paraesthesia and hemiparesis, déjà vu and dreamlike states, olfactory and gustatory hallucinations (temporal lobe), distortions of body image (parietal lobe), diplopia, vertigo, ataxia, and dysarthria (brainstem). The hemiparesis is often described as a sense of heaviness without true weakness of the limbs and is usually associated with sensory symptoms beginning in the hand and then spreading to the arm, face, lips, and tongue. As with visual aura, these sensory symptoms may take 10–20 minutes to evolve and positive symptoms (tingling) are typically followed by negative symptoms (numbness). The aura in migraine may precede or accompany the headache, or may occur in isolation (a so-called migraine equivalent) often seen in middle age. In some patients, migraine aura may be difficult to distinguish from transient ischaemic attack (TIA) or epilepsy. However, migraine aura is usually positive, of gradual onset (5–10 minutes) and accompanied or followed by migraine headache. Although a TIA may be accompanied by headache, it is distinguished by its negative symptoms (loss of vision, weakness, or numbness), abrupt, nonevolving/spreading onset and its confinement to a single blood vessel territory. Photophobia, phonophobia, dizziness, and vertigo are also commonly reported. However, in patients with long-standing migraine, the development of new or more severe headache with vomiting, particularly if related to positional change or accompanied by acute vertigo, should be treated with suspicion, and scanning to exclude a posterior fossa lesion carried out.

Specific forms of migraine can be identified symptomatically:

Hemiplegic migraine

Hemiplegic migraine is a rare, but frequently over diagnosed, autosomal dominantly inherited disorder. The migraine aura is often associated with transient focal weakness or other cortical symptoms (e.g. dysphasia, dysarthria, drop attacks) that resolve within 24 hours, usually without evidence of infarction. These transient deficits may occur without aura or headache and diagnosis of migraine may be difficult unless there is a clear family history.

Vertebrobasilar migraine

This is associated with prodromal symptoms arising from the vertebrobasilar territory: brainstem (vertigo, tinnitus, diplopia, ataxia, dysarthria, cranial neuropathies, pyramidal dysfunction); mid brain reticular formation (fainting, sudden loss of consciousness, agitation, acute confusion, or prolonged stupor and coma); occipital lobe (bilateral visual disturbance). These prodromal symptoms may also occur without subsequent headache.

Ophthalmoplegic migraine

Here patients present with unilateral, periorbital headache followed within hours by a third nerve palsy with an enlarged pupil. Less commonly, the fourth or sixth cranial nerve may be involved or a partial Horner's syndrome may occur. The resultant double vision usually outlasts the headache by days or weeks and can even become permanent.

Retinal migraine

Patients experience recurrent monocular visual loss lasting <30 minutes, normally limited to the same eye and associated with a dull ipsilateral ache.

Cluster headache

Cluster headache may begin at any age, although more commonly it occurs in the third and fourth decades. Males are more affected then females in a ratio of 7:1. Patients are affected by attacks usually in clusters lasting 6–12 weeks, with variable periods of remission. During each cluster the attacks are usually of rapid onset and start with a prickling or tingling sensation in the orbit and nostril. This is followed within minutes by severe pain ('like a red hot poker' or 'acid') in the same area, lasting 15–180 minutes. The pain is strictly unilateral, although the side may vary; the affected eye is bloodshot and the nose congested with a watery discharge. The initial attacks are usually nocturnal, waking patients from sleep several times, and are usually at the same time each night. Daytime attacks are less frequent, but again occur at the same time of the day. Alcohol, exercise, and heat may precipitate an attack during a cluster period but not during remissions. A full range of migrainous symptoms has been reported in patients with cluster headache. However, unlike migraine patients, cluster sufferers are usually restless and prefer to move around rather than lie still.

Chronic paroxysmal hemicrania

Attacks of pain and associated autonomic features are similar to cluster headache. However, females are predominantly affected, attacks are shorter (lasting 2–45 minutes), more frequent (>5 per day on most days) and are responsive to treatment with indomethacin.

Hypnic headache

This benign headache disorder occurs mainly in elderly patients. The attacks occur during sleep and patients wake with a medium or severe generalized headache, unaccompanied by autonomic features. Attacks typically occur at fixed times each night, last for 1 hour and respond well to indomethacin or lithium (cautiously used).

Secondary headache disorders

Sinusitis

Sinusitis may cause pain in the affected sinus, and be referred to other areas of the face and head. However, pain in the affected sinus should be identifiable and there should be evidence of nasal discharge or nasal blockage. Chronic, subclinical sinus infection as a cause of recurrent severe headache does not occur, although so often headache is attributed to this.

Refractory errors

Refractory errors may cause mild periorbital or frontal headache, but cannot account for intermittent severe headache that is not linked to prolonged visual tasks at a distance or angle where vision is impaired. Apart from pain, patients will have evidence of an uncorrected refractive error and may also complain of visual blurring, 'swimming', or double vision.

Cervical spine

A number of conditions affecting the cervical spine, such as osteo- and rheumatoid arthritis, cervical instability following trauma, and Paget's disease may irritate the upper three cervical roots; pain arises in the neck and back of the head on the ipsilateral side with forward radiation to the orbits and frontal regions. Certain neck movements may be painful and restricted. Careful palpation of the occipital nerves may produce local tenderness and induce the occipital headache.

Post-traumatic headache

Post-traumatic headache may vary from mild to severe. The intensity and duration of the headache do not correlate with the severity of the head injury and, indeed, some studies have suggested an inverse relationship with mild head injury causing more problems. The headache may be either acute or chronic (persisting >8 weeks) and begins within 2 weeks of the injury (or termination of post-traumatic amnesia). The chronic form evolves into a daily headache and can be complicated by analgesia misuse headache. The headache is variably characterized as a tension type headache, a migraine type headache, or a combination of both. It is often associated with other post-traumatic problems such as dizziness, depression, and cognitive impairment.

Analgesia misuse headache

This is perhaps the most common association with chronic daily headache. Patients report that their headache is frequently improved by analgesia, only to return (rebound) as the drug effect wears off. This leads to a vicious cycle, and it is not uncommon for patients with chronic daily headache to end up taking large doses of analgesia. Most analgesics have been implicated, particularly over-the-counter treatments containing aspirin or paracetamol with caffeine or codeine phosphate, as well as triptan preparations. After stopping the offending drug, the headache can take some weeks to settle down.

Giant cell arteritis

Giant cell arteritis (or temporal arteritis) is an inflammatory disorder affecting medium-sized, extra cranial arteries, and should be considered in any patient presenting with new headache over 50 years of age. The affected arteries are painful, tender, swollen, and pulseless. Although the temporal arteries are commonly affected, other scalp arteries may be involved and occipital pain with tenderness is not uncommon. Tenderness of the scalp may cause difficulty with washing or brushing the hair. Patients may complain of 'jaw claudication' when talking or chewing, with pain in masseter muscles. General unwellness with muscle aching, anorexia, weight loss, and even low-grade pyrexia is common. Patients may also develop monocular blindness or carotid and vertebrobasilar territory transient ischaemic attacks. Blindness occurs in 50% of patients if untreated, and urgent investigations and treatment with steroids are indicated. A raised erythrocyte sedimentation rate (ESR) can help confirm the diagnosis but a near normal ESR does not exclude it. Temporal artery biopsy (**140**) may confirm the diagnosis, but a normal biopsy again will not completely exclude it, as vessel involvement is patchy. A dramatic immediate response to steroids is also diagnostic.

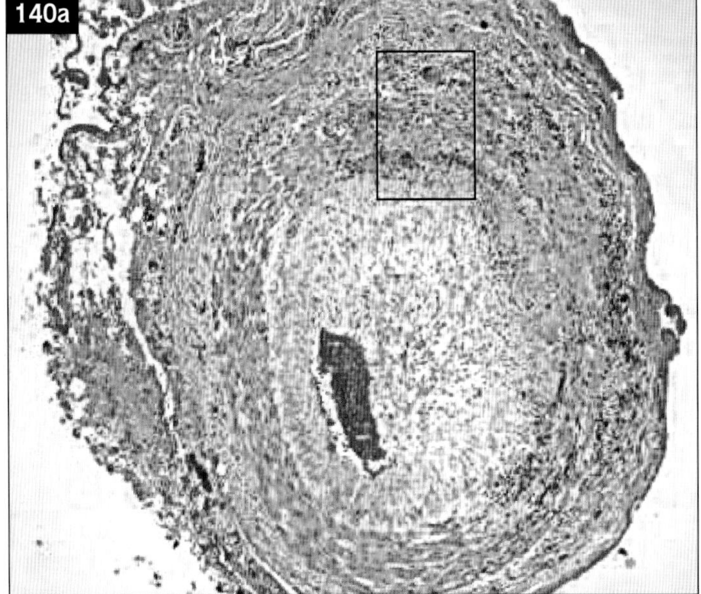

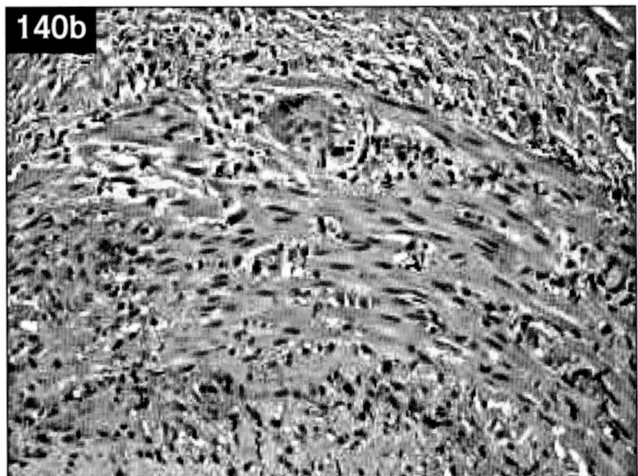

140 Temporal arteritis. **a:** biopsy of a temporal artery in transverse section, showing thickening of the intimal layer with stenosis of the vessel lumen. There is also disruption of the internal elastic lamina with thickening of the inner layers of the media (haematoxylin and eosin, low power); **b:** higher power magnification of the vessel wall at the junction between intima and media, showing disruption of the internal elastic lamina, multinucleated giant cell formation, and a chronic inflammatory cell infiltrate.

Raised crebrospinal fluid pressure headache

Raised intracranial (cerebrospinal fluid [CSF]) pressure headache is characterized by a bursting sensation in the head that is normally present on waking, aggravated by bending or coughing and associated with visual obscuration (*Table 51*). It responds poorly to analgesia. Although patients presenting with these symptoms need further investigation to exclude potentially serious disease (*Table 43*), many of these features occur in migraine and many patients with new onset migraine are extensively investigated without any abnormality being found. There are a number of 'red flags' or warnings (*Table 49*) which should raise suspicion but particular pointers to serious intracranial pathology are the presence of very short-lived headaches with a pounding quality related to changes in position or straining, with no headache at other times, and recent onset headache associated with positional vertigo and repeated vomiting. Focal signs or papilloedema may or may not be present but must always be examined for.

Table 51 Causes of raised cerebrospinal fluid (CSF) pressure headache

Mass lesions	Tumours Haematomas Abscess
CSF circulation block	Aqueductal stenosis Intraventricular tumour Fourth ventricular outflow block
Cerebral oedema	Post head injury Post cerebral anoxia Benign intracranial hypertension
Raised CSF protein	SAH Post meningitis GBS Spinal cord tumours
Disorders of circulation	Lateral sinus thrombosis Jugular vein thrombosis Superior vena cava obstruction
Systemic causes	Malignant hypertension Hypercapnia

GBS:Guillain–Barré syndrome; SAH: subarachnoid haemorrhage.

Posterior fossa lesions

An evolving mass lesion in the posterior fossa (**141**), with foramen magnum herniation, may present with continuous neck and occipital pain. This can be associated with neck stiffness, head tilt (for comfort and to offset double vision), paraesthesia of the shoulders, dysphagia, and loss of upper limb reflexes. In more acute lesions, there may be episodes of tonic extension and arching of the neck and back, extension and internal rotation of the limbs, respiratory disturbances, cardiac irregularity, and loss of consciousness.

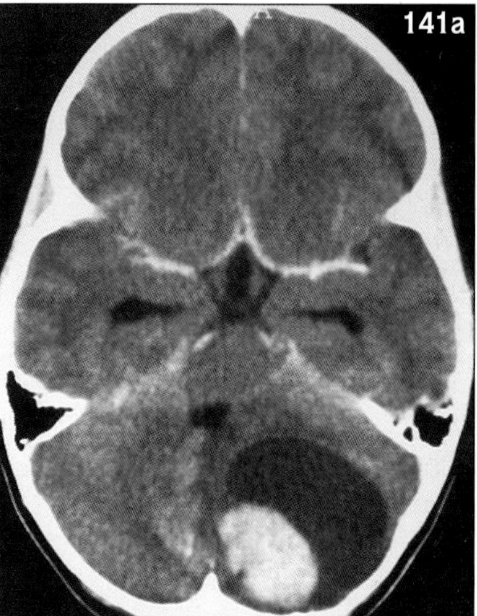

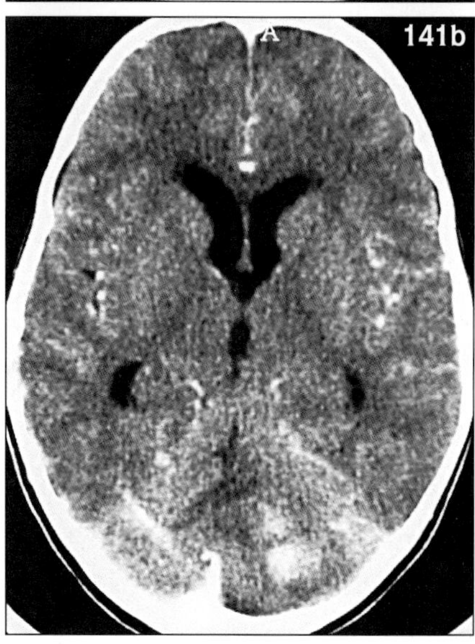

141 Axial computed tomography scans with contrast, showing a left posterior fossa tumour with obstructive hydrocephalus (**a**). There is enlargement of the temporal horns, lateral, third, and fourth ventricles (**b**). There is also mid-line shift, with the fourth ventricle pushed to the right and effacement of the normal sulcal pattern.

Low cerebrospinal fluid pressure headache
Although spontaneous CSF leaks can occur in patients with low CSF pressure headache, most develop after a lumbar puncture (LP), epidural injection, or Valsalva manoeuvre (during lifting, straining, coughing, or clearing the eustachian tubes). The headache occurs daily, is not present on waking but increases towards evening, and is relieved by lying down to be aggravated again by standing up.

Benign intracranial hypertension
Benign intracranial hypertension typically occurs in young, overweight females. Patients present with raised intracranial pressure headache, visual obscuration or loss, bilateral papilloedema and, occasionally, a sixth nerve palsy (**142**). The neurological examination is otherwise normal. Alternative diagnoses such as mass lesions, ventricular enlargement, and venous sinus thrombosis must be excluded by imaging. CSF pressure is >200 mm of CSF, with a normal or low protein concentration and normal cell count. Weight gain and drugs (e.g. tetracycline) may be incriminated, but the majority of patients have no identifiable underlying cause. However, other secondary causes (*Table 52*) should be considered, particularly in patients who do not fit the normal expected phenotype.

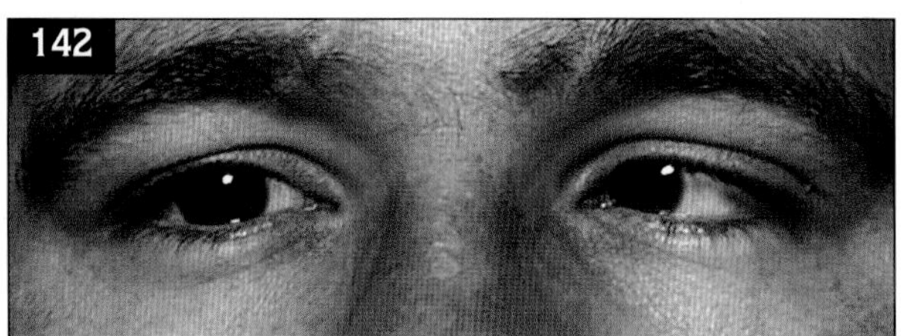

142 Right VI nerve palsy, with failure of the eye to abduct.

Table 52 Secondary causes of benign intracranial hypertension

Vascular	Cerebral venous sinus thrombosis Jugular vein thrombosis
Drugs	Tetracycline Vitamin A Anabolic steroids Growth hormone Nalidixic acid Lithium Norplant levonorgestrel implant
Endocrine	Addison's disease Hypoparathyroidism
Renal	Renal failure
Cardiovascular	Right heart failure
Respiratory	COPD
Haematology	Severe iron deficiency anaemia
Other	Sleep apnoea

COPD: chronic obstructive pulmonary disease.

ACUTE ONSET HEADACHE

Acute onset headache which is normally encountered in the Accident and Emergency Department, with or without neurological deficit and, regardless of the severity, needs urgent assessment and investigation. A third of these patients will have a potentially fatal or disabling intracranial condition. Although subarachnoid haemorrhage (SAH) is the immediate concern of most clinicians, a number of causes should be considered (*Table 53*). Many of these conditions can be excluded on the basis of the history, examination, and investigations. However, some patients require more directed investigations, such as computed tomography (CT) or magnetic resonance imaging (MRI) venography in patients suspected of having cerebral venous sinus thrombosis.

Table 53 Causes of acute onset headache

- ❑ Subarachnoid haemorrhage
- ❑ Cerebral venous sinus thrombosis
- ❑ Spontaneous intracranial hypotension
- ❑ Pituitary apoplexy
- ❑ Carotid or vertebral artery dissection
- ❑ Migraine
- ❑ Acute hypertensive crisis
- ❑ Coital/cough/exertional/weight lifter's headache
- ❑ Thunderclap headache

Subarachnoid haemorrhage

SAH (**143**) presents with headache, reaching its maximum intensity instantaneously or at most over a couple of minutes. The pain usually lasts more then 1 hour. Apart from headache, patients can be otherwise well and the absence of neck stiffness, reduced level of consciousness, focal deficit, vomiting, or photophobia is no indication of a more benign condition. In the investigation of SAH (**144**) the sensitivity of both CT and LP is largely dependent on the timing of the tests and the methods used in acquiring and analyzing the CSF sample. CT scanning should always be done before a LP is performed. CT is reported to be 95–98% sensitive in detecting SAH if performed within 12–24 hours of clinical onset. However, this sensitivity decreases rapidly with time and by the end of the first week is <50%. It is therefore important that all patients with suspected SAH who have a normal CT scan should go on to have CSF examination. When blood is detected in the CSF following a LP it is important to distinguish between SAH and blood from a 'traumatic tap'. When red blood cells enter the CSF they start to lyse rapidly and release pigments giving the appearance of xanthochromia. These pigments such as oxyhaemoglobin, methaemoglobin, and bilrubin may be detected in CSF when spun down and the red cells are removed. Detection of xanthochromia by visual inspection alone has <50% sensitivity; however, detection by spectrophotometry is reported to be 100% accurate if performed on samples taken between 12 hours and 2 weeks after ictus. Diagnostic confusion may still arise if delay occurs in removing the red cells from the CSF sample before performing spectrophotometric analysis, as this may allow time for traumatic red cell to lyse and release xanthochromia. It is therefore important that samples of CSF are processed urgently.

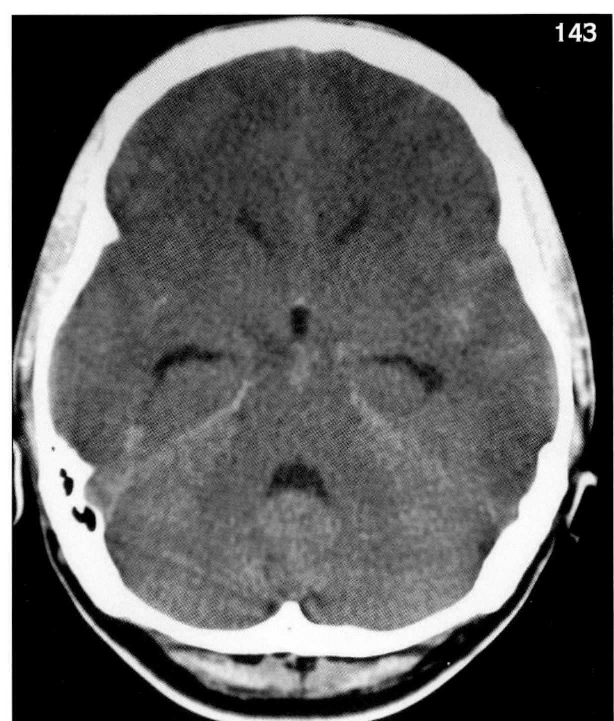

143 Computed tomography scan of subarachnoid haemorrhage with early hydrocephalus.

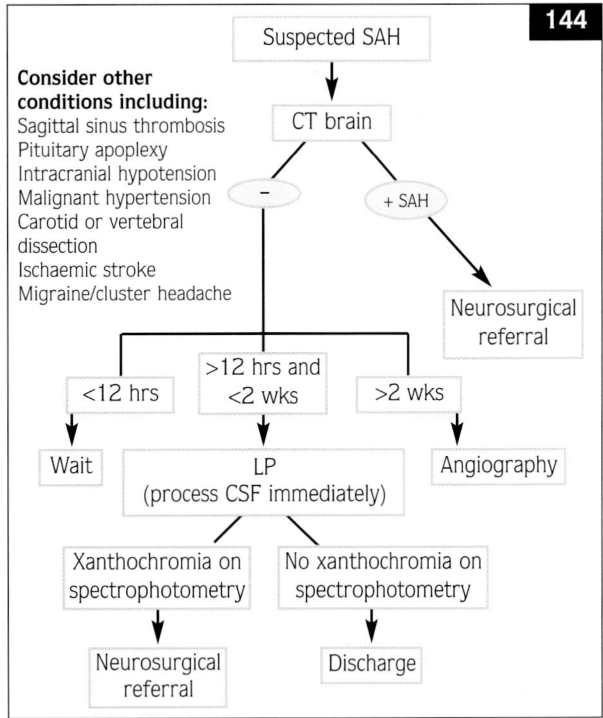

144 Algorithm for the investigation of suspected subarachnoid haemorrhage.

Cerebral venous sinus thrombosis

Cerebral venous sinus thrombosis (**145**) should be suspected in any patient with a hypercoaguable state or infection of the paranasal sinuses, middle or inner ear presenting with features of stroke or raised intracranial pressure without ventricular enlargement (*Table 54*). The presence of multiple cerebral infarcts outwith arterial territories, the slower evolution of symptoms, seizures, and a clotting disorder favour venous over arterial thrombosis. In some patients, thrombosis of a particular venous sinus can be suggested from the clinical presentation.

Cavernous sinus thrombosis (**146**) presents with chemosis, proptosis, and multiple cranial nerve involvement (III, IV, VI, and ophthalmic division of V). **Saggital sinus thrombosis** presents with headaches, seizures, and a hemiparesis that predominantly affects the leg. Later in the course of the disease both lower limbs are often involved. **Posterior cavernous sinus and inferior petrosal sinus thrombosis** may present with multiple cranial nerve palsies (V, VI, IX, X, and XI).

Pituitary apoplexy syndrome

When a pituitary adenoma has outgrown its own blood supply it infarcts. This life-threatening condition presents with acute onset headache, ophthalmoplegia, bilateral blindness, reduced level of consciousness, and pituitary failure. A CT scan shows infarction and often haemorrhage within the tumour (**147**).

Table 54 Causes of cerebral vein thrombosis

Infections	Ear (middle and inner ear) Paranasal sinuses
Haematological	Sickle cell anaemia Polycythaemia Thrombocytopenia Paroxysmal nocturnal haemoglobinuria Antiphospholipid antibody syndrome Protein S and C deficiency
Cancer	
Cardiac	Cyanotic congenital heart disease
Drugs	Oral contraceptive pill
Others	Post partum Post operative states

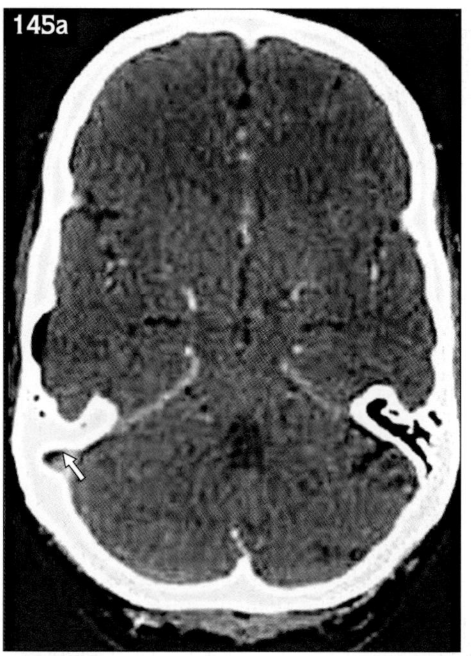

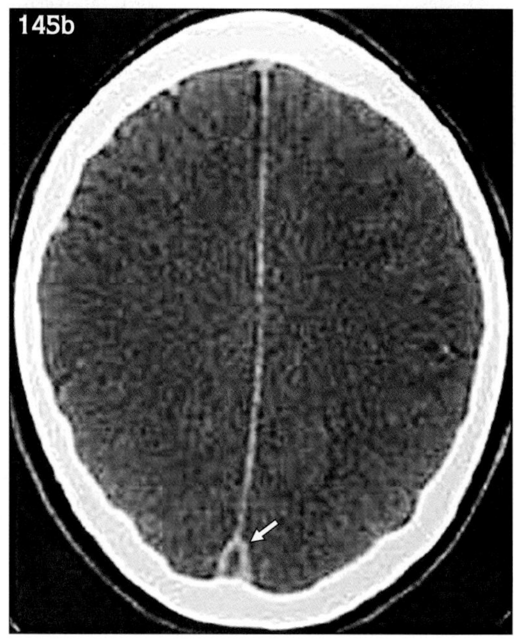

145 Axial contrast-enhanced computed tomography scans, showing cerebral venous sinus thrombosis. Note the filling defects within the right transverse sinus (**a**, arrow) and superior sagittal sinus (delta sign) (**b**, arrow), diagnostic of venous thrombosis.

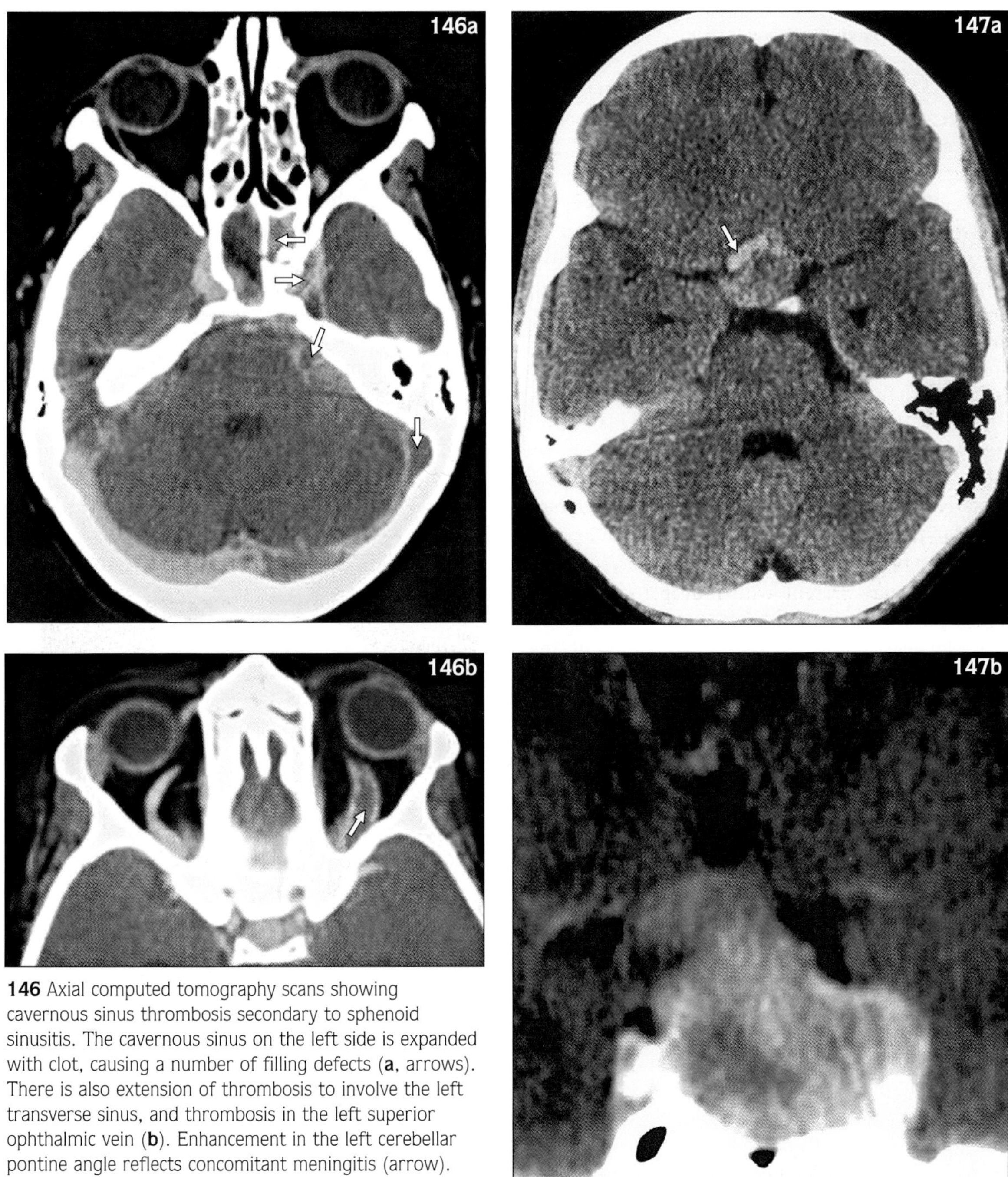

146 Axial computed tomography scans showing cavernous sinus thrombosis secondary to sphenoid sinusitis. The cavernous sinus on the left side is expanded with clot, causing a number of filling defects (**a**, arrows). There is also extension of thrombosis to involve the left transverse sinus, and thrombosis in the left superior ophthalmic vein (**b**). Enhancement in the left cerebellar pontine angle reflects concomitant meningitis (arrow).

147 Pituitary apoplexy. **a:** axial postcontrast computed tomography (CT) scan, showing a pituitary and suprasellar high attenuation mass with focal haemorrhage (arrow); **b:** postcontrast corneal CT scan confirming the pituitary and suprasellar mass with invasion of the left cavernous sinus.

Acute hypertensive crisis

Chronic arterial hypertension of mild or moderate degree does not cause headache. However, hypertension may be a cause of headache in circumstances where there is an acute, severe, and prolonged elevation in diastolic blood pressure. In **malignant hypertension,** diastolic blood pressure is >120 mmHg (16 kPa), there is evidence of grade 3 or 4 retinopathy, the patient may be encephalopathic, and the headache is temporally related to the rise in blood pressure and disappears within 2 days of the blood pressure normalizing (7 days if encephalopathy is present). Patients with a **phaeochromocytoma** may present with headache when there is an acute rise (>25%) in diastolic blood pressure. This may be associated with sweating, palpitations, or anxiety. The headache disappears within 24 hours of blood pressure normalization. Patients with **pre-eclampsia and eclampsia** may also present with headache which is associated with oedema or proteinuria, and a blood pressure rise of 15 mmHg (2 kPa) from the pre-pregnant level or a diastolic pressure of 90 mmHg (12 kPa). The headache disappears within 7 days of blood pressure normalization or termination of the pregnancy. Some toxins or medications may cause an acute rise (>25%) in diastolic blood pressure associated with headache. The headache will disappear within 24 hours of blood pressure normalization.

Stroke

Carotid and vertebral artery dissection may cause a stroke or TIA and is commonly associated with sudden onset headache ipsilateral to the affected artery.

Coital headache

Coital headache is bilateral at onset, precipitated by sexual excitement, prevented or eased by ceasing sexual activity before orgasm, and is not associated with intracranial pathology such as an aneurysm. There are three forms: dull, explosive, and postural types. The dull form is characterized by a dull ache in the head and neck that intensifies as sexual excitement increases. In the explosive form, there is a sudden severe headache that occurs at the time of orgasm, and in the postural form the headache develops after coitus and resembles that of low CSF pressure headache.

Benign cough headache

Cough headache is bilateral, of sudden onset, and is precipitated by coughing. It may be diagnosed only after structural lesions have been excluded by neuroimaging.

Benign exertional headache

Benign exertional headache is specifically brought on by any form of physical activity. Patients complain of bilateral, throbbing pain that normally lasts between 5 minutes and 24 hours. It is prevented by avoiding excessive exertion and is not associated with any systemic or intracranial disorder.

Idiopathic stabbing headache

Idiopathic stabbing headache is predominantly felt in the orbit, temporal or parietal region. It is stabbing in nature, lasts a fraction of a second, and recurs at irregular intervals. It should only be diagnosed after structural lesions have been excluded by neuroimaging.

Thunderclap headache

Thunderclap headache refers to patients who present with suspected SAH but who have a normal CT scan and CSF examination performed within the appropriate time window. This is considered to be a relatively benign condition, which does not require any further investigations.

Summary

- ❏ Headache is common and for most is a benign self-limiting symptom.
- ❏ It is crucial to determine if the headache is new or the exacerbation of an existing headache, which has become more frequent or severe.
- ❏ The possibility of having a serious cause does not increase in proportion to the severity, frequency, or duration of the headache.
- ❏ Patients with tumours rarely present with headache alone.
- ❏ History and examination should identify those patients with red flag symptoms and signs who need investigation.
- ❏ Sudden onset headache should be investigated urgently.
- ❏ All patients over the age of 50 years with new onset daily headache should have their ESR checked.

CLINICAL SCENARIOS

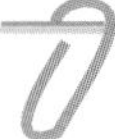

CASE 1

A 69-year-old woman presented to Accident and Emergency with a 12-day history of pain and tenderness diffusely affecting her scalp and associated with jaw claudication.

This elderly woman is presenting with new daily persistent headache (Table 50). Scalp tenderness and jaw claudication suggest an extracranial vascular cause.

Five days later she developed diplopia and complete ptosis of the right eyelid.

Diplopia and complete ptosis of the right eyelid suggest III cranial nerve palsy. This may be due to compression of the nerve by an aneurysm or ischaemia of the nerve due to narrowing of the blood vessel that supplies it.

On examination, she had a right III nerve palsy with pupillary sparing. The right temporal artery pulsation was absent, but there was no overlying tenderness.

A III nerve palsy with pupillary sparing suggests ischaemia of the nerve rather then compression, and taken together with absence of the temporal artery pulsation suggests temporal arteritis.

On investigation, she had a normal full blood count and glucose. Her C-reactive protein (CRP) was 17 mg/l (normal <10 mg/l) and her ESR, which was repeated on a number of occasions, ranged between 8 and 27 mm/hr. A CT scan of her brain and a CT angiography were both normal.

Neuroimaging has excluded a compressive lesion and the raised inflammatory marker supports the diagnosis of temporal arteritis. She had a temporal artery biopsy and immediately following this she was started on prednisolone 60 mg daily. In 24 hours her headache had gone and the diagnosis of temporal arteritis was confirmed a few days later by histology. Her CRP normalized and her third nerve palsy gradually recovered completely.

The diagnosis of temporal arteritis is confirmed on biopsy and by the rapid clinical response to steroids.The ESR is not always significantly raised and a normal reading does not exclude this important diagnosis. Failure to diagnose and treat can lead to permanent visual loss and may be fatal.

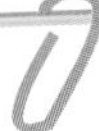

CASE 2

A 39-year-old female presented to the out patient clinic with increasingly frequent headache. She first developed headaches in her early teens; these were mild and infrequent and seemed to be associated with the time of her periods. Her headaches then stopped for a few years but restarted again at the age of 24 years and gradually increased in severity. At the time of her presentation she had a generalized headache which was constant and dull and had episodes of more severe headache occurring up to eight times a month. The severe headaches were similar although more severe than those she experienced in her teens. They usually began in the left occipital region and radiated forward to the left frontal region and behind both eyes. They were throbbing in character and aggravated by any type of movement. They were associated with nausea and frequently with vomiting, photophobia, and phonophobia. There was no history of visual disturbance. Although these headaches could occur at any time she frequently woke up with a headache. There were no obvious precipitating features.

She seems to have a combination of two headache types. The first, chronic tension type headache is constant, generalized, dull, and featureless. The second, migraine, is intermittent, severe, with focal throbbing, and is associated with nausea, vomiting, photophobia, and phonophobia.

She was taking two tablets of naratriptan per attack without any benefit. She was also on a serotonin antagonist (pizotifen) 1.5 mg twice daily, which although initially reducing the frequency of attacks was now having little impact. Over the previous year she had started taking increasingly frequent doses of Solpadol (codeine phosphate/paracetamol) and was now on six to eight tablets a day. This gave her good symptomatic control but her headaches normally returned after several hours.

(Continued overleaf)

Case 2 *(continued)*

She is over-using both naratriptan and Solpadol medication. Although Solpadol is giving her good symptomatic relief, she has developed rebound headache and is requiring increasing doses of analgesia to control her headache.

On examination there was no focal neurological deficit and fundoscopy was normal.

She was diagnosed with migraine headaches complicated by analgesic and naratriptan misuse. She was advised to stop both her naratriptan and Solpadol medication. After 4 months her headaches had improved significantly and she was having only two attacks of migraine a month. Subcutaneous sumatriptan was added to her prophylactic treatment and she was advised to limit its use to twice a month.

Case 3

A 55-year-old male, admitted to his district general hospital, was referred to the visiting neurologist with a history of new onset headache that had been constant for 10 days, with only temporary relief from simple analgesia. There was no history of head injury. He had a past history of rheumatic fever and had a prosthetic heart valve replacement 10 years earlier for which he was on warfarin. He was also being investigated for a raised prostate specific antigen.

This man is presenting with new daily persistent headache (Table 50). Although there is no history of head injury, he is at risk of intracranial haemorrhage and subdural haematoma because of his anticoagulation therapy. He is under investigation for raised prostate specific antigen (a tumour marker) and the headache may be a presentation of cerebral metastasis.

His headache had come on instantaneously while watching television with his wife. There were no associated symptoms, precipitating, or aggravating features. On examination he was alert and orientated. There was no neck stiffness and Kernig's sign was negative. Cranial nerves, fundoscopy, and upper and lower limb examination were normal. A CT scan of his brain performed on admission was normal.

The sudden onset suggests a vascular cause and SAH needs to be excluded urgently. The normal CT scan and lack of focal deficit, neck stiffness, and reduced level of consciousness are not totally reassuring and do not exclude SAH.

Following the administration of fresh frozen plasma to temporarily reverse his warfarin, he had a LP performed which was abnormal and consistent with a late diagnosis of SAH. Four-vessel cerebral angiography was performed, but no evidence of cerebral aneurysm or arteriovenous malformation was found. His headache settled spontaneously and completely.

Some patients with proven SAH do not have a radiologically demonstrable aneurysm or vascular malformation; prognosis here is favourable with negligible recurrence rates.

REVISION QUESTIONS

1 In the assessment and investigation of subarachnoid haemorrhage, which of these statements is true?
   a The headache reaches its maximum intensity instantaneously or at most over a couple of minutes.
   b Meningism is an important sign.
   c A normal CT scan done within the first 12 hours of ictus excludes the diagnosis.
   d A normal lumbar puncture done within the first 12 hours of ictus excludes the diagnosis.
   e A normal lumbar puncture done a week after the ictus excludes the diagnosis.
   f A patient who presents with coital headache for the first time can be reassured.

2 In patients with chronic daily headache, which of these statements is true?
   a Patients presenting to Casualty with chronic daily headache are unlikely to have migraine.
   b Patients over the age of 50 years who present with a new-onset, focal, daily headache should be considered to have temporal arteritis until proven otherwise.
   c Migraine prophylactic medication is effective in patients with migraine and analgesia-induced headache.
   d Analgesia-induced headache may take up to 6 months to settle down after stopping the offending agent.
   e All analgesic and triptan medications can be associated with analgesia-induced headache.
   f Migraine may present with chronic daily headache.

3 Which of these statements is true?
   a Subarachnoid haemorrhage may present with new-onset, chronic, daily headache.
   b Sudden-onset, unilateral headache associated with ipsilateral Horner's syndrome and contralateral hemiparesis suggests carotid dissection ipsilateral to the headache.
   c A normal temporal artery biopsy excludes the diagnosis of temporal arteritis.
   d Patients with cluster headache prefer to lie still.
   e Alcohol may precipitate a cluster headache during periods of remission.
   f Chronic arterial hypertension of moderate degree does not cause headache.

Answers
1 a, e
2 b, d, e, f
3 a, b, f

SPINAL SYMPTOMS: NECK PAIN AND BACKACHE

John Paul Leach

INTRODUCTION

Neck pain and backache are common causes of self-referral in primary care, but are much less frequent visitors to neurology outpatients, being seen mainly in orthopaedic clinics. Almost anyone over the age of 40 years will be able to give a history of back or neck pain at some point in their lives, as it would appear that one of the flaws inherent in the design of the human spine is the frequency with which it will produce pain, stiffness, and a general creaking as age advances. Among men over the age of 50 years, 90% will display radiographic evidence of degenerative changes.

As a result of the profusion of frequent, often nonspecific symptoms, spinal disease is one of the few areas in clinical neurology where history taking seems secondary to examination in terms of importance. Since neck and back pain are common enough to be almost physiological states, the role of the neurologist is to determine which patients warrant further investigation and which require reassurance alone.

Most cases of neck and back pain will have no demonstrable neurological deficit. Localization of spinal pathology on the basis of neurological findings can be challenging, despite the common anatomy (a bundle of nerves and nerve roots encased in a segmented bony canal) (**148**). The patterns of deficit caused by cervical, thoracic, and lumbar spinal disease are different, and here will be addressed as upper (cervical and thoracic) and lower (lumbar and sacral) spinal syndromes.

CLINICAL ASSESSMENT

While patients' histories may dwell on limb symptoms and localized pain, care should be taken to elicit any complaint of sphincter disturbance or truncal sensory disturbance. General examination is absolutely essential as this may identify features suggesting generalized conditions in which the spinal cord may be secondarily involved, e.g. neurofibromatosis, adrenal insufficiency, or primary neoplasm. Such findings expand the differential diagnosis of underlying spinal pathology. As with all patients referred for an opinion, while the emphasis is on possible spinal disease, a full neurological examination is mandatory.

Cranial nerve examination

In patients with arm and/or leg symptoms, cranial nerve examination may seem irrelevant. However, it may provide vital clues to multilevel neurological disease, or the intracranial masquerading as spinal pathology. Abnormal eye movements, fundal changes, pupillary abnormalities, and lower cranial nerve/cerebellar signs should be particularly sought. Subtle eye movement disorders may betray the existence of multiple sclerosis presenting with myelopathy, while cerebellar ataxia suggests posterior fossa disease. Horner's syndrome can be a helpful localizing sign, ipsilateral to weakness at the cervical level while contralateral at the cranial level.

Upper limb examination

If there is significant cervical root compression, motor system examination may show signs of lower motor neurone (LMN) involvement (wasting, weakness, poor reflexes) which will vary with the level of the lesion (*Table 55*).

Sensory examination can help elucidate the level (**149**) although it should be stressed that it is motor involvement (weakness and wasting) and radiology

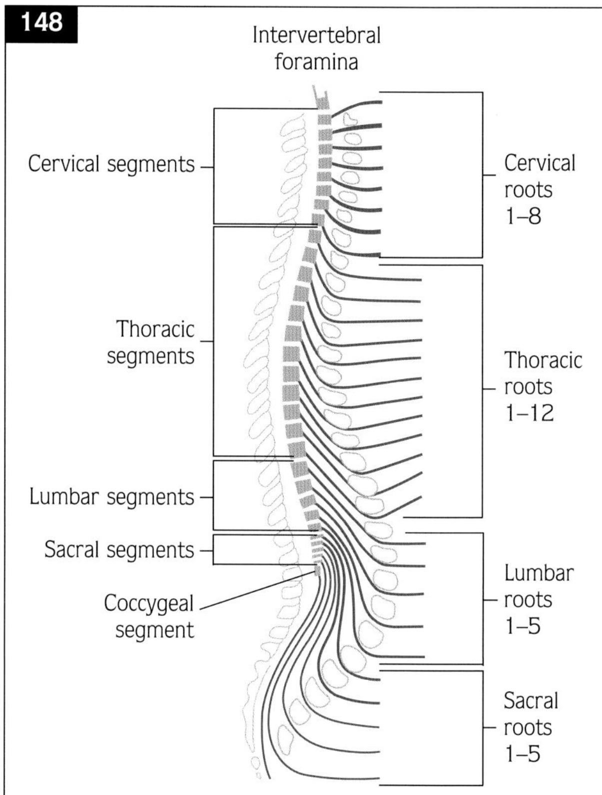

148 Diagram of sagittal spinal cord, illustrating nerve roots in relation to vertebral bodies.

that will motivate the surgeon when to operate. Any lesion above C8 may be associated with some evidence of upper motor neurone (UMN) dysfunction in one or both arms. In general, the higher the cervical lesion, the more probable that there will be UMN signs in the arms, often with a clear reflex level (absent or reduced at the level, and brisk below the level).

Lower limb examination

Assessment of lower limbs in patients with upper spinal cord lesions will show UMN signs. These take the form of brisk reflexes, spread of reflexes both above and below the tested level, clonus with increased tone, and extensor plantar responses. It would seem logical (although not definitive) that patients with cervical vertebral problems will be more likely to experience lumbar spine disease. Widespread spinal degenerative disease is one of the recognized causes of mixed UMN and LMN signs.

An additional test of lower spine function involves stretch testing to indicate nerve root compression/irritation. The commonest such test is straight leg raising. This involves an assessment of the discomfort and pain induced by hip flexion, when the knee is either flexed or fully extended. When the leg is raised and the knee extended, stretching of the nerve roots will cause a shooting pain in the distribution of the affected nerve roots. This pain will not occur (or will be much less) when the knee is flexed during leg raising.

Table 55 Reflexes and roots

Reflex	Level
Jaw jerk	Trigeminal nerves
Pectoral jerks	C3, C4
Triceps	C6, C7
Biceps	C5, C6
Supinators	C5, C6
Abdominal reflexes	Thoracic roots
Crossed adductors	L2, L3
Knees	L3, L4
Ankles	L5, S1

Sphincter and perineal examination

In patients with sacral root lesions, anal sphincter tone may be lost. When there is suspected involvement of these lower spinal roots, assessment of anal tone is necessary. Where a central (within the cord) spinal lesion is present, the positioning of the spinothalamic pathways (more caudal fibres lying most peripherally within the spinal cord) will mean that there is widespread caudal loss of pinprick sensation that spares the perianal region. This is called 'sacral sparing'. The reverse pattern of sensory

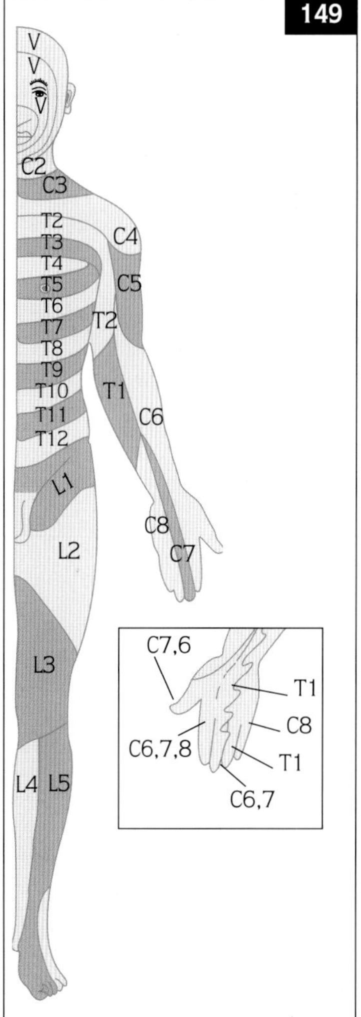

149 Dermatomal map showing lesion localization.

loss occurs when the cord is compressed from without (**150**).

When there are symptoms suspicious of spinal disease with accompanying neurological symptoms, the main questions to be addressed are:

- ❑ At what level in the neuraxis is the lesion? (Use of cord and radicular signs.)
- ❑ Where is the lesion: intramedullary, extramedullary intradural or extradural (see page 207)?
- ❑ What is the lesion (see page 209)?

Lesion level localization

This may be ascertained by differentiating the cord or nerve roots signs. The constellation of symptoms will vary depending on the region affected. In upper spinal disease (cervical and thoracic spine), the spinal cord or nerve roots may be affected.

At upper levels, therefore, the potential effects are:

- ❑ Upper motor problems in the legs.
- ❑ Lower motor neurone problems in the arms.
- ❑ Truncal sensory level changes.
- ❑ Sphincter disturbance.
- ❑ Horner's syndrome (with cervical lesions).

The spinal cord finishes at approximately L1 level. As a result, neurological effects of lumbar or sacral spine disease almost exclusively involve a radicular pattern.

Pressure on the lower spinal cord and cauda equina causes:

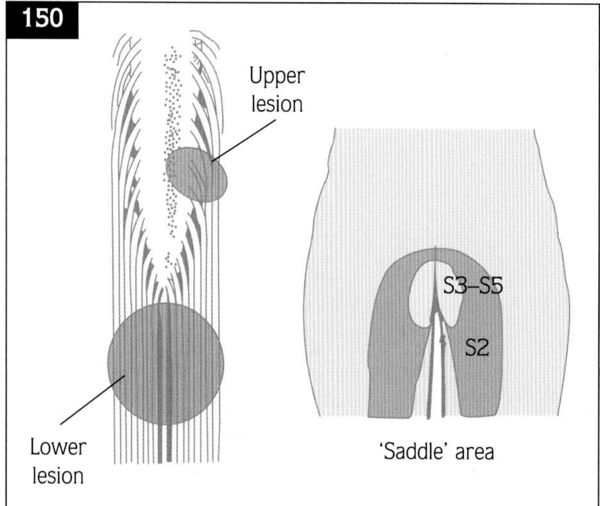

150 Diagram of cauda equina lesions, illustrating the affected saddle area.

- ❑ LMN problems in the legs, with clinical features dependent on the particular roots affected.
- ❑ Truncal or sacral sensory level changes.
- ❑ Sphincter disturbance.

Cord involvement will cause LMN lesions at the level of the lesion, with UMN signs below. Involvement of the cauda equina (i.e. below the level of L1) will cause only LMN symptoms.

Localization by cord symptoms

A lesion produces neurological deficit at or below its level. Sometimes, however, a lesion may be at a higher level than is apparent clinically, i.e. a sensory level suggesting a thoracic level may be being produced by a cervical lesion (a 'dropped level'). At the level of the lesion, motor signs may be of a LMN type, given the direct destructive effect on anterior horn cells. Sensory signs may be soft or absent, but there may be a band of dysaesthesia round the truncal circumference at the level of spinal involvement. Below the lesion, sensory changes will usually become more likely and more severe. Motor signs will be of UMN type below the level of any spinal lesion.

Bladder symptoms only occur where the cord is affected bilaterally. Such cord lesions will initially leave an atonic bladder, with absence of sensation of fullness. With time, the bladder begins to undergo

Table 56 Pitfalls in root/peripheral nerve lesion differentiation

L5–S1 versus peroneal nerve:

- ❑ Both will cause weakness of ankle dorsiflexion and sensory changes over anterior shin and foot
- ❑ Peroneal nerve lesion may be associated with Tinel's sign round the fibular neck
- ❑ L5–S1 lesion may cause reduced ankle jerk and weakness of foot inversion (and possibly a positive straight leg raising test)

C8–T1 versus ulnar nerve

- ❑ Both will cause weakness of intrinsic muscles of the hand
- ❑ Isolated ulnar lesions should cause only hypothenar eminence and interossei wasting. Sensory changes are usually confined to the hand
- ❑ C8–T1 lesions may cause wasting also at the thenar eminence and may have associated sensory change along the medial border of the forearm

reflex emptying causing urinary urgency and urge incontinence. In general, a hypertonic bladder indicates a UMN lesion, e.g. a lesion affecting the spinal cord or brain.

Autonomic fibres in the cervical cord supply sympathetic function which can be clinically assessed by checking sweating in limbs, trunk, and face. Another measure of spinal sympathetic function is the presence or absence of a Horner's syndrome. There will sometimes be a localized pain or even tenderness overlying cord pathologies which can help with localization.

Localization by radicular symptoms

Radicular localization can be done on the basis of sensory or motor changes. Knowledge of the basic dermatomal pattern (see below) will allow inference to be drawn on the level of involvement. Sensory change is usually a subjective electric shock-like pain along the affected dermatome, although more chronic lesions can lead to numbness in the affected area. Motor changes will usually involve reduction or loss of the relevant reflexes on the affected side (*Table 55*).

Differentiation of radicular symptoms from peripheral nerve-related symptoms can only be done when there is a knowledge of the characteristic patterns of innervation of each of the peripheral nerves and the functions supplied by each spinal root. This can be difficult, however, and some characteristic pitfalls are listed (*Table 56*). Direct pressure on the sacral roots by a lumbar or sacral lesion causes a LMN bladder, with loss of sensation of fullness and an atonic overfilling bladder.

Lesion anatomical localization

The extent and pattern of involvement of the spinal cord in disease may result in characteristic patterns of deficit, which can give further clues to the nature of the pathological process (**151**).

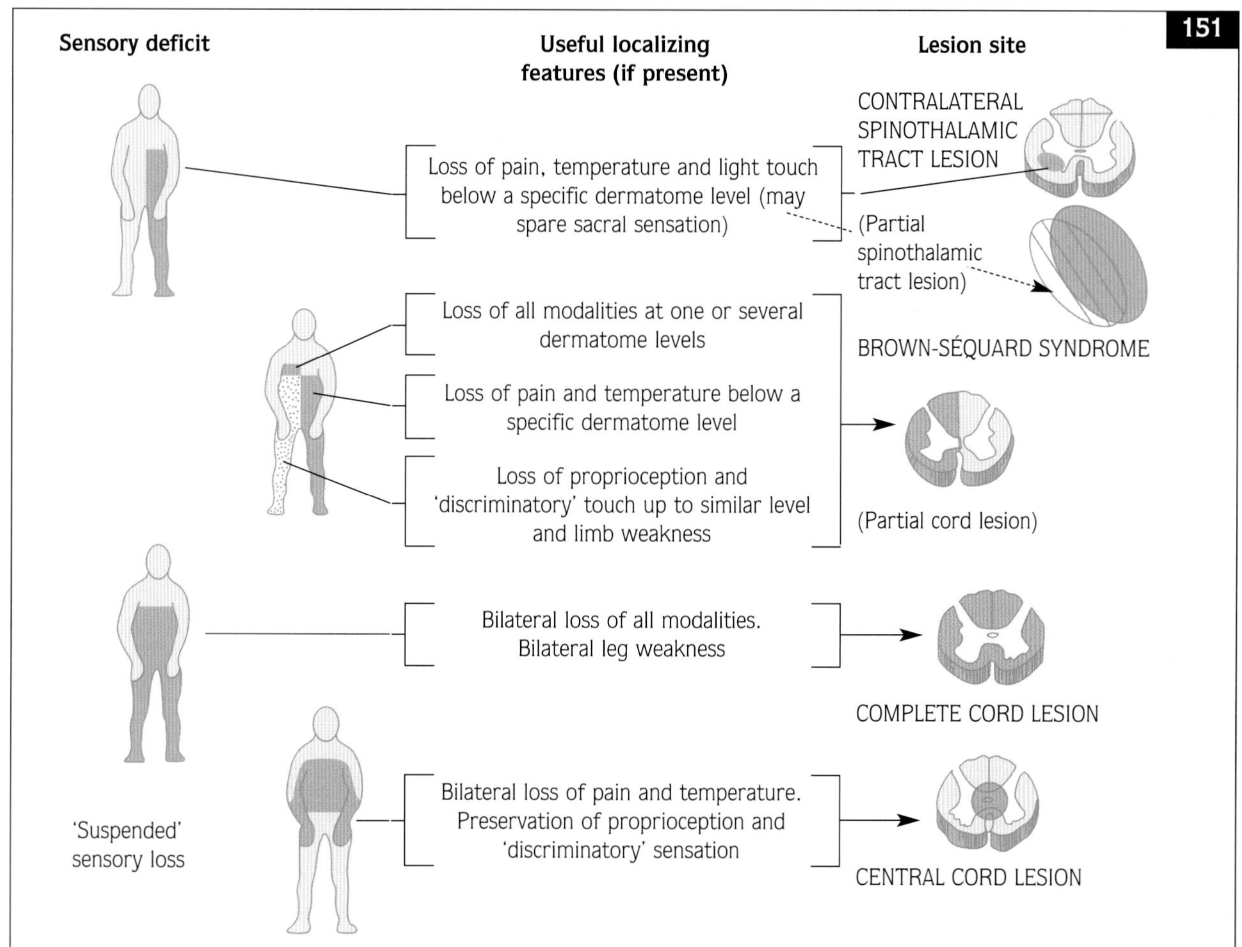

151 Diagram to show the characteristic patterns of sensory loss in various spinal cord lesions.

Brown-Séquard syndrome
Lesions affecting one or other half of the spinal cord will cause UMN weakness and spasticity below the lesion. There occurs typically a mixed bilateral sensory deficit of spinothalamic loss (pain and temperature) below and contralateral to the lesion, and dorsal columnar loss (proprioception and vibration) below and ipsilateral to the lesion (**152**).

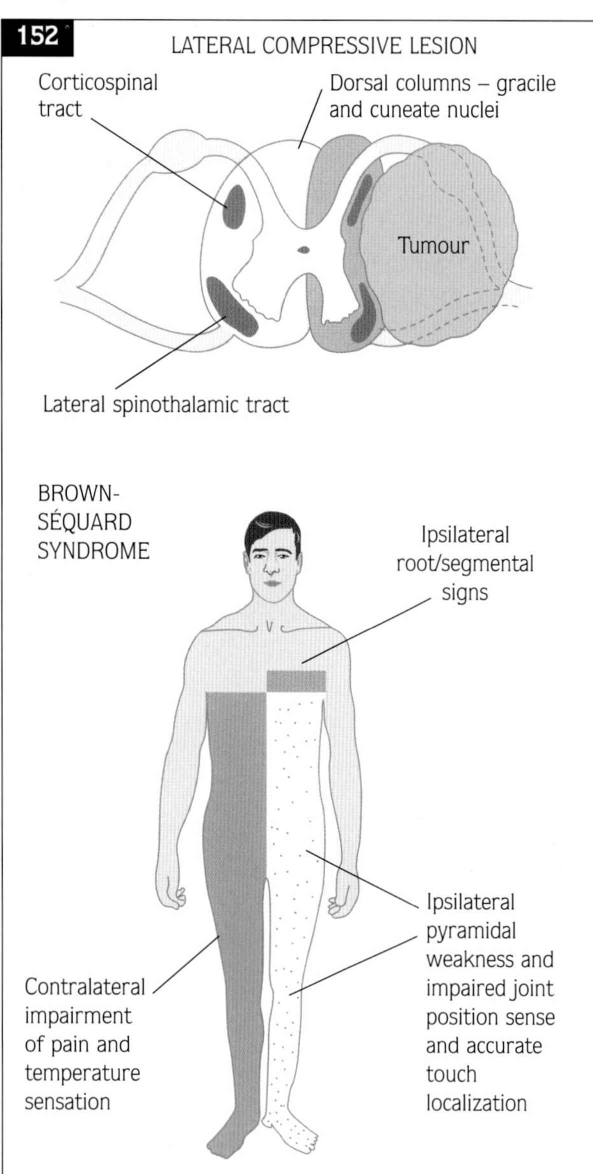

152 Diagram of an incomplete lateral compressive lesion, with the attendant pattern of sensory impairment.

Complete transverse lesions
These result in bilateral UMN weakness and spasticity below the lesion. There may be LMN signs at the level of the lesion which can help in localization. Corticospinal, spinothalamic, and dorsal column tracts are affected (**153**). All modalities are affected (there may frequently be sphincter involvement, and sometimes Lhermitte's sign).

Central cord lesions
Earliest motor effects of central cord lesions will involve anterior horn cells at the levels of the lesion, with a resultant LMN lesion pattern. Later, with further expansion, the corticospinal tracts can be involved and can cause caudal UMN signs. Early decussation near the point of entry by spinothalamic fibres means that more rostral fibres layers tend to be more centrally placed in the cord. This explains why central cord lesions may therefore spare spinothalamic fibres below the level of the lesion (sacral or abdominal pinprick) (**154**). Central cord lesions which extend anteriorly may also affect second order spinothalamic fibres as they decussate in front of the anterior ventral commissure.

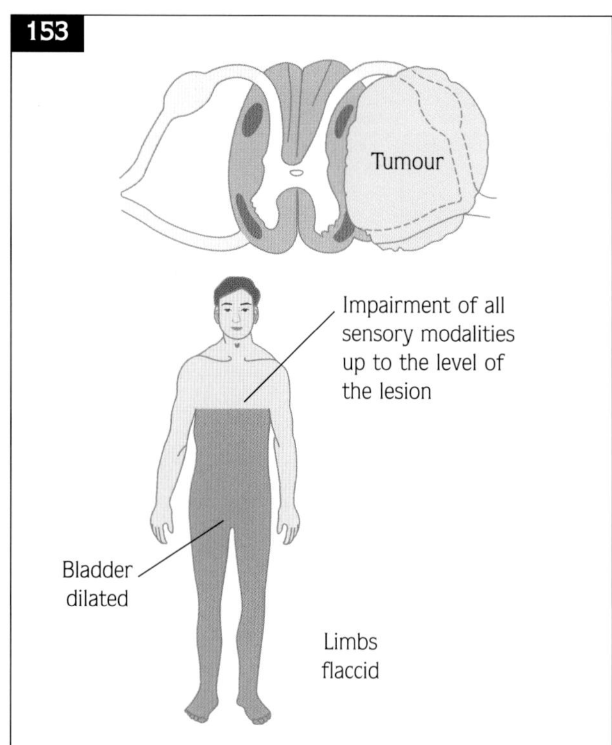

153 Diagram of a complete extrinsic spinal cord lesion, with attendant clinical features.

Anterior spinal cord

Thrombosis of the anterior spinal artery damages anterior spinal cord only. The effects on corticospinal tracts leave bilateral spasticity and weakness below the lesion with, sometimes, LMN weakness at the level of the lesion. There is a dissociated sensory loss, i.e. there is a bilateral decrease in pinprick and temperature sensation with sparing of light touch, joint position sense, and vibration sense. This is because of selective damage to the spinothalamic tracts: dorsal column sensation is supplied by the posterior spinal arteries, and is therefore unaffected.

Nature of the lesion

The nature of onset and rate of progression will suggest the nature of the lesion; for example, vascular lesions will occur abruptly, while demyelinating lesions may demonstrate a more subacute onset. Metastatic lesions will usually be slowly progressive, and may cause pain secondary to local destruction. Pathologies around the spinal cord may be referred to as either intrinsic to the spinal cord (intramedullary) or extrinsic to the cord (extramedullary) (*Table 57*). Extramedullary lesions may in turn be intradural or extradural.

154 Diagram of a central cord lesion, with sensory findings.

Investigations

As stated above, minor 'wear and tear' is seen in the majority of plain X-rays of cervical and lumbar spine in middle age. Plain X-rays of spine will be useful where there has been acute spinal trauma, but not otherwise. The imaging regime of choice is magnetic resonance imaging (MRI). This will give both axial (transverse cuts) and sagittal (longitudinal cuts) views of the affected region, which will allow a good assessment both of any spinal cord compression and any root canal stenosis that may correlate with radicular symptoms. In patients where MRI is contraindicated (e.g. patients with prostheses *in situ*) then computed tomography myelogram is a helpful alternative. In differentiation of peripheral nerve and root lesions, nerve conduction studies and electromyography can be useful.

SUMMARY

- ❑ Minor spinal symptoms are common, neurological sequelae are not.
- ❑ Imaging is best done where there is a possibility of surgery; or where symptoms or signs suggest serious neurological disease.

Table 57 Causes of spinal cord pathology

Pathology around the cord

Vertebral/spinal column disease:
- ❑ Degenerative
- ❑ Infiltrative (neoplastic)
- ❑ Infective
- ❑ Dural disease
- ❑ Neoplastic

Pathology within the cord:
- ❑ Inflammatory
- ❑ Neoplastic (primary or secondary)
- ❑ Ischaemic/haemorrhagic
- ❑ Developmental (syringomyelia)
- ❑ Degenerative

CASE 1

A 66-year-old female was referred for an inpatient neurology review. She had a long history of back and neck pain over the previous 30 years, but had sustained a fall the week previously. Prior to the fall, she could do her own shopping, but was now unable to walk. She was unable to dress herself and could not brush her hair as her arms were so weak. She complained of dyspnoea on mild exertion. She was also being treated for a presumed urinary tract infection on account of urinary symptoms. The attending physicians were concerned initially that she had sustained a stroke and had organized a CT scan of brain, which proved normal.

The sudden deterioration in walking was originally thought to be due to stroke; the involvement of both legs and both arms, however, should immediately raise suspicion of a cervical spinal lesion. The onset of dyspnoea in the absence of any history of chest disease may also relate to an upper cervical lesion compromising diaphragmatic function. Her bladder symptoms may represent a hyperactive bladder secondary to spinal pathology rather than being indicative of infection.

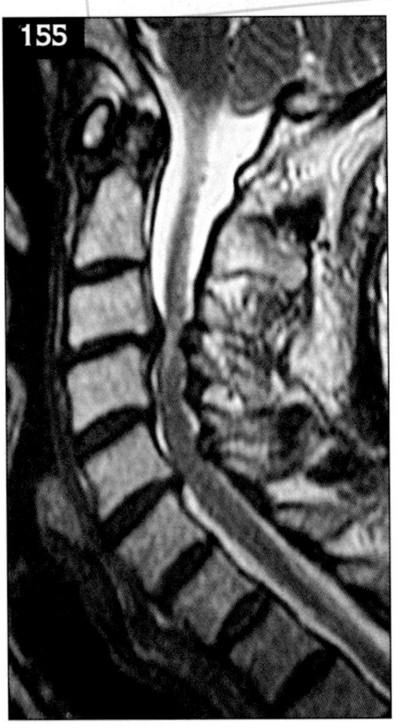

155 Sagittal magnetic resonance image of cervical spine, showing severe cord compression at C3–C5 levels.

The patient was alert and fully orientated. Cardiovascular and respiratory examinations were normal although the patient was breathless on minimal exertion. Cranial nerve examination was unremarkable. Examination of the upper limbs revealed increased tone bilaterally, symmetrically reduced power of all movements, and brisk biceps, supinator, and triceps jerks. Sensory testing was normal. In the lower limbs, tone was increased, and there was mild weakness of all movements with increased reflexes and upgoing plantars.

Examination confirmed UMN signs involving all four limbs: together with the sphincter disturbance (mid-stream specimens of urine were consistently sterile) this would immediately alert the clinician to a spinal cord lesion at the cervical level. Dyspnoea had become prominent and was another localizing symptom (muscles of respiration are supplied at C3,4, and 5 levels). Speed of onset was quicker than would be expected for a demyelinating or inflammatory lesion. (In any event, demyelination is rare at this age.) The timing of the weakness, coming immediately after a fall, was felt to be more than coincidental, and it appeared likely that there had been significant mechanical damage to the cervical spine sustained during (or perhaps contributing to) her fall.

MRI of cervical spine showed there to be severe spondylitic and degenerative changes, most pronounced at higher levels (**155**). Referral was made to the neurosurgeons, who initially refused to offer operation in view of the risk of exacerbation. She deteriorated over the next few weeks, with increasing weakness in both arms and a worsening in respiratory function.

It was decided that a conservative policy posed an unacceptably high risk to her respiratory function. Decompression was carried out in order to prevent further deterioration, but she did surprisingly well; she regained her mobility, and has now begun to mobilize outdoors with the aid of a zimmer frame.

Case 2

A previously well 45-year-old female was admitted to the medical wards after a collapse at home. She remembers having a sudden onset of neck pain followed by a weakness on the right side. She had been diagnosed as having a stroke and had undergone a (normal) CT of brain. She complained of some weakness and numbness of both legs and her right arm, which had been ascribed to her stroke. She gave no history of previous back or neck problems.

The sudden onset of symptoms would be consistent with cerebrovascular disease, but a crucial part of the history was the initial neck pain: the abrupt onset of this pain without preceding trauma is suggestive of a vascular lesion or a haemorrhage.

Cardiological and respiratory examinations were normal. The patient was alert and orientated. The pupil was smaller on the right side, but both pupils were reactive to light and accommodation. There was a slight right-sided ptosis, but a full range of eye movements. Acuities were normal and cranial nerve function was otherwise normal. She had a spastic catch in the right arm and had grade 4 weakness of her right arm and mild weakness in the right leg. Sensory testing was inconsistent. Pinprick was altered in all limbs, but less noticeably in the left leg. Vibration testing was absent to the left ankle and right knee.

A helpful localizing sign was the Horner's syndrome: it would be very unusual for a stroke to cause an isolated Horner's syndrome. The dissociated sensory loss (not quite the classical pattern) was clue to the spinal origin of her symptoms.

MRI scanning showed very marked degenerative cervical spine disease (**156**).

After surgical review, the patient underwent cervical spine decompression with good effect. The Horner's syndrome eventually resolved.

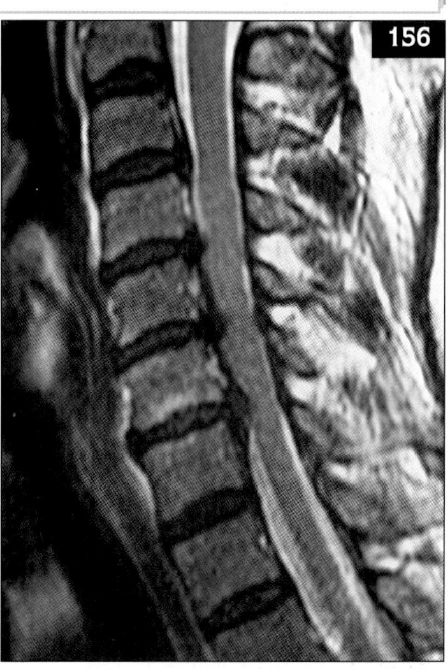

156 Sagittal magnetic resonance image of cervical spine, showing severe cord compression at level C4–C7, with marked bulging of disc at C6–7.

Case 3

A 61-year-old male presented to the neurology services after a subacute onset of leg weakness 10 days previously. After the leg weakness had evolved, he began to notice some terminal dribbling on micturition. There was no recent onset of altered sensation, although 3 years previously he had been diagnosed as having a peripheral neuropathy 'of abrupt onset' which affected the legs. There were no cranial or upper limb symptoms, and no history of back pain or trauma.

The limitation of symptoms to legs and bladder is a clue to a spinal pathology. The history of previous leg symptoms suggests that current symptoms may be a further manifestation of a pre-existing lesion. Stepwise progression of such deficits can occur due to piecemeal infarction caused by dural arteriovenous fistulae.

(Continued overleaf)

CASE 3 *(continued)*

Examination revealed normal cranial nerve and upper limb function. Tone was reduced in the legs, with weakness of hip flexion to grade 3, and grade 4 weakness elsewhere. The right knee jerk and both ankle jerks were lost and both plantars were upgoing. Sensory testing showed subjective distal sensory change; there was a loss of vibration to both knees and lost pinprick to mid shins.

Abrupt onset of neuropathy is rather rare. The mixture of LMN and UMN signs limits the diagnosis to a short list of possibilities. Given these signs, imaging of the spine is essential.

Nerve conduction studies appeared to confirm the presence of a peripheral neuropathy, but other tests did not reveal any systemic or nutritional cause of such a neuropathy. MRI and CT scanning showed some serpiginous flow voids over the lower thoracic cord and cauda equina (**157–159**).

Such changes were consistent with the presence of a dural arteriovenous fistula. Glue embolism was attempted with some radiographic success, but it had no effect on his clinical symptoms. Further scans showed a recurrence. Further surgical ligation was undertaken with good effect.

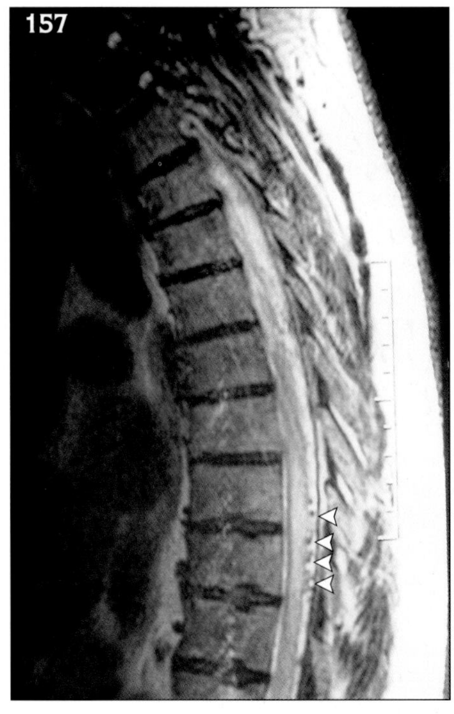

157 Sagittal magnetic resonance image, showing dural fistula (arrowheads).

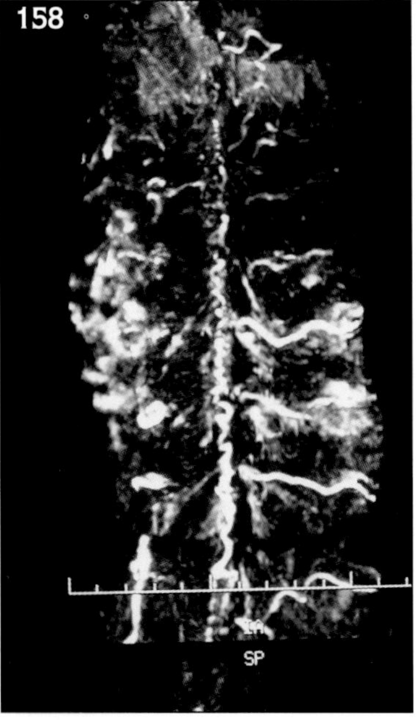

158 Magnetic resonance angiogram of spinal vasculature, hunting for the source of dural fistula.

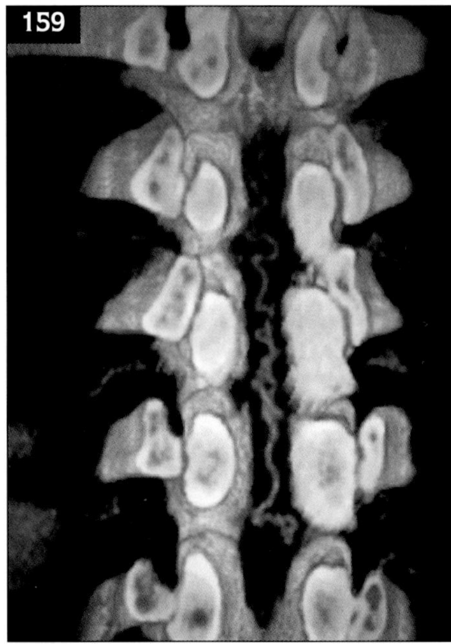

159 Computed tomography angiogram illustrating the length of dural fistula.

Revision questions

1 In cervical spine disease which of the following statements are true?
  a A ‘clicking’ or ‘crunching’ sensation experienced by the patient is a symptom of serious pathology.
  b Bony change on X-ray is unusual in patients of middle age.
  c Cranial nerve examination can provide useful information.
  d Jaw jerk is a sign of cervical myelopathy.
  e Hyper-reflexia in the legs is a reliable sign of myelopathy.

2 In thoracic spine disease which of the following statements are true?
  a The sensory level is a reliable pointer to the level of the involvement.
  b Urinary urgency and incontinence is a sign of radiculopathy.
  c Loss of perianal sensation is a sign of pathology in the central cord.
  d Unilateral cord pathology causes loss of pain and temperature sensation inferior and ipsilateral to the lesion.
  e Anterior cord lesions cause loss of vibration and proprioception.

3 In lumbar and thoracic spine disease which of the following statements are true?
  a Hyper-reflexia is a common sign of lumbar spine involvement.
  b A normal straight leg raising test precludes surgical intervention.
  c Loss of knee jerks is a sign of L5 radiculopathy.
  d Unilateral lesions commonly cause bladder symptoms.
  e A lower motor neurone bladder is small and has a small residual volume when catheterized.

Answers

1 c, e
2 None, all false.
3 None, all false.

NUMBNESS AND TINGLING

Colin O'Leary

INTRODUCTION

Numbness and tingling are frequently reported symptoms. They occur not only in neurological disorders, but are a feature of metabolic disturbances such as hypocapnia (e.g. due to over-breathing in panic attacks) or hypocalcaemia; most people have experienced these symptoms following either a dental or other local anaesthetic, or resulting from lying awkwardly on a limb. Thus, these are familiar sensations. In neurological disorders, sensory symptoms are frequent presenting complaints, even though on examination patients may have evidence of extrasensory involvement, or may subsequently develop extrasensory symptoms. There are, however, some disorders that can singularly or predominantly affect the sensory system.

ANATOMY AND PHYSIOLOGY

A detailed consideration of the complexities and function of sensory pathways is beyond the remit of this chapter; what follows is a simplified overview pertinent to clinical practice in facilitating the localization and nature of a lesion(s). Special senses (sight, hearing, smell, taste) are not considered here.

Sensation begins as a stimulus to a sensory receptor; this message is then conveyed by peripheral and central neuronal pathways back to the brain. Disorders of sensation can be due to lesions at any point along these pathways. Within this sensory network, there are anatomical and physiological divisions, a working knowledge of which permits clinical localization. These factors are considered below from a physiological viewpoint.

Sensory receptors

There are many different sensory receptors subserving superficial and deep sensation. These include touch and pressure receptors, Pacinian corpuscles (vibration), pain and temperature receptors, and stretch receptors in muscle spindles. These receptors are the starting points of the sensory pathways and convey different sensory information from the skin (touch, pain, temperature), and deep structures such as muscles, joints, ligaments, and organs (proprioception [joint position sense], pressure, pain). The receptors synapse with sensory nerve endings that merge to form peripheral nerves.

Peripheral nerves

Peripheral nerves comprise many thousands of individual nerve axons, and are mainly mixed, i.e. contain motor nerves supplying muscles, sensory nerves, and autonomic nerves. These axons vary in diameter and in their degree of myelination, factors which determine the speed at which impulses are conducted through the nerve; the largest and most heavily myelinated fibres conduct most quickly (up to 130 m/second), and unmyelinated fibres are the slowest (2 m/second) (*Table 58*). Different sensations are subserved by differing populations of nerves and this determines how quickly these sensations are perceived, e.g. proprioception is conveyed very quickly and pain/temperature relatively slowly. A practical example of this is that when touching something very hot, one appreciates the sensation of touch before one is aware of the temperature. Many peripheral nerves lie deep and are well protected, but some are prone to pressure damage at particular sites, e.g. the median nerve at the wrist (deep to the flexor retinaculum), the ulnar nerve at the elbow (medial epicondyle), and the common peroneal nerve behind the knee (neck of the fibula).

Nerve plexuses

The innervation of limbs and limb girdles is via plexuses (brachial and lumbo-sacral) formed by spinal nerves, which allows nerves from several different spinal levels to form peripheral nerves. The trunk (cage) is supplied by spinal nerves only: viscera are supplied by the vagus nerve (X cranial nerve).

Spinal nerves and roots

At each level of the spinal cord, a pair of nerve roots emerge on both sides, posterior and anterior. These join together to form spinal nerves that then exit the spinal canal as a pair at each level, right and left. The anterior spinal nerve root conveys motor axons only. All sensory nerves enter the spinal cord via the posterior roots. The nerve cell bodies of all peripheral sensory axons are in a ganglion protruding from each posterior spinal root, the dorsal root ganglion (DRG). These nerve roots and spinal nerves are particularly prone to injury within the spinal canal and as they exit it via the intervertebral foramina.

Table 58 Classification of sensory nerve fibres

Fibre type	Maximum diameter (μ)	Maximum conduction velocity (m/second)	Degree of myelination	Function
Ia	22	120	+++	Muscle spindle primary afferents
Ib	22	120	+++	Golgi tendon organs, touch and pressure receptors
II	13	70	++	Muscle spindle secondary afferents, touch and pressure receptors, Pacinian corpuscles (vibratory receptors)
III	5	15	+	Touch, pressure, pain, temperature
IV	1	2	-	Pain, temperature

Spinal cord

Up to the spinal cord, sensation follows a common pathway (although the differing morphology of peripheral axons renders them susceptible to different pathological processes). In the spinal cord, the nerves entering via the posterior spinal root (via the posterior root entry zone) divide into two main bundles. Those nerves subserving proprioception ascend in the ipsilateral (same side) posterior columns to the mid medulla oblongata, where they terminate in the cuneate and gracile nuclei. From these nuclei, second order neurones decussate and ascend to the contralateral thalamus in the medial lemniscus. Fibres subserving touch, pain, and temperature synapse with second order sensory nerves and traverse the spinal cord, anterior to the central canal. The fibres ascend to the thalami as the anterior spino-thalamic tracts, those nerves entering the more distal spinal cord most, lying more superficially. Thus, within the cord, there is functional and anatomical separation that is of significance in localizing lesions (160).

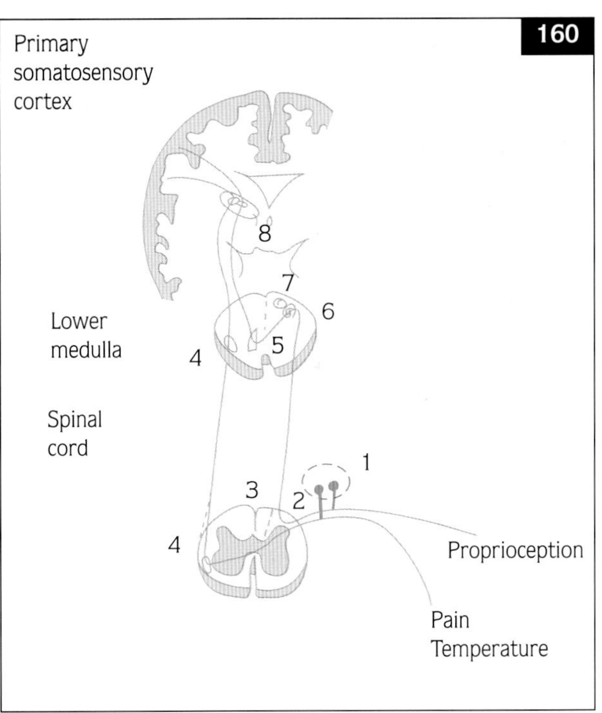

160 Diagram to show a simplified outline of major sensory pathways. **1:** dorsal root ganglion; **2:** fasciculus cuneatus; **3:** fasciculus gracilis; **4:** lateral spino-thalamic tract; **5:** medial lemniscus; **6:** nucleus cuneatus; **7:** nucleus gracilis; **8:** thalamus.

Facio-cranial sensation

The face and deep cranial structures receive their sensory supply via the V (trigeminal) cranial nerve (also motor to the muscles of mastication) (**161**). The upper cervical roots supply the posterior scalp. The cell bodies of the sensory afferents of the trigeminal nerve are contained in the trigeminal (gasserian) ganglion, the equivalent of the spinal nerve DRG. The trigeminal nerve enters the brainstem at the level of the mid pons where the proprioceptive (and motor) nuclei are located, and the second order sensory axons then traverse the pons to ascend to the thalamus. Fibres subserving pain, temperature, and touch descend as the spinal tract of the trigeminal nerve to the ipsilateral medulla and upper cervical cord where they form the nucleus of the spinal tract of V. Second order sensory neurones then traverse the cord/medulla and ascend to the thalami. Thus, unilateral lesions in the upper cervical spine/medulla can give rise to contralateral trunk and limb pain, temperature and touch loss (ascending spino-thalamic tract), as well as facial loss of the same sensory modalities (descending spinal tract and nucleus). This feature is characteristic of lower brainstem lesions.

Thalami

These large, deep-brain nuclei are the first level at which one becomes conscious of sensory stimuli. Unilateral lesions here and above, give rise to partial or complete hemi sensory syndromes. Lesions of the thalami are often associated with pain (thalamic syndrome). Third order neurones project from the thalami to the ipsilateral sensory cortex via the posterior limb of the internal capsule.

Sensory cortex

The primary sensory cortex is located at the postcentral gyrus, and is where integrated fine sensation (i.e. the texture and temperature of objects) is appreciated (**162**). Associated sensory areas in the parietal cortex are responsible for integrated sensations such as stereognosis (the ability to recognize objects through touch), graphaesthesia (the ability to identify characters traced on the skin), and two-point discrimination (the ability to recognize two adjacent stimuli as separate). Clearly, these functions depend on intact peripheral sensation.

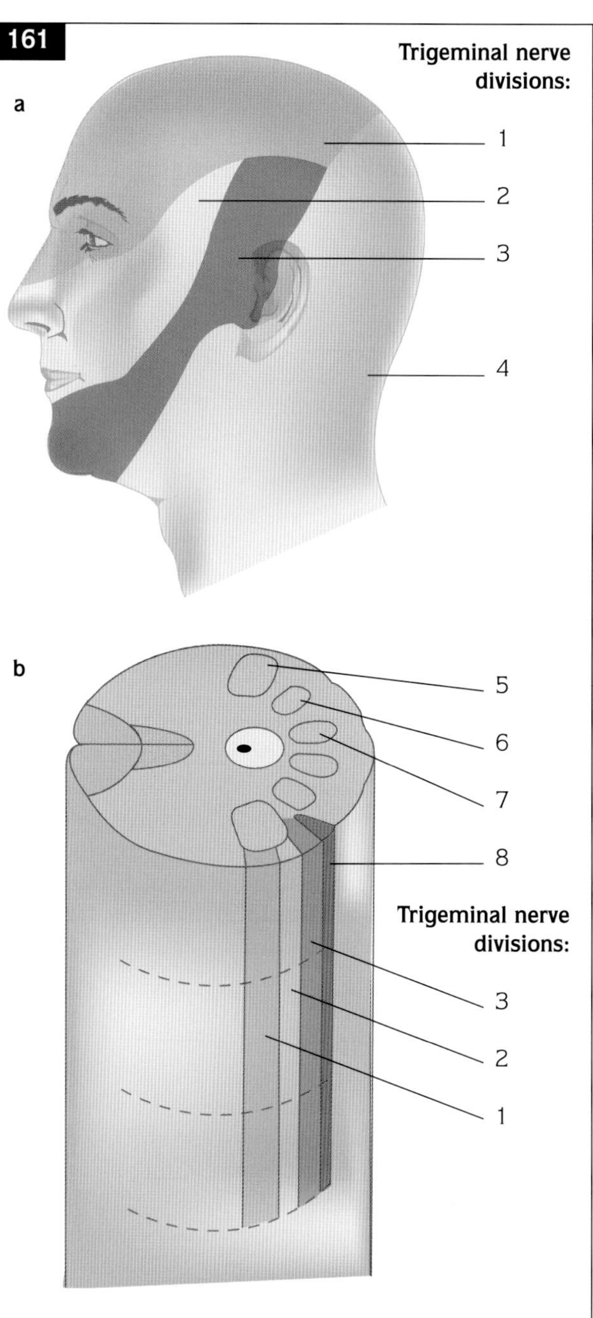

161 Diagram to show the somatotrophic organization of the trigeminal system. **a:** peripheral innervation territories of the trigeminal nerve. **1:** ophthalmic; **2:** maxillary; **3:** mandibular trigeminal nerve; **4:** innervation by cervical sensory roots. **b:** organization of the spinal trigeminal tract in relation to the three trigeminal nerve divisions and the glossopharyngeal nerves for the portion of the medulla that includes the caudal nucleus. **5:** spinal trigeminal nucleus; **6:** cuneate nucleus; **7:** gracile nucleus; **8:** glossopharyngeal nucleus.

Other sensory pathways

The brainstem and cerebellum also receive sensory input via specific spinal tracts. These subserve the maintenance of smooth movements, balance, and coordination, and are subconscious. These are not considered further here.

CLINICAL ASSESSMENT

History and examination

History taking is particularly important when it comes to elucidating sensory symptoms, as in many cases there may be few, if any, objective neurological signs. Although the history should focus on the presenting complaint(s), it is important to ask about other neurological symptoms, as well as encompassing non-neurological causes. It is also important to be aware that patients may describe nonsensory symptoms in sensory terms: a common example is the patient who describes weakness of a limb as numbness. Equally, it is important to complete a full neurological examination.

It is important to interrogate the patient as to the precise nature of their sensory symptoms. As sensory symptoms are often vague in nature, a superficial history will lead to imprecise localization and differential diagnosis. Armed with basic anatomico-physiological concepts, it is important to detail important negatives in the history, in addition to recording the positive findings. For example, in someone presenting with symptoms suggestive of

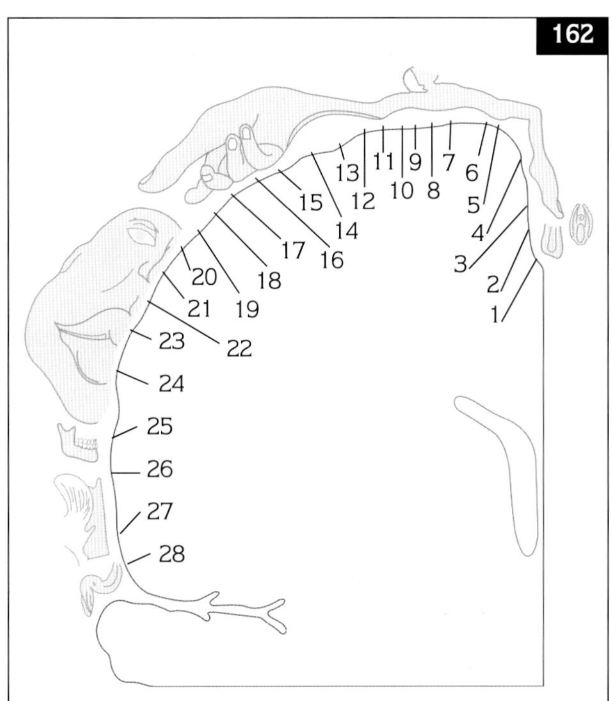

162 Penfield homunculus: the primary somatic cortex (postcentral gyrus). **1:** genitalia; **2:** toes; **3:** foot; **4:** leg; **5:** hip; **6:** trunk; **7:** neck; **8:** head; **9:** shoulder; **10:** arm; **11:** elbow; **12:** forearm; **13:** wrist; **14:** hand; **15:** little finger; **16:** ring finger; **17:** middle finger; **18:** index finger; **19:** thumb; **20:** eye; **21:** nose; **22:** face; **23:** upper lip; **24:** lower lip; **25:** teeth, gums, jaw; **26:** tongue; **27:** pharynx; **28:** intra-abdominal.

spinal disease, it is vital to enquire about bladder function. The main points of the history are as outlined in *Table 59*. Thus, for example, with a patient presenting with tingling of the hand, it is important to describe what part of the hand is affected, which digits, the frequency and duration of the symptoms, whether the patient awakes at night with the symptoms, or whether it is worsened by certain wrist postures (as in carpal tunnel syndrome).

Sensory examination can be laborious. It should follow a general neurological examination and be directed to the presenting complaint. *Table 60* indicates the main features of the sensory examination. The following points should be considered when carrying out a sensory examination:

- ❑ Ensure the patient is relaxed and not distracted.
- ❑ Explain to the patient what to expect and what is expected of them prior to each component of the examination; demonstrate initially (on an area of normal sensation).

Table 59 Sensory history and loss

History	Define	Additional	Examples
Where?	Focal	Specify	Root or peripheral nerve lesion
	Multifocal	Timing: simultaneous, evolutionary, migratory	❑ Mononeuritis multiplex ❑ Polyradiculopathy
	Distal limb	Ascending, which limbs?	Polyneuropathy
	Truncal level	Upper level, lower level, pain?	❑ Spinal cord lesion ❑ Suspended sensory level with central cord lesion
	Hemisensory	Face involved?	❑ Stroke ❑ Tumour
	Face/contralateral limb	Other brainstem features?	Stroke
Onset/progression	How long?		
	Acute	How sudden, pain?	❑ Trauma ❑ Vascular lesion
	Subacute	Rate of evolution?	Inflammatory processes
	Chronic	Stable, progressive, stepwise?	Degenerative processes
	Improving monophasic		
Nature	Episodic	Frequency, duration, nocturnal?	❑ Multiple sclerosis ❑ Carpal tunnel syndrome
	Constant	Variability?	
	Precipitating/provoking factors	Postural, coughing, exercise, temperature?	❑ Compressive radiculopathy ❑ Uhthoff's phenomenon
Associated features	Pain	At onset, distribution?	❑ Radiculopathy – 'sciatica' ❑ Thalamic syndrome
	Weakness		
	Bladder symptoms		❑ Cord/cauda equina lesion ❑ Uncommon with peripheral neuropathies
	Ataxia		❑ Large fibre polyneuropathy ❑ Posterior column disease ❑ Vitamin B_{12} deficiency
	Trauma	Acute, chronic?	❑ Saturday night radial nerve palsy ❑ Ulnar nerve palsy at elbow
	Others		

Table 60 Testing for sensory loss

Modality	Tool/technique	Testing	Comments
Touch	Fingertip	❑ Medium-large, myelinated peripheral nerves	❑ Light touch only, otherwise testing pressure receptors
	Cotton wool	❑ Spino-thalamic tract	❑ Do not stroke
Pain	Neuro-tip	❑ Small, lightly myelinated peripheral nerves ❑ Spino-thalamic tracts	❑ Avoid too much pressure ❑ Do not use hypodermic needles ❑ Do not reuse neuro-tips ❑ Never use hat pins
Temperature	Universals with hot and cold water Tuning fork	❑ Small, lightly myelinated peripheral nerves ❑ Spino-thalamic tracts	❑ Do not use very hot water
Joint position sense	Fingers and toes		❑ Avoid using pressure ❑ Start with small joints, e.g. ring finger DIP, 2nd toe
Vibration	128 Hz tuning fork	❑ Medium-large, myelinated peripheral nerves ❑ Posterior columns	❑ Start distally, use bony eminences ❑ Unilateral loss on rib cage and cranium is suspicious of nonorganic disease
Pseudoathetosis	Arms extended, fingers abducted, eyes closed	❑ Large, myelinated peripheral nerves ❑ Posterior columns	❑ Observe spontaneous athetotic movements of the fingers
Pronator drift	Arms extended, hands supine, eyes closed	❑ Contralateral fronto-parietal lobe	❑ Observe slow, downward drift of affected arm, with pronation of the wrist ❑ Lack of pronation reduces the strength of the sign
Sensory inattention	Eyes closed, stimulate each side independently, then simultaneously	❑ Contralateral parietal lobe	❑ Subject will report stimulus from both sides when tested independently ❑ Only from unaffected side when tested simultaneously
Stereognosis	Eyes closed, present key or similar to hand	❑ Contralateral parietal lobe	❑ Assumes normal peripheral sensation
Graphaesthesia	Eyes closed, draw letter/ digit on palm	❑ Contralateral parietal lobe	❑ Use continuous characters, e.g. S, O, 3, 8 ❑ Assumes normal peripheral sensation
2-point discrimination	Dividers	❑ Contralateral parietal lobe	❑ Light touch only ❑ Varies <5 mm on index finger to >1 cm on back
Reflexes	Tendon hammer	❑ Large, myelinated peripheral nerves, sensory (afferent)and motor (efferent)	❑ Frequently lost early in peripheral neuropathies ❑ Retained or exaggerated with central sensory loss (due to associated UMN disease)
Romberg's sign	Stands with feet together, hands by side, then closes eyes	❑ Large, myelinated peripheral nerves ❑ Posterior columns	❑ Subject falls (prevent fall): a sign of sensory (not cerebellar) ataxia
Finger–nose	Extended arm, touches nose with index finger, repeats on eye closure	❑ Large, myelinated peripheral nerves ❑ Posterior columns	❑ Stop if at risk of injuring eyes
Heel–shin	Lifts heel onto opposite knee and runs down shin, lifts and repeats with eyes closed	❑ Large, myelinated peripheral nerves ❑ Posterior columns	❑ Avoid letting subject use shin as a guide, i.e. repeated passes up and down

DIP: distal inter-phalangeal; UMN: upper motor neurone.

- ❑ The following line of questioning is useful – 'Can you feel this? Does it feel normal? Does it feel the same on both sides?'.
- ❑ Avoid using excessive pressure when testing light touch, pain, and proprioception.
- ❑ Testing superficial sensation should be random, and encompass radicular (nerve root) and peripheral nerve territories.
- ❑ Remember that there is considerable overlap between root territories and, to a lesser extent peripheral nerve territories, resulting in areas of sensory loss less than anticipated; e.g. a single truncal root lesion may not result in demonstrable sensory loss.
- ❑ Also, there is some crossover at the mid line, such that in a unilateral lesion sensory impairment may not reach the mid line.
- ❑ Always map an area of sensory loss from the centre of the deficit outwards; doing the opposite tends to underestimate the area of disordered sensation.
- ❑ Always repeat the examination of a deficit, preferably in a different order/direction to confirm the findings.
- ❑ When testing proprioception:
  - Ask the patient to close their eyes (or look away).
  - Start with small joints to elucidate the most subtle deficits (e.g. ring finger, distal interphalangeal joint or second toe) before moving on to larger joints or joints with greater cortical representation (e.g. the index finger).
  - After demonstrating, ask the patient to indicate the last direction of movement, not the final position.
  - Avoid applying too much pressure on the digit to indicate the direction of movement.
  - Move the digit by holding it by the sides.
- ❑ The majority of the sensory examination depends on the patient's replies, and is therefore subjective and relatively soft; associated motor signs and reflex changes are therefore valuable.
- ❑ Certain sensory tests are useful as a screen before embarking on a more detailed examination, especially pain and proprioception.

Recording the history and findings is important. It is usually best to record the patient's own description, especially when this is particularly illustrative. The terminology of sensory symptoms is extensive and there is an overlap between what is reported and what is found on examination (*Table 61*). In general terms, sensory modalities may be normal, reduced, absent, altered, or increased. Some of these are described in *Table 61*, in addition to those outlined in *Table 60*. *Table 62* provides a list of useful anatomical reference points.Classification of sensory nerves is presented in *Table 63*.

Table 61 Sensory disturbance terminology

Term	Meaning	Example
Hypoaesthesia, anaesthesia	Reduced/loss of sensation	Numbness
Hypodynia/allodynia	Reduced/loss of pain sensation	Can result in painless burns, Charcot joints
Paraesthesiae	Positive sensory phenomena	Pins and needles
Dysaesthesia	Altered interpretation of sensory stimulus	Feeling hot as cold, touch as pain
Astereognosis	Unable to recognize an object through touch alone	Subject unable to find keys in pocket, correct coins
Agraphaesthesia	Unable to recognize a character traced on the skin	Examined for: e.g. trace a figure 8 on patient's palm
Sensory neglect	Ignores sensory stimuli to one side, with intact peripheral sensation	Parietal lobe infarct

Nonorganic sensory loss

Sensory loss is a frequent manifestation of nonorganic or elaborated disease, either as a feature of conversion syndromes or in the malingerer. The lack of objective clinical signs often makes this difficult to exclude, and making a diagnosis of nonorganic sensory loss depends a lot on clinical experience. The clinician should beware of discounting sensory symptoms too rapidly; nonorganic disease should be a diagnosis of exclusion. However, there are a few useful pointers:

- ❑ Nonorganic sensory loss frequently:
  - Is complete, i.e. totally numb.
  - Affects all modalities of sensation, i.e. small and large fibre, spino-thalamic, and posterior column.
  - Does not respect anatomical/physiological boundaries.
  - Has circumferential cut-off on the limbs.
  - Completely respects the mid line.
  - Respects patients' modesty!
  - Is associated with unusual (nonorganic) postures and movements.
  - Has absent associated features/signs.
- ❑ On examination it is worth checking for:
  - Vibration loss that respects the mid line on face and thorax; in genuine sensory loss vibration can be appreciated by the contralateral (normal) side.
  - Nonpronating arm drift.
  - Withdrawal or an emotional response to painful stimuli, while denying appreciation.
  - Lack of trophic changes.
  - Consistent reporting of the direction opposite to the direction of actual movement when testing proprioception.

None of these features individually points to nonorganic sensory loss, and some are features of true sensory loss. In addition, patients often try to help or impress the examiner by elaborating their signs. Also, patients manifesting gross nonorganic features may have a genuine, often minor underlying disorder. However, usually an overall pattern emerges suggesting nonorganic disease.

Patterns of sensory disturbance

Patterns of sensory loss, taking into account their distribution and evolution, suggest the site and nature of the lesion. Single-site focal loss suggests a root or peripheral nerve lesion. Compressive causes are frequently painful (e.g. sciatica). Associated

Table 62 Selected sensory localization reference points

Site	Area subserved	Additional
C4 root	Shoulder	
C7	Middle finger	Triceps reflex
T4	Trunk: nipple level	
T8	Trunk: costal margin	
T10	Trunk: umbilical level	
L3	Leg: over knee	
S1	Foot: sole	Ankle reflex
S2	Buttocks: over ischial tuberosities	Stand on S1; sit on S2

Table 63 Classification of sensory nerve fibres

Type	Maximum fibre diameter (μ)	Maximum conduction velocity (m/sec)	Degree of myelination	Function
Ia	22	120	+++	❑ Muscle spindle primary afferents
Ib	22	120	+++	❑ Golgi tendon organs ❑ Touch and pressure receptors
II	13	70	++	❑ Muscle spindle secondary afferents ❑ Touch and pressure receptors ❑ Pacinian corpuscles (vibratory sense)
III	5	15	+	❑ Touch, pressure, pain, and temperature
IV	1	2	-	❑ Pain and temperature

weakness, wasting, or reflex loss should be assessed for. Nerve stretching manoeuvres (e.g. straight leg raising) may exacerbate pain, as may certain postures (bending over). Percussion or compression of nerves over entrapment sites (Tinel's sign) may increase paraesthesiae or numbness, and/or cause pain.

Multiple focal sites can be affected in mononeuritis multiplex, often sequentially, sometimes flitting, and it is frequently due to vasculitis. Multiple spinal roots can be affected by infiltrative disease within the spinal canal/dura, often affecting the lumbo-sacral roots as in lepto-meningeal carcinomatosis.

Distal limb sensory loss, progressing proximally, is a feature of dying-back polyneuropathies, such as those due to vitamin deficiencies and diabetes. Pathologically, there is axonal degeneration affecting the axon most distal to the cell body initially. Usually there is sensory loss to the level of the knee before the upper limbs are involved. Exceptions to this rule include the sensory neuronopathy associated with the sicca syndrome and paraneoplastic sensory neuropathy (dorsal root ganglionopathies). Reflexes are frequently lost early in peripheral polyneuropathies. A pseudo-neuropathic (peripheral) pattern can be seen in cervical cord compression whereby patients present with distal limb paraesthesiae. On examination however, there will be upper motor neurone signs (i.e. brisk reflexes rather than depressed or absent reflexes). Distal limb paraesthesiae can also be a feature of multiple sclerosis.

Sensory loss affecting the perineum suggests a conus medullaris or cauda equina lesion. This is associated with loss of sphincter control, i.e. bladder and bowel dysfunction. Sensory loss with a level on the trunk indicates spinal cord disease. Often patients complain of pain or heightened sensation at the upper level. Causes include cord compression (e.g. tumour or disc protrusion), inflammation (transverse myelitis), and vascular disease (anterior spinal artery syndrome, posterior column function preserved). Hemicord syndromes can present with ipsilateral posterior column (proprioceptive loss), and contralateral spino-thalamic loss (Brown-Séquard syndrome); there may be ipsilateral motor loss. Central cord lesions (e.g. intrinsic cord tumours and syringomyelia) tend to cause bilateral spino-thalamic loss initially, due to interruption of the decussating fibres, followed by motor loss. These lesions may present with a suspended sensory loss, i.e. with preserved sensation distally. An example of this is a syrinx affecting the cervical spinal cord that presents with 'cape' distribution spino-thalamic sensory loss.

The hallmark of brainstem sensory loss is crossed spino-thalamic sensory loss, i.e. trigeminal (facial) sensory loss ipsilateral to the lesion, with limb/trunk loss on the contralateral side. The lateral medullary syndrome of Wallenburg is a good example of this. Thalamic lesions are associated with hemipain disturbances (thalamic syndrome, is often burning in nature), often with retained simple sensations. Cortical sensory syndromes are again characterized by unilateral symptoms (unless bilateral cortical lesions), intact simple sensations (appreciated at the thalamic level), but impaired integrated sensory modalities (*Table 60*).

The hand

Sensory examination of the hand deserves particular attention. Peripheral nerve lesions, especially those due to trauma (acute and chronic), and less frequently as a result of vasculitis and granulomatous disorders, are especially common in the upper limb. Partial and chronic lesions often present with sensory symptoms prior to the onset of weakness and wasting. Radicular and brachial plexus lesions are more unusual, and often have coexisting motor features at presentation. The hand receives its sensory innervation from three peripheral nerves: median (C5–T1), ulnar (C8, T1), and radial (C6, 7, 8) nerves, derived from three spinal roots (C6, 7, 8) (**163**, **164**). The median nerve supplies the radial three and a half digits and associated palmar surface; the ulnar nerve the little and half of the ring finger, as well as the ulnar surface of the palm. Sensation from the dorsal surface of the hand and digits as far as the distal phalanges is mediated via the radial nerve (may be more proximal in ulnar innervated digits).

Sensory loss splitting the ring finger is a useful feature to distinguish median and ulnar nerve lesions from more proximal lesions (plexus and root), but in a small percentage of people the ring finger is supplied by either nerve completely. The median and ulnar nerves supply the intrinsic muscles of the hand: the median nerve supplies the two radial lumbrical muscles and the muscles of the thenar eminence bar the adductor pollicis and flexor pollicis brevis muscles; these and the rest of the intrinsic hand muscles are supplied by the ulnar nerve. The myotomal innervation of the hand muscles is via the C8 and T1 nerve roots. Thus, wasting in specific muscle groups may be an aid to diagnosing focal lesions and may precede frank symptomatic weakness. Advanced ulnar nerve lesions will produce

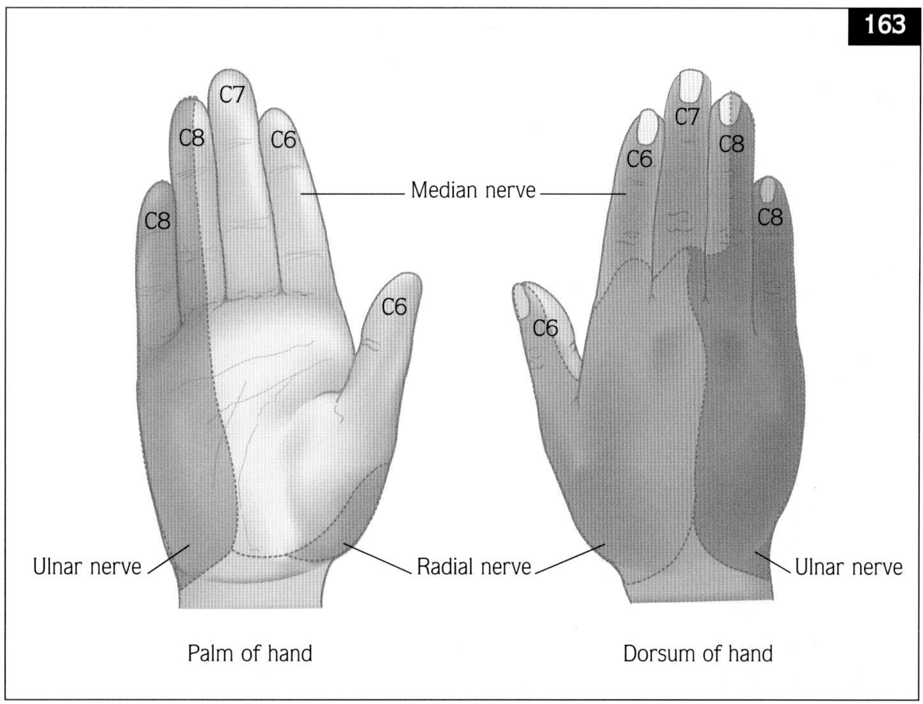

163 Diagram to illustrate somatic innervation of the hand.

characteristic clawing of the hand; median nerve lesions cause wasting of the thenar eminence.

The commonest median nerve lesion is carpal tunnel syndrome, where the median nerve is chronically compressed under the flexor retinaculum at the wrist. This condition can occur spontaneously, be bilateral, is more common in women, and is associated with a number of conditions, e.g. hypothyroidism, pregnancy, rheumatoid arthritis, and acromegaly. It typically presents as a painful sensory syndrome, patients often complaining initially of pain and paraesthesiae in the median innervated digits and hand, awakening them at night. As the condition progresses, patients complain of exercise- or posture-induced pain and numbness, often radiating into the radial aspect of the forearm and centred about the index finger in the hand. Typically, these symptoms progress over many months or years. Patients may have objective median territory sensory loss on examination. Percussion over the flexor retinaculum (Tinel's sign) may reproduce the symptoms, as may hyperextension of the wrist. Nerve conduction studies confirm the diagnosis by demonstrating slowing of conduction in the median nerve across the wrist. Conservative management includes treating any underlying disorder and wrist splinting; surgical division of the flexor retinaculum will relieve the symptoms.

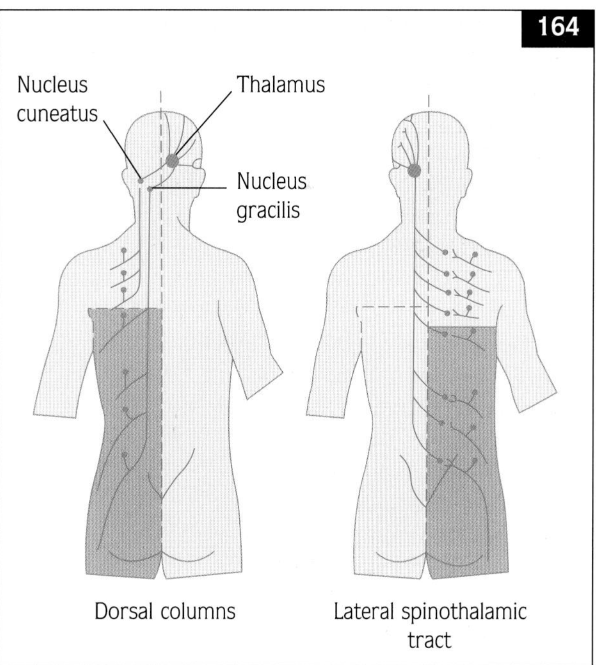

164 Schematic diagram of the spinal cord sensory pathways.

The ulnar nerve is most prone to injury where it passes across the medial epicondyle at the elbow (the 'funny bone'). Elbow fractures or repeated chronic trauma (e.g. leaning on the elbows) can cause ulnar distribution sensory symptoms and loss, progressing to ulnar weakness. Compressing the ulnar nerve at the medial epicondyle may reproduce these symptoms. Radial nerve lesions rarely present as sensory syndromes.

Summary

- Numbness and tingling may arise from lesions directly affecting the neuraxis, from the level of the peripheral nerve and sensory receptor through the spinal cord to cortical level: these symptoms may be secondary to non-neurological disorders.
- Distinct patterns of sensory loss and associated features facilitate clinical localization of the lesions: an understanding of the basic neuroanatomical pathways subserving sensation and their physiology enables this.
- Separation of sensation into large fibre/posterior column function versus small fibre/ spino-thalamic function helps in considering peripheral nerve and spinal lesions; assessment of proprioception and pain are useful screening examinations.
- Cortical and subcortical lesions produce loss of integrated sensory functions but these functions depend on intact spinal and peripheral sensory pathways: gross sensation may be intact with these higher level lesions.
- Sensory symptoms must not be considered in isolation: enquiry regarding motor and autonomic symptoms should be made where appropriate, and a full neurological examination should be conducted.
- An accurate sensory assessment may avoid unnecessary investigation.

CLINICAL SCENARIOS

Case 1

A 60-year-old, right-handed female presented to the neurology clinic with a 6-month history of ascending paraesthesiae, affecting her feet initially, but then progressing to a level below the knees. These symptoms were most noticeable in bed at night. She had also become aware of being slightly unsteady, especially in the dark. She denied any weakness, upper limb symptoms, or bladder symptoms. Past medical history was unremarkable, and she was not taking any regular medications. She was a nonsmoker, and drank <4 units of alcohol per week. Her mother suffered from maturity-onset diabetes.

The history is of a slowly progressing sensory disorder affecting the legs only, suggesting a peripheral 'dying-back' polyneuropathy. The lack of bladder and motor symptoms makes a spinal/cauda equina lesion unlikely. The slow progression suggests a metabolic/deficiency state; note family history of diabetes. Inflammatory, vascular, and neoplastic causes seem less likely. Her age makes congenital/genetic causes unlikely.

Neurological examination of the cranial nerves and upper limbs was normal. In the legs there was no wasting or fasciculation, tone was normal, and power was well maintained. Both ankle jerks were absent and the knee jerks were just present with reinforcement. Sensory testing showed loss of vibratory sensation at up to the knees. There was blunting of pinprick sensation over both feet. Joint position testing suggested a subtle deficit.

The examination confirms peripheral nerve disease with impaired/absent reflexes and distal sensory loss; there are no upper motor neurone signs. Both large and medium sized sensory axons are affected. Thus, clinically, the features are best explained by a peripheral polyneuropathy. The areflexia would be difficult to explain on the basis of a chronic spinal process, and although the sensory symptoms could be explained by combined posterior column and spino-thalamic damage, the lack of any motor or bladder features would make this unusual.

(Continued on page 225)

CASE 1 *(continued)*

The differential diagnosis of peripheral neuropathy is extensive, but clinical features help to narrow the field. Neuropathies are classified according to aetiology (e.g. diabetes, vitamin B_{12} deficiency), pathological process (demyelinating, axonal, neuronal) and functional loss (motor, sensory, mixed, autonomic). Demyelinating neuropathies usually have prominent motor features. Predominantly or purely sensory neuropathies tend be axonopathies or, less commonly, neuronopathies. Frequently these are subacute or chronic processes.

The investigation of peripheral neuropathy is initially directed towards the most likely causes. Electrophysiological examination (nerve conduction studies and electromyography [EMG]), although more useful in motor neuropathies, can provide information about the pathophysiology of the neuropathy facilitating the targeting of subsequent investigations. However, delays in obtaining electrodiagnostic studies often result in blood tests being requested first. In brief, nerve conduction studies can demonstrate slowing of conduction (due to demyelination), or conduction block (demyelination or vasculitis), or reduction in the amplitude of the compound muscle action potential (CMAP) with normal velocities (axonopathy) and loss of sensory nerve action potentials (SNAPs) (axonopathy/neuronopathy).

In this case, the nerve conduction studies demonstrated loss of distal lower limb SNAPs, with relatively normal motor studies and EMG. Initial investigations demonstrated a high random serum glucose that was confirmed on a fasting sample. Haemoglobin A1c was raised and glucose tolerance test was abnormal, confirming a diagnosis of diabetes.

Thus, a diagnosis of diabetic neuropathy was confirmed and the patient was initiated on appropriate medical treatment.

CASE 2

A 45-year-old, right-handed male plumber presented with a 2-year history of slowly evolving numbness and pain affecting both hands, beginning on the ulnar borders and progressing up the forearms. He noted impaired dexterity in carrying out his occupation, which he considered threatened by his disability. He was still able to feel objects but found it difficult to discern texture. On questioning, he also described loss of temperature sensation, and had unknowingly burnt his right index and middle fingers while smoking. He did not describe any positive sensory symptoms such as pain or paraesthesiae. He did not describe any weakness, or neurological symptoms elsewhere.

Progressive symmetric distal upper limb only, spino-thalamic (pain, temperature, and touch) sensory loss is being described. This would be an unusual pattern for a peripheral sensory polyneuropathy (legs spared; other poorly myelinated/ unmyelinated fibres not symptomatically affected as no autonomic features, e.g. bladder/postural hypotension). However, rare sensory neuronopathy associated with Sjögren/ sicca syndrome frequently affects the upper limbs first. Consider degenerative/metabolic/deficiency state, given the slow evolution. A possible diagnosis is spinal cord disease, but there are no long tract symptoms, e.g. mobility/bladder features.

Neurological examination of the cranial nerves and lower limbs was normal. Examination of the upper limbs showed normal tone and power, with some suggestion of early intrinsic hand muscle wasting. Upper limb reflexes were reduced. Sensory testing showed preserved proprioception and vibratory sensation. However, pain (sterile neurotip), was reduced bilaterally from the shoulders to nipple level (C4–T4), including the upper limbs. Temperature sensation was also reduced in this distribution, with lesser impairment of touch (**165**).

(Continued overleaf)

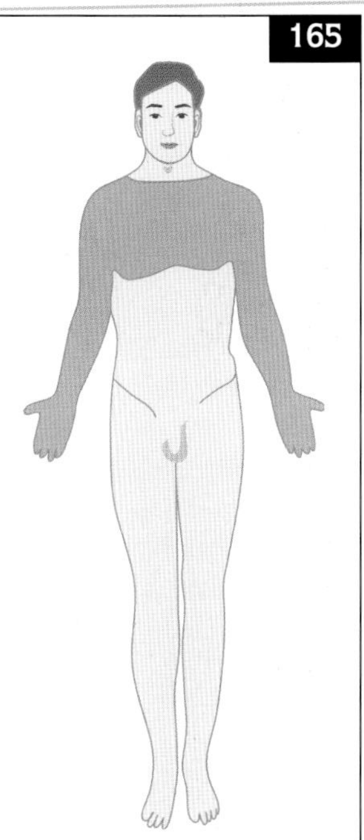

165 Diagram to illustrate suspended sensory loss in syringomyelia. Syringomyelia results in cape-like sensory impairment selectively for pain and temperature, often accompanied by loss of reflexes in the upper limbs.

CASE 2 *(continued)*

Examination confirms a suspended sensory loss, which is strongly indicative of central spinal cord disease. The signs extend over multiple adjacent dermatomes. Truncal sensory loss is unusual in polyneuropathies (but sometimes seen in obese people in the periumbilical area). The confluence of the signs and slow evolution suggest a slowly progressive structural lesion. Clinically, the lesion is now localized to the upper dorsal and cervical cord. Thus, the most appropriate investigation is to image this area and this is best achieved by MRI.

The MRI (**166**) demonstrates a central cavity within the spinal cord and herniation of the cerebellar tonsils through the foramen magnum (a Chiari malformation).

*These conditions are frequently associated and it is believed that the congenital cranio-cervical malformation (the Chiari malformation) predisposes to the development of the syrinx. As the syrinx (the fluid filled cavity positioned centrally in the cord) expands and extends, it transects the decussating spino-thalamic fibres resulting in the suspended spino-thalamic pattern sensory loss (**165**). With further expansion anterior horn cells are destroyed, resulting in muscle wasting, weakness, and areflexia. At this stage the ascending and descending long tracts become involved, giving rise to lower limb upper motor neurone signs and sensory loss. This patient was referred for neurosurgical decompression of the foramen magnum, and his condition subsequently stabilized.*

On cranial nerve examination, she had unsustained end-gaze nystagmus on lateral gaze bilaterally. Ophthalmoscopy showed pallor of the temporal portion of the right optic disc and colour vision testing (Ishihara chart) demonstrated impairment in the right eye. Jaw jerk was positive. Examination of the upper limbs showed hyper-reflexia only. In the legs, the reflexes were brisk, with minimal weakness of left ankle dorsiflexion and an extensor left plantar response. Sensory testing showed impaired vibratory sensation at both ankles only. Gait was normal, apart from minor difficulty with tandem walking (heel–toe) and Romberg's sign was negative. Abdominal reflexes were absent.

The examination findings 'outweigh' the clinical symptoms and provide evidence for multifocal disease: right optic neuropathy (pale disc and impaired colour vision), upper motor neurone signs (hyper-reflexia and extensor left plantar response), and sensory impairment (impaired distal lower limb vibratory sensation). In addition, the history suggests disordered bladder control.

As the history suggests a multifocal disorder of the central nervous system, involving at least an upper level of the brainstem (eye movement control), an MRI of brain was requested. This demonstrated multiple white matter lesions, both recent (gadolinium enhancing) and established (**167**). This provided strong supportive evidence for the diagnosis of multiple sclerosis. Visual evoked responses demonstrated significant slowing of conduction in the right visual pathways, consistent with demyelination. Cerebrospinal fluid (CSF) examination (obtained by lumbar puncture) demonstrated 7 lymphocytes per mm^3, normal protein and glucose, but the presence of isolated oligoclonal bands in the CSF alone, a finding consistent with and supportive of a diagnosis of MS (**168**).

In the 6 months following presentation, the patient suffered two further relapses (symptomatic left optic neuritis and mild partial transverse myelitis), and was commenced on interferon-beta therapy.

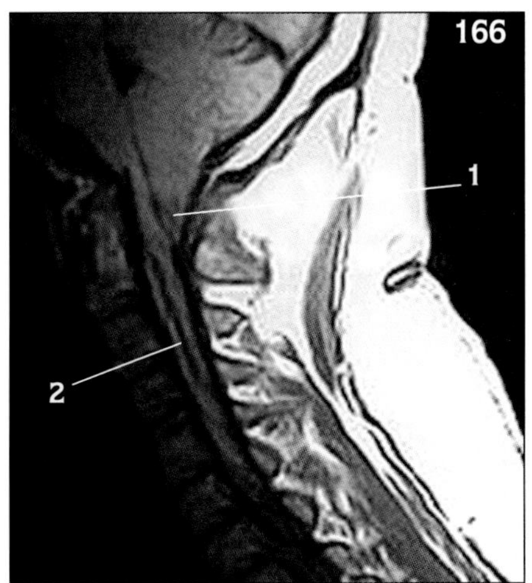

166 Magnetic resonance image of syringomyelia. 1, descended cerebellar tonsils; 2, syrinx.

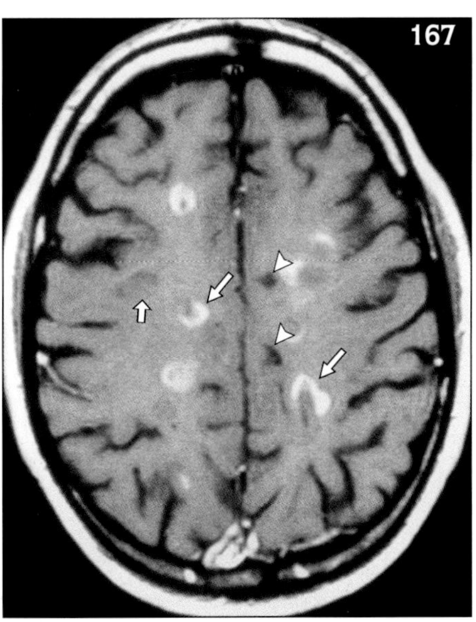

167 Gadolinium-enhanced T1-weighted magnetic resonance image of the brain in multiple sclerosis, demonstrating enhancing (acute) lesions (arrows), established lesions (short arrow), and 'black holes' (arrowheads).

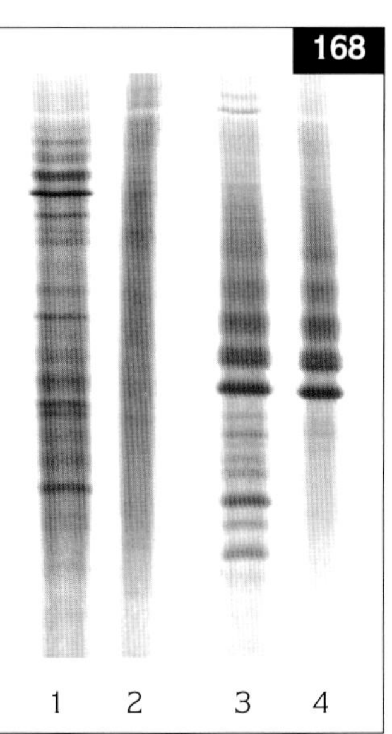

168 Cerebrospinal fluid (CSF) IgG oligoclonal banding patterns. Lanes 1 and 2 demonstrate isolated oligoclonal bands, consistent with an intrinsic central nervous system response, the usual response indicative of multiple sclerosis. Lanes 3 and 4 show both paired and isolated bands. (Lanes 1, 3: CSF; lanes 2, 4: serum.) (Courtesy of Mrs J Veitch, Neuroimmunology Laboratory, INS, Southern General Hospital, Glasgow.)

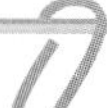

CASE 3

A 25-year-old, left-handed, Caucasian female presented with a 3-month history of intermittent tingling affecting both hands and feet. She was most aware of this in the evenings, especially on retiring to bed. However, she has also noted a worsening of her symptoms following a jog or a hot bath. These symptoms did not interfere with her normal activities. On questioning, she did admit to some urinary urgency that had persisted following the birth of her first (only) child 3 years earlier. She also recalled an episode of transient left leg heaviness (possibly weakness), in her late teens, which resolved over a couple of weeks. She had no other significant past medical history, and there was no relevant family or social history. She was taking no regular medication, apart from the oral contraceptive pill.

In addition to the presenting sensory symptoms, a number of potentially important other symptoms are described: previous leg weakness and on-going bladder symptoms. The intermittent nature of the sensory symptoms, together with heat sensitivity (Uhthoff's phenomenon), is more suggestive of a central rather than a peripheral cause. Bladder symptoms suggest spinal cord disease. The history suggests remitting disease, possibly at different sites within the central nervous system. Her age (gender), race, and symptoms postpartum suggest multiple sclerosis (MS).

REVISION QUESTIONS

1 Pain is mediated by fast-conducting, peripheral sensory neurones.
2 Proprioception is impaired early in central cord disease.
3 A (lateral) hemicord lesion will cause loss of spino-thalamic sensation ipsilaterally below the lesion.
4 Sensation can only be appreciated at a cortical level.
5 Stereognosis depends on intact peripheral sensory pathways.
6 Dorsal root ganglia contain the nuclei of proprioceptive nerves.
7 Romberg's sign is a test of proprioceptive function.
8 Sensory loss in the ulnar two digits with weakness of finger flexion suggests an ulnar neuropathy.
9 In sensory inattention, the patient is unable to appreciate a sensory stimulus when presented to the affected side only.
10 Pseudoathetosis can be caused by a dorsal root ganglionopathy.
11 In suspended sensory loss, pain and temperature sensation are retained until advanced disease.
12 C7 root usually mediates sensation from the ring finger.
13 An infarct of the anterior limb of the internal capsule causes contralateral hemisensory loss.
14 Lateral pontine lesions may cause ipsilateral limb sensory loss.
15 Ataxia worsening on eye closure suggests a sensory cause.

Answers

1 False.
2 False.
3 False.
4 False.
5 True.
6 True.
7 True.
8 False.
9 False.
10 True.
11 False.
12 False.
13 False.
14 False.
15 True.

Chapter 4 Multiple Choice Questions

Note: answers are on page 234

Blackouts: epileptic seizures and other events

1 Vasovagal syncope:
  a Presents with lateralized visual aura.
  b Causes biting of the tip of the tongue.
  c Is usually infrequent.
  d May cause myoclonic jerks.
  e May be provoked by exercise.

2 True petit mal seizures:
  a Are associated with a generalized spike-wave discharge.
  b Usually last 30–60 seconds.
  c Usually originate in the temporal lobe.
  d May occur many times per day.
  e May occur in juvenile myoclonic epilepsy.

3 Psychogenic nonepileptic seizures:
  a Are usually frequent.
  b May cause injury.
  c Are not stereotyped.
  d Are associated with synchronous clonic movements.
  e Are associated with head injury.

Acute confusional states

1 In an acute confusional state the stream of thought can be either slowed or accelerated.
2 A lesion of the ascending reticular activating system may cause a confusional state.
3 Fluctuations in a confusional state may occur by day and by night, but are more marked by night.
4 In an acute confusional state, remote memory is intact.
5 There is no universal susceptibility to developing an acute confusional state.
6 The predominant EEG rhythm in an acute confusional state is fast theta or alpha rhythm.
7 Autonomic hyperactivity, e.g. a tachycardia, is usually present.
8 The acute confusional state is always accompanied by increased psychomotor activity.
9 Visual hallucinations are rarely seen in the acute confusional state.
10 In an acute confusional state there is disorientation for time before that for place or person.
11 The two subtypes of a confusional state never coexist in the same patient.
12 Following recovery from an acute confusional state, the patient has an amnesia for the period of confusion.
13 There are specific features found at postmortem following the acute confusional state.
14 Emotional lability is a frequent accompaniment to the acute confusional state.
15 The acute confusional state lasts <24 hours.

Memory disorders

1 All memories reach conscious awareness.
2 Remembering last month's holiday is short-term memory.
3 Premorbid intelligence does not affect bedside cognitive performance.
4 It is easy to determine the time of onset of neurodegenerative disease.
5 A normal Mini-Mental State Examination score excludes Alzheimer's disease.
6 Digit span is a useful bedside test of short-term memory.
7 Korsakoff's syndrome results in a significant retrograde amnesia.
8 With memory impairment, loss of personal identity usually indicates a nonorganic cause.
9 Herpes encephalitis may selectively impair either episodic or semantic memory.
10 Insight may be retained early in Alzheimer's disease.
11 Depression can superficially resemble early dementia.
12 Hippocampal pathology primarily results in an anterograde rather than retrograde amnesia.
13 Short-term memory relies on the frontal lobes.
14 Retrograde memory can be tested both by asking about autobiographical memories and also by asking about famous public events.
15 Semantic memory can become impaired only if there is also episodic memory impairment.

Speech and language disorders

1 The right hemisphere is dominant for language in the majority of left-handers.
2 Phonemic paraphasias (spoonerisms) tend to occur with Broca's aphasia.
3 Repetition ability allows discrimination between conduction aphasia and the transcortical aphasias.
4 Reading ability is often spared in the aphasias.
5 The ability to write, yet be unable to read what has been written, indicates functional rather than organic disease.
6 Slow monotonous speech occurs in extrapyramidal disease.

7 Language impairment cannot be due to stroke unless there is also evidence of hemiparesis.
8 If a patient cannot write, yet has preserved oral spelling, then their symptoms are not organic in origin.
9 The ability to converse by phone is a very sensitive marker of early language dysfunction.
10 Analysis of the type of naming error can identify which part of the language system is impaired.
11 If reading aloud is impaired, then reading comprehension must be impaired.
12 The ability to correctly read irregular words is linked with knowledge of meaning of the word.
13 Normal performance on the Mini-Mental State Examination excludes the possibility of language impairment.
14 Difficulty naming objects occurs in most aphasias.
15 Clinical classification of an aphasia renders subsequent imaging unnecessary.

VISUAL LOSS AND DOUBLE VISION

1 Five lesion sites (a–e) and five visual loss patterns (1–5) are stated below. Match the site with the visual deficit that a lesion at that site commonly produces:

a Right optic nerve.	1 Left incongruous homonymous hemianopia.
b Optic chiasm.	2 Left macular sparing homonymous hemianopia.
c Right optic tract.	3 Right central scotoma.
d Right temporal optic radiation.	4 Bitemporal hemianopia.
e Right visual cortex.	5 Left superior homonymous quadrantinopia.

2 The following statements about the medical history of a patient with visual loss are true:
   a Binocular visual loss will be abolished by shutting one eye.
   b Optic neuritis characteristically occurs in patients over 60 years.
   c Tumours tend to cause progressive visual disturbance over days or months.
   d Migraine causes monocular or binocular visual disturbance normally followed by severe headache.
   e Temporal arteritis usually causes a hemianopic visual disturbance.

3 During a focused assessment for visual disturbance:
   a A left relative afferent pupillary defect suggests disease of the left optic nerve.
   b Visual field testing may be omitted if visual acuity is normal.
   c An enlarged blind spot and constriction of the visual field are features of papilloedema.
   d Finding associated lateralized motor weakness and upper motor neurone signs suggests that the lesion lies in the optic chiasm.
   e ESR and carotid Doppler should be ordered to investigate acute monocular visual loss in a 70-year-old male.

4 Neurological diplopia:
   a Is abolished by shutting either eye.
   b Always results in images appearing side by side.
   c Can be caused by a lesion affecting the oculomotor, trochlear, or abducens nerves, or the muscles that they supply.
   d Occurs only as a symptom of brainstem disease.
   e Remains a lifelong problem for patients with congenital strabismus ('squint').

5 Which of the following statements about the history of a patient with diplopia are true?
   a Isolated trochlear palsy causes vertical diplopia maximal when looking down.
   b Myaesthenic symptoms will be most marked when the patient wakes up.
   c Proptosis suggests aneurysmal expansion causing diplopia.
   d Unilateral ptosis indicates that the patient must be suffering from an oculomotor nerve palsy.
   e Diplopia is maximal in the direction of action of a paralysed muscle.

6 Which of the following investigation and management plans, formulated by a Casualty officer, would you agree with?
   a A patient with a painful complete oculomotor nerve palsy (pupil involved) was reassured and sent home for review in the neurology clinic the following week.
   b A patient with diplopia and ophthalmoplegia which worsened as the day progressed was referred for a Tensilon Test.
   c A patient with a sudden abducens nerve palsy and a history of hypertension, whose CT scan was normal, was started on aspirin, given a patch to wear over his right eye, and reassured. Plans were made for clinic review.
   d A 20-year-old patient was found on examination to have a left internuclear ophthalmoplegia and a relative afferent pupillary defect in the right eye. The patient was told that he had probably suffered a stroke and was referred for a CT scan.
   e A patient with symptoms of unilateral pain behind the eye, and a combined oculomotor and abducens palsy and tingling on their forehead, was referred for an MRI scan of their orbital apex and cavernous sinus.

Dizziness and vertigo

1 Which of the following statements are true?
  a Dizziness often coexists with vertigo, but is not the same as vertigo.
  b Dizziness always implies neurological disease.
  c The vestibular apparatus projects sensory information to the cerebellum and parieto-temporal cortex.
  d Peripheral vertigo is often rotational and in a yaw plane.
  e Vestibular sensory information is conveyed with sensory information from the cochlea (hearing) in the VIII cranial nerve.

2 Five 'symptom complexes' and five common 'disease processes' are shown below. Match each symptom complex with a disease process that is a common cause:

a Acute severe vertigo.	1 Migraine with aura.
b Positional vertigo.	2 Ménières disease.
c Vertigo with headache.	3 Postural hypotension.
d Hydrops (hearing disturbance, vertigo, tinnitus).	4 Acute peripheral vestibulopathy.
e Medical dizziness.	5 Benign paroxysmal positional vertigo.

3 The following statements about the assessment of a patient complaining of dizziness are true:
  a Cardiovascular examination may be omitted if there is no history of altered consciousness.
  b Weber's test lateralizes to the right in a patient with conductive hearing loss on the right.
  c In a patient with benign paroxysmal positional vertigo, Hallpike's test usually reproduces the symptoms.
  d A history of imbalance in the dark is suggestive of a proprioceptive (joint position sense) deficit.
  e Sudden severe vertigo in combination with diplopia is most likely to be caused by acute peripheral vestibulopathy.

Weakness

1 A lesion of the left S1 root would be expected to reduce or abolish the left ankle jerk reflex.
2 Muscle wasting is a characteristic feature of lower motor neurone weakness.
3 An elevation of serum creatine kinase activity to twice the upper limit of normal invariably indicates neuromuscular disease.
4 Extensor plantar responses are not a feature of upper motor neurone weakness.
5 A motor nerve always innervates a single muscle fibre.
6 A defect in oxidative muscle metabolism would be expected to produce limitation of sustained exercise rather than brief intense exercise.
7 Disorders of neuromuscular transmission may be associated with fatigue.
8 Cramps may be a prominent feature of motor neurone disease.
9 A lesion of the right C5 sensory root would be expected to be associated with sensory loss in the axilla.
10 A lesion in the spinal cord may produce both upper and lower motor neurone features.
11 It is appropriate to image the lumbar spine of a patient with spastic leg weakness and numbness involving the legs and up to just below the umbilicus.
12 Transection of the ulnar nerve at the elbow will cause weakness of all the intrinsic hand muscles.
13 Diseases of the motor unit would be expected to give rise to sensory symptoms.
14 Some inherited neuromuscular disorders are so mild affected individuals may never seek medical advice.
15 Steroid administration may cause muscle weakness.

Tremor and other involuntary movements

1 Parkinson's disease typically presents with unilateral postural arm tremor.
2 Essential tremor typically presents with bilateral postural arm tremor.
3 Huntington's disease is inherited in an autosomal recessive manner.
4 Wilson's disease often presents in patients aged over 50 years.
5 A fine bilateral postural arm tremor can be caused by sodium valproate.
6 An ischaemic lesion in the subthalamic nucleus could be the cause of acute onset hemiballism.
7 Imaging of the presynaptic dopaminergic neurone is expected to be abnormal in essential tremor.
8 Everybody with chorea should undergo genetic testing for Huntington's disease.
9 Thyroid function tests are indicated in a patient presenting with bilateral postural tremor and weight loss.
10 Structural brain imaging is not indicated when pyramidal signs (e.g. hyper-reflexia and extensor plantars) are found in conjunction with parkinsonian signs.
11 Antiemetic medications may cause parkinsonism.
12 Dopamine-depleting medications may cause Huntington's disease.
13 Beta-blockers may cause tremor.
14 Lithium may cause tremor.
15 Essential tremor responds to levodopa.

Poor coordination

1 The final common pathway in the cerebellar output involves:
   - a Red nucleus.
   - b Purkinje cell.
   - c Dentate nucleus.
   - d Granule cell.

2 Ataxia on eye closure but not with open eyes is suggestive of:
   - a Cerebellar ataxia.
   - b Sensory ataxia.
   - c A positive Romberg's test.
   - d Middle ear disease.

3 Neurological symptoms of vitamin B_{12} deficiency may present:
   - a As noncompressive myelopathy, i.e. spinal cord disease.
   - b With symptoms of burning feet.
   - c Without haematological changes of megaloblastic anaemia.
   - d With cerebellar symptoms.

4 Paraneoplastic neurological diseases affecting coordination may manifest as:
   - a Weakness of neuromuscular junction (antivoltage gated calcium channel antibody).
   - b Subacute sensory neuropathy (anti-Hu antibody).
   - c Opsoclonus, truncal ataxia (anti-Ri antibody).
   - d Cerebellar ataxia (anti-Yo antibody).

5 Blood supply of the cerebellum is derived from the branches of:
   - a Carotid artery.
   - b Vertebral artery.
   - c Basilar artery.
   - d All of the above.

6 Within the spinal cord, fibres carrying proprioception are located in the:
   - a Spinocerebellar tract.
   - b Spinothalamic tract.
   - c Posterior column.
   - d None of the above.

7 Ataxic hemiparesis refers to:
   - a Ipsilateral corticospinal weakness and contralateral ataxia.
   - b Corticospinal weakness and ataxia on the same side.
   - c Neither (**a**) nor (**b**).
   - d Both (**a**) and (**b**).

8 Sudden dizziness and vomiting, along with marked truncal ataxia in a hypertensive patient who is unable to stand upright, suggests a diagnosis of:
   - a Ménière's disease.
   - b Cerebellar haemorrhage.
   - c Internal capsular haemorrhage.
   - d Subarachnoid haemorrhage.

9 Ataxic neuropathies may be associated with:
   - a Monoclonal or polyclonal gammopathy.
   - b Paraneoplastic antibody.
   - c Sjögren's syndrome.
   - d Inflammatory demyelinating neuropathy.

10 Cerebellar features present in conjunction with rapidly deteriorating level of consciousness are suggestive of:
   - a Expanding posterior fossa mass.
   - b Posterior inferior cerebellar artery infarct.
   - c Anterior inferior cerebellar artery infarct.
   - d Viral encephalitis.

11 The following clinical signs would suggest a diagnosis of acoustic neuroma (vestibular Schwannoma):
   - a Hearing loss.
   - b Cerebellar ataxia.
   - c Nystagmus.
   - d Decreased facial sensation.

12 Cerebellar ataxia is inherited as an autosomal recessive disorder in:
   - a Hypothyroidism.
   - b Friedreich's ataxia.
   - c Spinocerebellar ataxia.
   - d Ataxia-telangiectasia.

13 A combination of cerebellar and sensory ataxia may be seen in:
   - a Coeliac disease.
   - b Alcohol abuse.
   - c Lyme disease.
   - d B-vitamin deficiency.

14 Vertigo is a side-effect of toxicity from:
   - a Phenytoin.
   - b Aminoglycoside antibiotics.
   - c Salicylates.
   - d Alcohol.

15 The preferred neuroimaging for acute cerebellar ataxia is:
   - a MRI.
   - b CT.
   - c CT followed by MRI.
   - d Plain X-ray of the skull base.

Headache

1 In the assessment and investigation of subarachnoid haemorrhage, which of these statements is true?
   - a The headache reaches its maximum intensity instantaneously or at most over a couple of minutes.
   - b Meningism is an important sign.
   - c A normal CT scan done within the first 12 hours of ictus excludes the diagnosis.
   - d A normal lumbar puncture done within the first 12 hours of ictus excludes the diagnosis.
   - e A normal lumbar puncture done a week after the ictus excludes the diagnosis.

f A patient who presents with coital headache for the first time can be reassured.

2 In patients with chronic daily headache, which of these statements is true?
a Patients presenting to Casualty with chronic daily headache are unlikely to have migraine.
b Patients over the age of 50 years who present with a new-onset, focal, daily headache should be considered to have temporal arteritis until proven otherwise.
c Migraine prophylactic medication is effective in patients with migraine and analgesia-induced headache.
d Analgesia-induced headache may take up to 6 months to settle down after stopping the offending agent.
e All analgesic and triptan medications can be associated with analgesia-induced headache.
f Migraine may present with chronic daily headache.

3 Which of these statements is true?
a Subarachnoid haemorrhage may present with new-onset, chronic, daily headache.
b Sudden-onset, unilateral headache associated with ipsilateral Horner's syndrome and contralateral hemiparesis suggests carotid dissection ipsilateral to the headache.
c A normal temporal artery biopsy excludes the diagnosis of temporal arteritis.
d Patients with cluster headache prefer to lie still.
e Alcohol may precipitate a cluster headache during periods of remission.
f Chronic arterial hypertension of moderate degree does not cause headache.

Spinal symtoms: neck pain and backache

1 In cervical spine disease:
a A 'clicking' or 'crunching' sensation experienced by the patient is a symptom of serious pathology.
b Bony change on X-ray is unusual in patients of middle age.
c Cranial nerve examination can provide useful information.
d Jaw jerk is a sign of cervical myelopathy.
e Hyper-reflexia in the legs is a reliable sign of myelopathy.

2 In thoracic spine disease:
a The sensory level is a reliable pointer to the level of the involvement.
b Urinary urgency and incontinence is a sign of radiculopathy.
c Loss of perianal sensation is a sign of pathology in the central cord.
d Unilateral cord pathology causes loss of pain and temperature sensation inferior and ipsilateral to the lesion.
e Anterior cord lesions cause loss of vibration and proprioception.

3 In lumbar and thoracic spine disease:
a Hyper-reflexia is a common sign of lumbar spine involvement.
b A normal straight leg raising test precludes surgical intervention.
c Loss of knee jerks is a sign of L5 radiculopathy.
d Unilateral lesions commonly cause bladder symptoms.
e A lower motor neurone bladder is small and has a small or undetectable residue.

Numbness and tingling

1 Pain is mediated by fast-conducting, peripheral sensory neurones.
2 Proprioception is impaired early in central cord disease.
3 A (lateral) hemicord lesion will cause loss of spino-thalamic sensation ipsilaterally below the lesion.
4 Sensation can only be appreciated at a cortical level.
5 Stereognosis depends on intact peripheral sensory pathways.
6 Dorsal root ganglia contain the nuclei of proprioceptive nerves.
7 Romberg's sign is a test of proprioceptive function.
8 Sensory loss in the ulnar two digits with weakness of finger flexion suggests an ulnar neuropathy.
9 In sensory inattention, the patient is unable to appreciate a sensory stimulus when presented to the affected side only.
10 Pseudoathetosis can be caused by a dorsal root ganglionopathy.
11 In suspended sensory loss, pain and temperature sensation are retained until advanced disease.
12 C7 root usually mediates sensation from the ring finger.
13 An infarct of the anterior limb of the internal capsule causes contralateral hemisensory loss.
14 Lateral pontine lesions may cause ipsilateral limb sensory loss.
15 Ataxia worsening on eye closure suggests a sensory cause.

ANSWERS

Blackouts

1 b, c, d
  a False. Lateralized visual aura suggests epileptic seizure.
  b True. In tonic–clonic seizures, tongue biting is usually lateral, or the inside of the cheek is bitten.
  c True.
  d True.
  e False. Provocation by exercise should suggest cardiogenic syncope.

2 a, d, e
  a True.
  b False. Seizures last several seconds at most.
  c False. They are generalized seizures.
  d True.
  e True.

3 a, b, e
  a True.
  b True, though in a minority of patients.
  c False.
  d False. Movements are normally alternating or tremulous. Asynchronous jerks may occasionally occur.
  e True. A history of minor head injury is elicited in approximately 50% of patients.

Acute confusional states

1 True.
2 False.
3 True.
4 True.
5 False.
6 False.
7 True.
8 False.
9 False.
10 True.
11 False.
12 True.
13 False.
14 True.
15 False.

Memory disorders

1 False.
2 False.
3 False.
4 False.
5 False.
6 True.
7 True.
8 True.
9 True.
10 True.
11 True.
12 True.
13 True.
14 True.
15 False.

Speech and language disorders

1 False.
2 True.
3 True.
4 False.
5 False.
6 True.
7 False.
8 False.
9 True.
10 True.
11 False.
12 True.
13 False.
14 True.
15 False.

Visual loss and double vision

1 a with 3
  b with 4
  c with 1
  d with 5
  e with 2
2 c, d
3 a, c, e
4 a, c
5 a, e
6 b, c, e

Dizziness and vertigo

1 a, c, d, e
2 a with 4
  b with 5
  c with 1
  d with 2
  e with 3
3 b, c, d

Weakness

1 True.
2 True.
3 False.
4 False.
5 False.
6 True.
7 True.
8 True.
9 False.
10 True.
11 False.
12 False.
13 False.
14 True.
15 True.

Tremor and other involuntary movements

1 False.
2 True.
3 False.
4 False.
5 True.
6 True.
7 False.
8 False.
9 True.
10 False.
11 True.
12 False.
13 False.
14 True.
15 False.

Poor coordination

1 b
2 b, c
3 a, b, c
4 b, c, d
5 b, c
6 a, b, c
7 b
8 b
9 a, b, c, d
10 a
11 a, b, c, d
12 b, d
13 a, c
14 a, b, c, d
15 c

Headache

1 a, e
2 b, d, e, f
3 a, b, f

Spinal symtoms

1 c, e
2 All false.
3 All false.

Numbness and tingling

1 False.
2 False.
3 False.
4 False.
5 True.
6 True.
7 True.
8 False.
9 False.
10 True.
11 False.
12 False.
13 False.
14 False.
15 True.

Index

Note: page numbers in **bold** refer to the main discussion of a topic; those in *italic* refer to content of tables